LAST MINUTE PE

A CONCISE REVIEW FOR THE SPECIALTY BOARDS

Table 2-2
Table 4-14
Table 6-3
Table 6-13
Table 7-5

George Keith Meyer, MD
Clinical Fellow
Division of Pediatric Critical Care Medicine
New York–Presbyterian Hospital
Weill Medical College of Cornell University
New York, New York

Patricia A. DeLaMora, MD
Clinical Fellow
Division of Pediatric Infectious Diseases
New York–Presbyterian Hospital
Weill Medical College of Cornell University
New York, New York

McGraw-Hill
Medical Publishing Division

New York   Chicago   San Francisco   Lisbon   London
Madrid   Mexico City   Milan   New Delhi   San Juan
Seoul   Singapore   Sydney   Toronto

Last Minute Pediatrics: A Concise Review for the Specialty Boards

2 3 4 5 6 7 8 9 0   DOC/DOC   0 9 8 7 6 5 4

ISBN 0-07-142179-3

Notice

Medicine is an ever-changing science. As new research and clinical experience broaden our knowledge, changes in treatment and drug therapy are required. The authors and the publisher of this work have checked with sources believed to be reliable in their efforts to provide information that is complete and generally in accord with the standards accepted at the time of publication. However, in view of the possibility of human error or changes in medical sciences, neither the authors nor the publisher nor any other party who has been involved in the preparation or publication of this work warrants that the information contained herein is in every respect accurate or complete, and they disclaim all responsibility for any errors or omissions or for the results obtained from use of the information contained in this work. Readers are encouraged to confirm the information contained herein with other sources. For example and in particular, readers are advised to check the product information sheet included in the package of each drug they plan to administer to be certain that the information contained in this work is accurate and that changes have not been made in the recommended dose or in the contraindications for administration. This recommendation is of particular importance in connection with new or infrequently used drugs.

This book was set in Electra by McGraw-Hill Professional's Hightstown, NJ, composition unit.
The editor was James F. Shanahan.
The production supervisor was Richard Ruzycka.
Project management was provided by Andover Publishing Services.
RR Donnelley was printer and binder.
The index was prepared by Andover Publishing Services.
This book was printed on acid-free paper.

Cataloging-in-Publication Data is on file with the Library of Congress.

CONTENTS

AUTHORS AND CONTRIBUTORS

Authors

George Keith Meyer, MD
Clinical Fellow
Division of Pediatric Critical Care Medicine
New York-Presbyterian Hospital
Weill Medical College of Cornell University
New York, New York

Patricia A. DeLaMora, MD
Clinical Fellow
Division of Pediatric Infectious Diseases
New York-Presbyterian Hospital
Weill Medical College of Cornell University
New York, New York

Editorial Advisor

Bruce M. Greenwald, MD
Professor of Clinical Pediatrics
Vice Chairman for Clinical Affairs,
  Department of Pediatrics
Director, Division of Pediatric Critical
  Care Medicine
Weill Medical College of Cornell University
New York, New York

Associate Editors

Alexa B. Adams, MD
Chief Pediatric Resident
New York-Presbyterian Hospital
Weill Medical College of Cornell University
New York, New York

Dennis C. Coffey, MD
Assistant Professor of Pediatrics
Division of Pediatric Critical Care Medicine
Weill Medical College of Cornell University
New York, New York

Anna Grattan, MD
Chief Pediatric Resident
New York-Presbyterian Hospital
Weill Medical College of Cornell University
New York, New York

Kyriakie Sarafoglou, M.D.
Assistant Professor of Pediatrics
Division of Pediatric Endocrinology
  and Metabolism
Weill Medical College of Cornell University
New York, New York

Joseph Stavola, MD
Assistant Professor of Pediatrics
Division of Pediatric Infectious Diseases
Weill Medical College of Cornell University
New York, New York

Todd Sweberg, MD
Resident in Pediatrics
New York-Presbyterian Hospital
Weill Medical College of Cornell University
New York, New York

H. Michael Ushay, MD, PhD
Associate Professor of Pediatrics
Division of Pediatric Critical Care Medicine
Weill Medical College of Cornell University
New York, New York

Contributors

Marie Ambroise, MD
Clinical Fellow
Division of Pediatric Neonatology
New York-Presbyterian Hospital
Weill Medical College of Cornell University
New York, New York

Melanie Greifer, MD
Clinical Fellow
Division of Pediatric Gastroenterology
New York-Presbyterian Hospital
Weill Medical College of Cornell University
New York, New York

Stephen W. Gilheeney, MD
Clinical Fellow
Division of Pediatric Hematology/ Oncology
Memorial Sloan Kettering Cancer Center and
   New York-Presbyterian Hospital
Weill Medical College of Cornell University
New York, New York

Lara M. Gordon, MD
Clinical Fellow
Child Protection Team
New York-Presbyterian Hospital
Weill Medical College of Cornell University
New York, New York

Benjamin J. Lentzner, MD
Clinical Fellow
Division of Pediatric Cardiology
New York-Presbyterian Hospital
Columbia University College of Physicians
   and Surgeons
New York, New York

Rajeshwari Mahalingam, MD
Clinical Fellow
Division of Pediatric Neurology
   and Neuroscience
New York-Presbyterian Hospital
Weill Medical College of Cornell University
New York, New York

Marc N. Richman, MD
Chief Resident
Division of Urologic Surgery
University of North Carolina at Chapel Hill
Chapel Hill, North Carolina

Theresa Schlott, MS, RD, CDN
Registered Dietician
New York-Presbyterian Hospital
Weill Medical College of Cornell University
New York, New York

Jila Senemar, MD
Chief Resident
Department of Obstetrics and Gynecology
Long Island Jewish Medical Center
New Hyde Park, New York

Romina Wancier, MD
Resident in Pediatrics
New York-Presbyterian Hospital
Weill Medical College of Cornell University
New York, New York

Faculty Advisors

Mary F. DiMaio, MD
Associate Professor of Pediatrics
Division of Pediatric Allergy, Immunology
  and Pulmonology
Weill Medical College of Cornell University
New York, New York

Patrick Flynn, MD
Assistant Professor of Pediatrics
Division of Pediatric Cardiology
Weill Medical College of Cornell University
New York, New York

Joy D. Howell, MD
Assistant Professor of Pediatrics
Division of Pediatric Critical Care Medicine
Weill Medical College of Cornell University
New York, New York

Martha C. Kutko, MD
Assistant Professor of Pediatrics
Division of Pediatric Critical Care Medicine
Weill Medical College of Cornell University
New York, New York

Thomas J. A. Lehman, MD
Professor of Clinical Pediatrics
Chief, Division of Pediatric Rheumatology
Weill Medical College of Cornell University
New York, New York

A. Maurine Packard, MD
Assistant Professor of Neurology
Division of Pediatric Neurology
  and Neuroscience
Weill Medical College of Cornell University
New York, New York

Eduardo Perelstein, MD
Assistant Professor of Pediatrics
Division of Pediatric Nephrology
Weill Medical College of Cornell University
New York, New York

Dana I. Ursea, MD
Assistant Professor of Pediatrics
Division of Pediatric Gastroenterology
Weill Medical College of Cornell University
New York, New York

Illustrations

William B. Zucconi, DO
Resident
Department of Radiology
Stony Brook University Health Sciences Center
Stony Brook, New York

FOREWORD

Preparing for board examinations has become a lifelong challenge for physicians at all levels and in all disciplines. Nonetheless, passing the first one remains a critical first step. This book is a product of the many hours a group of fellows of the Department of Pediatrics at the Weill Medical College of Cornell University spent in preparing for the pediatric boards. It is a practical, focused approach to preparing for the exam that should make study hours more productive. It contains a tremendous amount of information in a concise, easy-to-use format. Considering the explosion in knowledge over the past decade, having a large amount of important information presented in such a fashion is a great boost to preparing for the exam.

I am confident that this book will have broad application and appeal and will be invaluable not only for first-time exam takers but also for those seeking to maintain their certification years after completing residency. Drs. Keith Meyer and Tricia DeLaMora, the forces behind this publication, should be complimented for their industry, creativity, and attention to detail. Future generations of test takers will applaud this effort.

Good luck with the test.

Gerald M. Loughlin, M.D.
Nancy C. Paduano Professor and Chairman
Department of Pediatrics
Weill Medical College of Cornell University

PREFACE

We are pleased to introduce a unique concept in board review preparation. While studying for our boards, we found that there are no books that efficiently prepare physicians to take the pediatric board examination. As we shared our opinion on the matter, it became immediately clear that many recent residency graduates and practicing physicians were similarly frustrated at the lack of options available to help them prepare for the exam.

Our goal in writing this book was to provide the reader with high-yield, easy-to-read, absolute-need-to-know information without the extraneous details that are frequently found in lengthy print reviews and in board preparation courses. This book is designed to arm you with the essential information required to pass the pediatric board exam. Our philosophy is based on the belief that it is more important to understand core concepts well, rather than attempt to be familiar with lots of little bits of very detailed information.

This book should be used *before* the initiation of studying to identify strengths and weaknesses, *during* studying to focus on the important details, and *at the end of* studying to solidify the most important concepts you will need to know for the examination.

We would like to thank the fellows and faculty of the Department of Pediatrics at Weill Medical College of Cornell University, New York-Presbyterian Hospital for the support and guidance in writing this book. We would also like to thank Jim Shanahan and Jennifer Cosgrove of McGraw-Hill for their encouragement during this project.

Keith Meyer
Tricia DeLaMora

CHAPTER 1

NEONATOLOGY

MATERNAL SCREENING

Maternal Serum Alpha-Fetoprotein (MSAFP)

- A glycoprotein analogous to albumin.
- Synthesized in the fetal yolk sac, liver, and gastrointestinal tract.
- Levels measured at 16 to 18 weeks gestation.
- Serum levels greater than 2.5 multiples of the median indicate the need for further assessment.

TABLE 1-1.	CONDITIONS ASSOCIATED WITH AN ELEVATED MSAFP
TABLE 1-2.	CONDITIONS ASSOCIATED WITH A LOW MSAFP

Chorionic Villous Sampling (CVS)

- Analysis of placental tissue.
- Performed in the first trimester (10-12 weeks).
- Detects only chromosomal abnormalities and metabolic disorders.
- Complications include fetal loss, limb abnormalities/amputations, and infection.

TABLE 1-1	CONDITIONS ASSOCIATED WITH AN ELEVATED MSAFP
Miscalculated fetal age	
Multiple gestation	
Neural tube defects (spina bifida, anencephaly)	
Omphalocele	
Gastroschisis	
Sacrococcygeal teratoma	
Gastrointestinal obstruction	
Turner syndrome	

TABLE 1-2	CONDITIONS ASSOCIATED WITH A LOW MSAFP

Chromosomal trisomies (13, 18, 21)
Intrauterine growth retardation
Fetal demise
Miscalculated fetal age

Amniocentesis

- Analysis of amniotic fluid.
- Performed in the second trimester (15-20 weeks).
- Detects chromosomal abnormalities, metabolic disorders, and neural tube defects.
- Complications include fetal loss, spontaneous rupture of membranes, and infection.

Indications for Amniocentesis and/or CVS

- Advanced maternal age (>35 years)
- Abnormal maternal serum alpha feto-protein (AFP)
- History of a previous child with chromosomal abnormalities
- History of a previous child with neural tube defects
- Family history of specific birth defects/abnormalities

Ultrasound

Ultrasound is typically performed at 18 to 20 weeks gestation. Common uses include:

- Detection of fetal heart tones
- Estimation of gestational age and weight
- Determination of gender
- Detection of fetal anomalies
- Assessment of placenta and amniotic fluid
- Assessment of fetal breathing and movement (biophysical profile)

PERINATAL ASSESSMENT

TABLE 1-3.	OLIGOHYDRAMNIOS VS. POLYHYDRAMNIOS

- **Gestational Period**: Defined as the period from conception to the day of delivery. The defined range for a full-term neonate is from 260 to 294 days (37-41 weeks). Approximately 10% of births occur at less than 37 weeks gestation (preterm) and another 10% occur after 41 weeks (postterm/postdate). There is an

| TABLE 1-3 | OLIGOHYDRAMNIOS VS. POLYHYDRAMNIOS |

OLIGOHYDRAMNIOS (↓AMNIOTIC FLUID)	POLYHYDRAMNIOS (↑AMNIOTIC FLUID)
• Renal agenesis (Potter's sequence) • Lung hypoplasia • Premature rupture of membranes	• Anencephaly • Duodenal atresia • Gastroschisis • Tracheoesophageal fistula • Congenital diaphragmatic hernia • Maternal diabetes mellitus

increased morbidity and mortality at both ranges when compared with the full-term infant.

• **Small for Gestational Age (SGA)**: Defined as a neonate weighing less than 2 standard deviations below the mean, or less than the 10th percentile for gestational age. Commonly seen in mothers with pregnancy-induced hypertension (PIH) and smokers.

• **Large for Gestational Age (LGA)**: Defined as a neonate weighing more than 2 standard deviations above the mean, or more than the 10th percentile for gestational age. Commonly seen in infants of diabetic mothers, hydrops fetalis, and Beckwith-Wiedemann syndrome.

• **Symmetric Intrauterine Growth Retardation (IUGR)**: Head circumference, weight, and length are all less than the 10th percentile. This is usually due to conditions occurring early in pregnancy, such as congenital infections and chromosomal abnormalities.

• **Asymmetric IUGR**: Head circumference and height are spared relative to low birth weight. It is usually secondary to maternal malnutrition or placental insufficiency.

PERINATAL EVALUATION

• **Nonstress Test**: Used to evaluate the variability of the fetal heart rate. Fetal heart rate variability is reassuring for viability.

• **Biophysical Profile (BPP)**: Ultrasound evaluation of fetal breathing, movement, amniotic fluid volume, fetal tone, and heart rate variability. Each parameter receives a score of 0 to 2 points. A score of 8 to 10 is reassuring. A score less than 4 may indicate the need for delivery.

• **Lecithin-to-Sphingomyelin Ratio**: Estimates fetal lung maturity. Lecithin is a basic component of surfactant that can be measured in amniotic fluid. A ratio higher than 2.0 is reassuring. Often measured before anticipated premature delivery.

TABLE 1-4	ANTEPARTUM FETAL HEART RATE MONITORING	
EARLY DECELERATIONS	**VARIABLE DECELERATIONS**	**LATE DECELERATIONS**
• Head compression	• Umbilical cord compression	• Uteroplacental insufficiency
• Increased vagal tone	• Increased vagal tone	• Fetal hypoxemia
• Mostly benign	• Mostly benign	• May indicate need for delivery

NEWBORN ASSESSMENT

- **Apgar Scores**: A useful evaluation of newborn well-being. Measured at 1 and 5 minutes after delivery. If the 5-minute score is less than 7, scoring should be repeated every 5 minutes until the score is greater than 7 or the newborn is 20 minutes old. A score of 3 or less at 15 minutes has been associated with a high mortality and poor neurologic outcome.

TABLE 1-5	APGAR SCORES		
	0	**1**	**2**
Appearance (color)	Blue or pale	Pink body/blue ext.	Completely pink
Pulse	Absent	<100 bpm	>100 bpm
Grimace	No response	Grimace	Cough/sneeze
Activity (tone)	Limp	Some flexion	Active motions
Respirations	Absent	Slow, irregular	Good, crying

NEWBORN SIGNS AND SYMPTOMS

TABLE 1-6   *CAUSES OF NEWBORN TACHYCARDIA/TACHYPNEA*

Fever
Pain
Congestive heart failure
Congenital heart disease
Hypovolemia
Sepsis
Metabolic acidosis
Hypoxia
Medications (albuterol, racemic epinephrine)
Pneumonia
Meconium aspiration
Transient tachypnea of the newborn

TABLE 1-7   *CAUSES OF NEWBORN BRADYCARDIA*

Prolonged head compression during birth (vagal response)
Prolonged hypoxia
Congenital heart block (systemic lupus erythematosus)
Electrolyte abnormalities

TABLE 1-8	*CAUSES OF NEWBORN HYPOTENSION*

Dehydration
Placental abruption
Sepsis
Intraventricular hemorrhage
Necrotizing enterocolitis
Anemia
Congenital heart disease

TABLE 1-9	*CAUSES OF NEWBORN CYANOSIS*

CONDITION	EXAMPLE
Respiratory disease	• Meconium aspiration syndrome • Respiratory distress syndrome • Hyaline membrane disease • Choanal atresia • Congenital diaphragmatic hernia
Cardiac disease	• Tetralogy of Fallot with pulmonary atresia • Transposition of the great arteries • Truncus arteriosus • Tricuspid atresia • Total anomalous pulmonary venous return • Hypoplastic left heart syndrome • Persistent pulmonary hypertension
Hematologic disease	• Methemoglobinemia
Neurologic disease	• Intraventricular hemorrhage • Central hypoventilation • Apnea of prematurity • Seizures
Infectious disease	• Sepsis
Gastrointestinal disease	• Gastrointestinal reflux

• **Acrocyanosis**: "Differential" cyanosis involving the distal extremities with the mucous membranes and trunk pink. Caused by peripheral vasoconstriction. A benign condition. Contrast this condition to the more ominous conditions associated with central cyanosis, listed in Table 1-9.

TABLE 1-10	*CAUSES OF NEWBORN HYPOGLYCEMIA*

Infant of a diabetic mother
Maternal obesity
Maternal drug abuse
Infection/sepsis
Stress
Prematurity
Beckwith-Wiedemann syndrome
Perinatal asphyxia

TABLE 1-11	*CAUSES OF NEWBORN HYPERGLYCEMIA*

Stress
Maternal drug abuse
Corticosteroid administration
Intraventricular hemorrhage
Perinatal asphyxia
Sepsis

TABLE 1-12	*CAUSES OF NEWBORN OLIGURIA*

The normal newborn should urinate within 24 hours of birth.

PRERENAL	RENAL	POSTRENAL
• Dehydration	• Polycystic kidney disease	• Ureteropelvic junction obstruction
• Congenital heart disease	• Acute tubular nephropathy	• Posterior urethral valves
• Sepsis	• Renal agenesis (Potter's)	• Congenital hydronephrosis
• Shock	• Nephrotoxic medications	• Abdominal compression (masses)

TABLE 1-13	*CAUSES OF AN ABDOMINAL MASS IN THE NEWBORN*

Congenital hydronephrosis
Polycystic kidney disease
Prune belly syndrome
Renal vein thrombosis
Adrenal hemorrhage
Neuroblastoma
Hydrometrocolpos

TABLE 1-14	*CAUSES OF NEWBORN HYPOTONIA*

Perinatal asphyxia
Intraventricular hemorrhage
Werdnig-Hoffman syndrome (spinal muscular atrophy)
Congenital myasthenia gravis
Spinal cord trauma
Myotonic dystrophy
Prader-Willi syndrome
Lowe syndrome
Mitochondrial disorders
Hypermagnesemia
Narcotic administration
Botulism
Congenital hypothyroidism

TABLE 1-15　　*CAUSES OF NEWBORN SEIZURES*

Perinatal asphyxia

Intraventricular hemorrhage

Traumatic brain injury

Hypoglycemia

Hyponatremia

Hypocalcemia

Pyridoxine deficiency

Inborn errors of metabolism

Mitochondrial disorders

Meningitis

Sepsis

Kernicterus

Toxins

Abstinence syndrome

TABLE 1-16　　*CAUSES OF NEWBORN/INFANTILE APNEA*

Apnea of prematurity

Perinatal asphyxia

Intraventricular hemorrhage

Arnold-Chiari malformation

Head trauma

Spinal cord trauma

Seizure

Gastrointestinal reflux

Sepsis

Meningitis

Pertussis

Botulism

Necrotizing enterocolitis

Hypoglycemia

Hypermagnesemia

Narcotics

Supraventricular tachycardia

Diaphragm dysfunction

Central sleep apnea (Ondine's curse)

TABLE 1-17	*CAUSES OF NEWBORN ANEMIA*	
DECREASED RBC PRODUCTION	**INCREASED RBC DESTRUCTION**	**INCREASED RBC LOSS**
• Diamond-Blackfan syndrome • Aplastic anemia • Malignancy	• ABO incompatibility • Rh disease (erythroblastosis fetalis) • Hereditary spherocytosis • G6PD deficiency • Vitamin E deficiency • Sepsis	• Placenta previa • Placental abruption • Twin-twin transfusion • Intraventricular hemorrhage • Vitamin K deficiency (hemorrhagic disease of the newborn) • Hemophilia • von Willebrand disease

COMMON NEONATAL CONDITIONS

Disorders of the Scalp

CAPUT SUCCEDANEUM

- A diffuse, edematous swelling of the scalp.
- Crosses the suture lines.
- A discoloration of the scalp is often present.
- Resolves spontaneously.

CEPHALOHEMATOMA

- A subperiosteal collection of blood.
- Does not cross the suture lines.
- Radiography is often necessary to rule out skull fractures.
- A large hematoma may lead to hyperbilirubinemia and jaundice secondary to blood resorption.

SUBGALEAL HEMORRHAGE

- A collection of blood above the periosteum, beneath the aponeurotic layer that covers the cranium.
- Presents with a boggy, firm swelling on the scalp following a traumatic delivery.
- Crosses the suture lines.
- A CT scan is often necessary to establish a diagnosis.

Respiratory Disorders

TRANSIENT TACHYPNEA OF THE NEWBORN

- Most commonly occurs after a cesarean delivery.
- Occurs secondary to excessive fluid in the interstitial space of the lungs.
- The patient presents with tachypnea, but is otherwise comfortable.

- Chest radiograph often reveals fluid in the right horizontal fissure.
- Requires only supportive therapy; usually resolves in 1 to 3 days.

RESPIRATORY DISTRESS SYNDROME (RDS)/HYALINE MEMBRANE DISEASE

DEFINITION: Respiratory distress and hypoxemia in the newborn period due to surfactant deficiency.

ETIOLOGY: The surfactant that is normally produced by type II alveolar pneumocytes is deficient or absent, resulting in increased surface tension of the alveolar sacs. The increased surface tension impairs expansion of the alveoli and oxygenation of blood.

TABLE 1-18. *RISK FACTORS FOR RESPIRATORY DISTRESS SYNDROME*

CLINICAL PRESENTATION: Most neonates with RDS are less than 35 weeks gestational age. There is usually respiratory distress at birth characterized by grunting, retractions, hypoxemia, and cyanosis. This condition may be indistinguishable from sepsis or pneumonia. Infants who experience stress in utero produce endogenous steroids, speeding maturation of the lungs and thereby decreasing the risk of RDS.

DIAGNOSIS: The amniotic fluid can be tested for the main components of surfactant (lecithin, phosphatidylglycerol) prior to anticipated delivery. A lecithin-to-sphingomyelin (L/S) ratio higher than 2.0 is a reliable indicator of fetal lung maturity. Postnatally, chest radiography reveals a reticulogranular, "ground-glass" appearance of the lungs.

TREATMENT: The prevention of preterm delivery is important. Intravenous glucocorticoid administration to the mother prior to premature delivery promotes endogenous surfactant production. Newborns who require intubation and mechanical ventilation may need exogenous surfactant administration to help decrease alveolar surface tension and promote improved oxygenation by the lungs.

COMPLICATIONS: Pneumothorax, air leak syndrome, chronic lung disease, and retinopathy of prematurity (as a consequence of O_2 administration).

TABLE 1-18 *RISK FACTORS FOR RESPIRATORY DISTRESS SYNDROME*

INCREASED RISK	DECREASED RISK
• Prematurity	• Pregnancy-induced hypertension
• Males	• Maternal drug abuse
• Caucasians	• Premature rupture of membranes
• Cesarean delivery	• Antenatal steroid use
• Infants of diabetic mothers	

MECONIUM ASPIRATION SYNDROME

DEFINITION: Acute lung injury secondary to aspirated meconium in the peripartum period.

ETIOLOGY: Fetal stress during labor may precipitate passage of meconium into the amniotic fluid. Aspiration of meconium during delivery causes subsequent asphyxia and hypoxemia.

RISK FACTORS: Pregnancy-induced hypertension (PIH), maternal diabetes, oligohydramnios, postterm delivery, and IUGR.

CLINICAL PRESENTATION: Thick meconium-stained amniotic fluid (often described as "pea soup") at delivery. Respiratory distress and hypoxemia are present immediately.

DIAGNOSIS: Visualization of meconium in the upper airway by laryngoscopy. Chest radiography reveals diffuse infiltrates and/or areas of consolidation.

TREATMENT: Prevention is most important. Oral suctioning of the neonate at the perineum once the head has been delivered is essential. Laryngoscopy and suctioning of particulate meconium from the upper airway is useful. Avoid positive-pressure ventilation prior to laryngoscopy. Supplemental oxygen, continuous positive-pressure ventilation (CPAP), and antibiotics are usually administered upon admission to the neonatal intensive care unit. Severe cases may precipitate persistent pulmonary hypertension necessitating high-frequency oscillatory ventilation (HFOV), inhaled nitric oxide therapy (iNO), and extracorporeal membrane oxygenation (ECMO).

CONGENITAL DIAPHRAGMATIC HERNIA

DEFINITION: Pulmonary hypoplasia due to migration of abdominal viscera into the affected hemithorax.

ETIOLOGY: There is incomplete closure of the diaphragmatic pleuroperitoneal hiatus secondary to defective development of the pleuropotential membrane. This results in movement of the abdominal viscera into the unilateral hemithorax with subsequent ipsilateral pulmonary hypoplasia. The foramen of Bochdalek defect is on the left. The foramen of Morgagni defect is on the right.

CLINICAL PRESENTATION: Most common in full-term male infants. Ninety percent occur on the left side. Respiratory distress, hypoxemia, and shock are present within the first few hours of life. Bowel sounds may be heard in the chest.

DIAGNOSIS: Chest radiography reveals air-filled bowel loops in the chest. Mediastinal shift is often present with pulmonary hypoplasia.

TREATMENT: Early surgical intervention. Aggressive respiratory support. HFOV, iNO, and ECMO are sometimes necessary.

TABLE 1-19	RISK FACTORS FOR PERSISTENT PULMONARY HYPERTENSION

Fetal distress

Meconium aspiration

Group B streptococcal sepsis

Cesarean section

Congenital diaphragmatic hernia

Hyaline membrane disease

Cardiac Disorders

PERSISTENT PULMONARY HYPERTENSION (PPHN)

DEFINITION: Pulmonary hypertension and high pulmonary vascular resistance producing persistence of the fetal circulation.

ETIOLOGY: Unknown.

TABLE 1-19.   RISK FACTORS FOR PERSISTENT PULMONARY HYPERTENSION

CLINICAL PRESENTATION: Most common in full-term infants. Respiratory distress and profound shock with significant hypoxemia are apparent within the first few hours of life. There is a differential of 10% to 15% between preductal and postductal oxygen saturations as measured by pulse oximetry. (Preductal oxygen saturation can be measured on the right hand, and postductal oxygen saturation can be measured on the lower extremities). Metabolic acidosis and cyanosis are common.

DIAGNOSIS: Suspect in full-term neonates presenting with shock and hypoxemia. Pre- and postductal differential saturations are useful. Preductal arterial blood gas reveals profound hypoxemia, metabolic acidosis, and an increased oxygenation index. Echocardiogram demonstrates a patent ductus arteriosus and a patent foramen ovale, both with left-to-right shunting.

TREATMENT: Airway, breathing, and circulation. Aggressive respiratory and hemodynamic support including iNO and ECMO.

Gastrointestinal Disorders

GASTROSCHISIS

- An abdominal defect to the right of the umbilicus with abdominal contents exposed at the time of delivery.
- The umbilical cord is intact.
- The usual treatment is aggressive fluid resuscitation and early surgical intervention.

OMPHALOCELE

- An abdominal wall defect through the midline at the umbilicus.
- Covered with peritoneum.
- Associated with Beckwith-Wiedemann syndrome, Edward syndrome, and myelomeningocele.

MECONIUM ILEUS

- Defined as obstruction of the distal small bowel by abnormal meconium.
- Almost always associated with cystic fibrosis.
- The infant presents with absent bowel movement, bilious emesis, and abdominal distention.
- Classic soap bubble appearance is seen on the abdominal radiograph.
- Barium enema is both diagnostic and therapeutic.

NECROTIZING ENTEROCOLITIS

DEFINITION: Necrosis of the bowel lumen with potential for bowel perforation and sepsis.

ETIOLOGY: Most likely secondary to intestinal immaturity and hypoxemia. Incidence increases with the degree of prematurity. Risk factors include prematurity, asphyxia, and rapid advancement in enteral feeds in infants at risk. Antenatal steroid administration for the prevention of hyaline membrane disease has recently been found to be protective.

CLINICAL PRESENTATION: The infant presents with abdominal distention, temperature instability, lethargy, feeding intolerance, occult stool blood, hypotension, and sepsis.

DIAGNOSIS: Pneumatosis intestinalis (air present in the bowel wall on radiography) is diagnostic. Intrahepatic portal venous gas may also be seen.

TREATMENT: Discontinuation of enteral feeds, gastric decompression, antibiotics, and possible surgical intervention (bowel resection and/or colostomy).

HYPERBILIRUBINEMIA

DEFINITION: Age-dependent elevation of bilirubin.

ETIOLOGY: Abnormal bilirubin production, metabolism, or excretion. Can be divided into indirect (unconjugated) and direct (conjugated) forms.

CLINICAL PRESENTATION: Unconjugated hyperbilirubinemia classically presents with jaundice beginning on the face (correlates to a level of 5 mg/dL), spreading to the abdomen (10 mg/dL) and finally to the extremities (20 mg/dL). In uncomplicated neonatal jaundice, bilirubin generally does not rise above 5 mg/dL per day. Differentiate from excess vitamin A, which spares the sclera.

| TABLE 1-20 | *CAUSES OF NEWBORN HYPERBILIRUBINEMIA* |

Over 50% of all newborns become jaundiced. Jaundice is caused by abnormal bilirubin production, metabolism, excretion, or a combination thereof.

UNCONJUGATED	CONJUGATED
• Physiologic	• Alpha 1 anti-trypsin deficiency
• Breast-feeding	• Galactosemia
• Breast milk	• Biliary atresia
• ABO incompatibility	• Choledochal cyst
• Rh disease	• Total parenteral nutrition administration
• G6PD deficiency	• TORCH infections
• Pyruvate kinase deficiency	
• Hereditary spherocytosis	
• Crigler-Najjar syndrome	

TORCH: **t**oxoplasmosis, **o**ther viruses, **r**ubella, **c**ytomegalovirus, **h**erpes simplex.

| TABLE 1-21. | *UNCONJUGATED HYPERBILIRUBINEMIA* |
| TABLE 1-22. | *CONJUGATED HYPERBILIRUBINEMIA* |

KERNICTERUS

Defined as encephalopathy secondary to increased levels of unbound bilirubin crossing the neonatal blood-brain barrier. Bilirubin commonly stains the basal ganglia resulting in choreo-athetosis. Risk factors include prematurity, sepsis, and malnutrition. Neurological damage is permanent. The infant presents with opisthotonus, high-pitched cry, seizures, hearing loss, developmental delay, and cerebral palsy. The level of bilirubin required for kernicterus is variable, generally greater than 20 mg/dL.

TABLE 1-21   *UNCONJUGATED HYPERBILIRUBINEMIA*

CONDITION	ETIOLOGY	CLINICAL PRESENTATION	DIAGNOSIS	TREATMENT
Physiologic jaundice	• Immature liver enzymes (deficient glucuronyl transferase) • ↑ Breakdown of RBCs releasing bilirubin • ↓ Bilirubin uptake by the liver • ↓ Life span of fetal hemoglobin	• Presents 24-72 h postdelivery • Mild jaundice • Bilirubin levels usually <15 mg/dL • No kernicterus	• History and clinical presentation	• Supportive • Reassurance • Phototherapy if severe
Breast-feeding jaundice	• Inadequate breast-feeding • Dehydration	• Mild jaundice • Onset 2+ d postdelivery	• History and clinical presentation	• Increase frequency of feedings • Fluid supplementation
Breast milk jaundice	• UDPG transferase inhibition by breast milk	• Mild jaundice • Onset 5+ d postdelivery	• History and clinical presentation	• Supportive • Temporary cessation of feeds
ABO incompatibility	• Antibody mediated • Maternal IgG crosses the placenta • Maternal blood type O (most frequent), A, or B • Fetal blood type A, B or AB	• Hemolytic anemia • Jaundice • Can present at 1st pregnancy	• Coombs positive • IgG anti-A or anti-B	• Supportive • Phototherapy if severe
Rh disease (erythroblastosis fetalis)	• Antibody mediated • Rh-negative mother • Antibody to the D antigen • Requires sensitization	• Hemolytic anemia • Jaundice • Hydrops fetalis • Spontaneous abortions • Kernicterus • Not with 1st pregnancy	• Coombs positive • IgG anti-D	• Phototherapy • Plasma exchange • Anti-D globulin (RhoGAM) administration to mother

TABLE 1-21	UNCONJUGATED HYPERBILIRUBINEMIA (CONTINUED)			
CONDITION	**ETIOLOGY**	**CLINICAL PRESENTATION**	**DIAGNOSIS**	**TREATMENT**
G6PD deficiency	• X-linked • Exposure to oxidant medications (e.g., sulfa drugs, antibiotics)	• Jaundice • Hemolytic anemia	• Measurement of G6PD enzyme activity	• Supportive • Phototherapy
Pyruvate kinase deficiency	• Autosomal recessive • Enzyme deficiency	• Jaundice • Hemolytic anemia • Splenomegaly	• Measurement of pyruvate kinase activity	• Supportive • Splenectomy
Hereditary spherocytosis	• Autosomal dominant • RBC membrane defect in spectrin • Osmotic damage to the RBC membrane leading to intravascular hemolysis • Sequestration in the spleen	• Anemia • Splenomegaly • Jaundice	• Osmotic fragility test • Coombs negative	• Splenectomy
Glucuronyl transferase deficiency (Crigler-Najjar syndrome)	**Type I:** • Autosomal recessive • Absence of UDPG transferase • No formation of bilirubin glucuronide	• Jaundice • Kernicterus • Pale stool • No hemolytic anemia	• Marked elevated unconjugated bilirubin • Liver biopsy • Indirect bilirubin >20 mg/dL	• Poor prognosis • Phototherapy • Exchange transfusion
	Type II: • Autosomal dominant • ↓ UDPG transferase	• Less severe form • Jaundice • No kernicterus • Pale stool	• ↓ Levels of bilirubin (<10 mg/dL) • Liver biopsy	• Responds well to phenobarbital • Phototherapy • Exchange transfusion

RBC, red blood cell; UDPG, UDP-glucuronyl.

TABLE 1-22   *CONJUGATED HYPERBILIRUBINEMIA*

CONDITION	ETIOLOGY	CLINICAL PRESENTATION	DIAGNOSIS	TREATMENT
Alpha 1 anti-trypsin deficiency	• Enzyme deficiency • A serum protease inhibitor • Incidence 1:2000 • PiZZ allele most common	• Jaundice • Hepatomegaly • Acholic stools • Cirrhosis	• Alpha 1 anti-trypsin phenotype • Liver biopsy	• Liver transplantation
Hepatitis B and C	• Liver cell injury	• Average age at presentation = 3 mo • Jaundice • Hepato-splenomegaly • Acholic stools • Hypoglycemia	• Elevated transaminases • Hepatitis antibody panel • Maternal history of disease • Liver biopsy	• Supportive • Therapy depends on severity of disease • Very rare in newborns

Galactosemia	• Deficiency of:
	  1. Galactose 1 phosphate uridylyl-transferase
	  2. Galactokinase
	• Incidence 1:60,000
		• Jaundice
		• Hepato-splenomegaly
		• Cataracts
		• Hypoglycemia
		• Seizures
		• FTT
			• Reducing substance in urine
			• Measurement of enzyme levels in red blood cells
			• Serum galactose levels
				• Lactose-free diet
				• Lactose = glucose + galactose

Biliary atresia	• Progressive obliteration of the biliary tree • Incidence 1:10,000	• Jaundice • Acholic stools	• Cholangiography • Liver biopsy	• Kasai procedure (anastomosis of porta hepatis to bowel) • High failure rate after age 3 mo associated with the need for transplantation

Neurologic Disorders

INTRAVENTRICULAR HEMORRHAGE (IVH)

DEFINITION: Intracranial hemorrhage originating from the vascular germinal matrix. Occurs most commonly in preterm, low birth weight (LBW) neonates. Grading system (see Fig.1-1):

- Grade I = Confined to the germinal matrix
- Grade II = without dilated ventricles
- Grade III = with ventricular dilatation
- Grade IV = with extension into the brain

FIGURE 1-1. *INTRAVENTRICULAR HEMORRHAGE.*

RISK FACTORS: Prematurity, birth asphyxia, seizures, pneumothorax, rapid intravascular expansion, positive-pressure ventilation, and sepsis.

COMPLICATIONS: Ventriculomegaly, hydrocephalus, cerebral palsy, developmental delay, and periventricular leukomalacia.

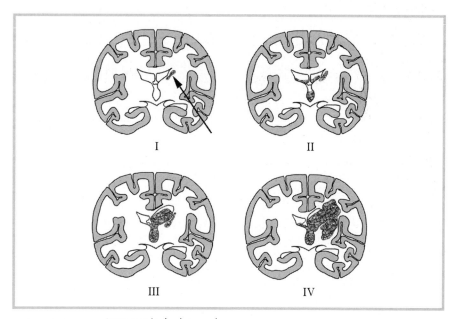

– FIGURE 1-1 – Intraventricular hemorrhage.

CLINICAL PRESENTATION: Variable. Symptoms include lethargy, irritability, pallor, anemia, apnea, bradycardia, cyanosis, and seizures. A bulging fontanel is often present on physical examination.

DIAGNOSIS: Head ultrasound is the most frequently employed imaging technique. CT and MRI may define the extent of the hemorrhage more precisely.

TREATMENT: Prevention is the most important treatment modality. Ventricular-peritoneal shunts are often needed secondary to the development of hydrocephalus.

Bleeding Disorders

HEMORRHAGIC DISEASE OF THE NEWBORN

DEFINITION: Vitamin K deficiency in the newborn infant.

CLINICAL PRESENTATION: Can present with bleeding anytime between birth and 3 months of age. The most common presentation is a breast-fed infant delivered at home with no subsequent medical care, including vitamin K prophylaxis. Poor feeding, apathy, and lethargy are common. In severe cases there are signs of IVH and bloody diarrhea.

DIAGNOSIS: History. Consider hemophilia if there is a history of vitamin K administration.

TREATMENT: Vitamin K. Fresh frozen plasma for clinical bleeding.

Ophthalmologic Disorders

RETINOPATHY OF PREMATURITY (ROP)

DEFINITION: Fibrosis of the developing retina and vasculature.

ETIOLOGY: Hyperoxygenation of premature retinal vasculature with subsequent fibrosis and scarring.

RISK FACTORS: Prematurity, RDS, IVH, long-term supplemental oxygen therapy, high-frequency ventilation, and sepsis. Children with a history of chronic lung disease are most at risk.

CLINICAL PRESENTATION: The onset of retinopathy is variable but generally occurs as the infant reaches term gestational age. Retinal scarring and detachment are serious consequences.

DIAGNOSIS: Ophthalmologic screening of high-risk and extremely low birth weight (ELBW) infants at 30 weeks gestational age and prior to discharge. Follow-up exams should be performed until the infant reaches term gestational age.

TREATMENT: Prevention. Most ROP regresses without treatment. Cryotherapy and laser photocoagulation are reserved for advanced stages. Long-term side effects include defects in visual acuity.

Maternal-Fetal Influences

TABLE 1-23   *MATERNAL CONDITIONS AND NEONATAL SEQUELAE*

IF MOM HAS...	BABY IS AT RISK FOR...
Systemic lupus erythematosus	• Congenital heart block • Thrombocytopenia
Insulin-dependent diabetes	• Large for gestational age • Hyperinsulinemia • Hypoglycemia • Polyhydramnios • Polycythemia • Pre-eclampsia • Renal agenesis • Duodenal atresia • Transposition of the great arteries • Respiratory distress (surfactant deficiency) • Caudal regression syndrome (maldevelopment of bowel, kidney, bladder and spine)
Hypertension	• Intrauterine growth retardation • Stillbirth • Hypoxia/asphyxia • Placental abruption
Urinary tract infection	• Premature rupture of membranes • Sepsis
Obesity	• Macrosomia • Hypoglycemia
PKU (uncontrolled)	• Microcephaly • Mental retardation
Graves disease	• Transient thyrotoxicosis
Pre-eclampsia	• Fetal hypoxia • Thrombocytopenia • Uteroplacental insufficiency • Fetal demise • Hypermagnesemia (from mother)

| TABLE 1-24 | *MATERNAL HABITS/INGESTIONS/MEDICATIONS AND NEONATAL MANIFESTATIONS* |

MATERNAL HABIT/INGESTION	NEONATAL MANIFESTATION
Smoking	• Intrauterine growth retardation • Small for gestational age
Alcohol	• Fetal alcohol syndrome • Intrauterine growth retardation • Microcephaly • Thin upper lip • Long philtrum • CNS dysfunction • Narrow palpebral fissures
Marijuana (THC)	• Intrauterine growth retardation • Behavioral problems
Cocaine	• Intrauterine growth retardation • Placental abruption
Opiates	• Yawning • Vomiting • Diarrhea • Tremors • Seizures • Irritability
Carbamazepine	• Spina bifida
Barbiturates	• CNS depression • Apnea • Hypotonia
Phenytoin	• Intrauterine growth retardation • Characteristic facies • Fifth fingernail or toenail hypoplasia • Neurodevelopmental abnormalities
Valproate	• Spina bifida, heart defect

(Continued)

TABLE 1-24   *MATERNAL HABITS/INGESTIONS/MEDICATIONS AND NEONATAL MANIFESTATIONS (CONTINUED)*

MATERNAL HABIT/INGESTION	NEONATAL MANIFESTATION
Benzodiazepines	• Seizures • Agitation • Tremors • Choreoathetoid movements
Tetracycline	• Enamel hypoplasia • Cataracts • Limb defects
Propranolol	• Hypoglycemia • Bradycardia • Respiratory distress
Coumadin	• Bleeding • Limb defects
Aspirin	• Bleeding • Antiplatelet effects
NSAIDs	• Renal failure • Oliguria • Necrotizing enterocolitis • Bleeding
Magnesium	• Hypotonia • Respiratory depression
Lithium	• Ebstein anomaly (downward displacement of tricuspid valve)
ACE inhibitors	• Renal failure • Hypotension
Thiazides	• Thrombocytopenia
Vitamin K	• Jaundice
Retinoids	• Congenital heart disease • Midfacial anomalies
Quinine	• Hearing loss • Thrombocytopenia

TABLE 1-25	*TORCH INFECTIONS*	
CONDITION	**CLINICAL PRESENTATION**	**NOTES**
Toxoplasmosis	• Chorioretinitis • Cerebral calcifications (scattered) • Mental retardation • Microcephaly • Intrauterine growth retardation • Hepatosplenomegaly	• Transmitted by infected cat/kitten/raw meat • Treatment with pyrimethamine + sulfadiazine • Infant serum IgA/IgE antibody is diagnostic
Rubella	• Deafness* • Cataracts* • Intrauterine growth retardation • Mental retardation • Microcephaly • Petechiae • Thrombocytopenia • Blueberry muffin skin	• Congenital rubella an important mechanism of transmission • Supportive treatment • Maternal serum IgG, fetal IgM diagnostic
Cytomegalovirus (CMV)	• Blueberry muffin skin* • Ventriculitis* • Periventricular calcifications • Inclusion disease • Chorioretinitis • Anemia • Thrombocytopenia • Hepatosplenomegaly • Jaundice • Deafness	• Most common congenitally acquired infection • Hearing loss is found in CMV and rubella, not toxoplasmosis • Urine culture is a helpful aid in diagnosis • IgM specific antibody test in infant • Treatment with ganciclovir is controversial
Herpes simplex virus (HSV)	• Temporal lobe seizures* • Microcephaly • Retinopathy • Vesicular skin lesions • Meningitis	• The only TORCH infection not transmitted by the placenta • Cesarean delivery if active maternal disease • HSV culture of lesions is specific for diagnosis • HSV polymerase chain reaction (PCR) of spinal fluid • Treatment with IV acyclovir

(Continued)

TABLE 1-25   *TORCH INFECTIONS (CONTINUED)*

CONDITION	CLINICAL PRESENTATION	NOTES

Syphilis	• Saber shins*
	• Hutchinson's teeth*
	• Saddle nose*
	• "Snuffles"*
	• Stillbirth
	• Intra-uterine growth retardation
	• Hepato-splenomegaly
	• Jaundice
	• Lymphadenopathy
	• Frontal bossing
		• VDRL/RPR screening test (nontreponemal)
		  - False positive: SLE, EBV, hepatitis, TB, and varicella
		• FTA-ABS for confirmation (treponemal)
		  - False positive: Lyme, yaws, and pinta
		• Treatment with penicillin G

Varicella	• Chorioretinitis • Optic atrophy • Cerebral atrophy • Limb hypoplasia • Vesicular lesions at birth* • Seizures	• Varicella IgG, IgM, Tzanck smear of lesions, DFA, viral culture for diagnosis • Viral culture is most specific • Treatment with IV acyclovir
Parvovirus	• Hydrops fetalis* • Anemia • Stillbirth	• Maternal IgM antibody diagnostic • Supportive treatment
Lyme disease	• Cortical blindness • Diffuse macular rash	• Lyme IgG, IgM titers for diagnosis • Treatment with ceftriaxone

DFA, direct fluorescent antibody; EBV, Epstein-Barr virus; FTA-ABS, fluorescent treponemal antibody absorption; SLE, systemic lupus erythematosus; TB, tuberculosis; TORCH, **t**oxoplasmosis, **o**ther viruses, **r**ubella, **c**ytomegalovirus, **h**erpes simplex; VDRL-RPR, Venereal Disease Research Laboratory/rapid plasma reagin.

*Most specific for condition.

NEURODEVELOPMENT

Neurologic development is a complex process that involves physical growth and environmental stimulation. Most of the physical development of the brain takes place before birth and continues for the first few years of life. Once the basic architecture of the brain has formed, it is dependent on the environment to stimulate biochemical pathways and synaptic impulses that allow for cognitive, motor, and sensory processes to grow. Neurologic development can be divided into four categories:

1. Motor
2. Cognitive
3. Language
4. Behavioral

It is uncommon for a child to have a single area of developmental impairment. Recognize that developmental deficiencies can manifest as behavioral problems. For example, children with language delay may present with aggressive behavior because they are unable to communicate their needs. Primary care physicians have an important role in screening children for possible developmental delay. The goal of developmental screening is to identify children who require formal testing. Parents will often overestimate their child's developmental abilities; therefore, any parental concern of developmental delay should be evaluated.

DEVELOPMENTAL MILESTONES

TABLE 2-1.   *DEVELOPMENTAL MILESTONES*

FIGURE 2-1.   *DEVELOPMENTAL AGE ASSOCIATED WITH DRAWING SHAPES.*

TABLE 2-1 *DEVELOPMENTAL MILESTONES*

AGE	GROSS MOTOR	FINE MOTOR	SOCIAL SKILLS/LANGUAGE
First 4 wk	• Tonic neck position • Moro reflex • Palmar grasp • Head lag	• Tracking to 90° across midline	• Regards face • Recognizes sound
1-2 mo	• Tonic neck position • Moro reflex • Palmar grasp • Improved head control	• Tracking to 180°	• Social smile • Recognizes parents • Cooing
4 mo	• Sits with support • Tonic position fades • Absent Moro reflex • Absent palmar grasp • Improved head control	• Reaches out for objects • Rolls from prone to supine • Hands to midline	• Laughs out loud • Recognizes objects
6 mo	• Sits without support • Stands with support • Creeps • No head lag	• Object transfer • Holds cracker	• Object permanence • Recognizes strangers without anxiety • Babbles "ba," "ga," "da"
8-9 mo	• Crawls • Walks with support • Pulls to stand (10 mo)	• Holds 1 object in each hand • Handles small objects • Throws objects • Plays patty cake • Holds bottle in one hand	• Babbles strings of syllables • Mama/dada, nonspecific • Understands "no" • Stranger anxiety begins
1 y	• Walks with hand held	• Pincer grasp • Plays ball • Drinks from a cup	• Speaks one word • Mama/dada specific • Self-play • Follows 1-step command
18 mo	• Climbs stairs with assistance • Runs	• Builds a tower of 3-4 cubes • Uses spoon to feed self	• Speaks 3-4 words • Recognizes body parts

TABLE 2-1   *DEVELOPMENTAL MILESTONES (CONTINUED)*

AGE	GROSS MOTOR	FINE MOTOR	SOCIAL SKILLS/LANGUAGE
2 y	• Climbs up stairs without assistance • Jumps	• Removes clothes • Draws a line • Builds a tower of 7 cubes	• 50-word vocabulary • Follows 2-step commands • 50% intelligible speech • Initiation of toilet training
3 y	• Alternates feet when climbing steps	• Throws a ball overhand • Rides a tricycle • Draws a circle • Builds a tower of 10 cubes	• Knows full name • Speaks complete sentences • 75% intelligible speech • Recognizes colors
4 y	• Hops • Skips (5 y)	• Brushes teeth • Dresses self • Draws a square • Catches ball	• Complex sentences • Names 4 colors • Initiates group play • 100% intelligible speech • Toilet training complete

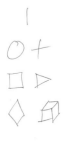

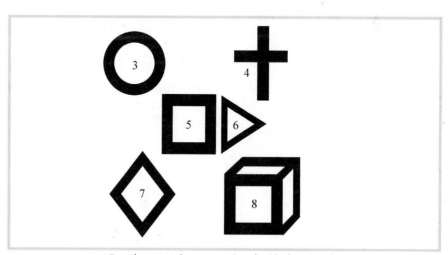

– **FIGURE 2-1** –   Developmental age associated with drawing shapes

Intelligence/Cognition

- **Intelligence Quotient (IQ)**: IQ is defined as mental age / chronological age × 100. The average range is 85 to 115, with a mean of 100. IQ testing is useful in evaluating overall intellectual ability. Historically it was developed to identify children who would benefit from school instruction. It is still the best predictor of academic success. IQ testing does not predict adult success. In infancy and early childhood, language is a better predictor of cognitive function than motor development.

Mental Retardation (MR)

MR is usually defined as an IQ of less than or equal to 70 with onset before age 18 years, and limitations in two or more of the ten following activities of daily living: communication, self-care, home living, social skills, community use, self-direction, health and safety, functional academics, leisure, and work. The incidence is approximately 1% to 3% of the general population. There are several categories of MR, best categorized by the IQ.

- **Mild Mental Retardation (IQ 55-70)**: The most common form of mental retardation. These individuals have mild defects in cognitive functioning that are very subtle. Most patients with mild MR are not usually recognized until they enter school. They possess the ability to be formally educated and can overcome their developmental deficiencies. They may function independently as adults.

- **Moderate Mental Retardation (IQ 40-55)**: These individuals have increased limitations in normal daily functions. They possess the ability to be trained to perform simple tasks and job functions. They may be able to function independently but often require some support.

- **Severe Mental Retardation (IQ 20-40)**: these individuals have significant limitations in all areas of cognitive development. They are usually not trainable. They are often dependent on a caretaker for daily support.

- **Profound Mental Retardation (IQ <20)**: These individuals have devastating limitations in all areas of cognitive development. They have minimal interaction with their environment and often require institutionalization.

TABLE 2-2.	*CONGENITAL ETIOLOGIES FOR MENTAL RETARDATION*
TABLE 2-3.	*ACQUIRED ETIOLOGIES FOR MENTAL RETARDATION*

TABLE 2-2	CONGENITAL ETIOLOGIES FOR MENTAL RETARDATION
Toxin exposure	• Fetal alcohol syndrome
	• TORCH infections
Metabolic disorders	• Mucopolysaccharidosis
	• Tay-Sachs disease
	• Hurler syndrome
	• Phenylketonuria
Brain malformations	• Anencephaly
	• Hydrocephalus
Genetic disorders	• Down syndrome
	• Edwards syndrome
	• William syndrome
	• Fragile-X syndrome
	• Klinefelter syndrome
	• Prader-Willi syndrome

TORCH, **t**oxoplasmosis, **o**ther viruses, **r**ubella, **c**ytomegalovirus, **h**erpes simplex.

TABLE 2-3	COMMON ACQUIRED ETIOLOGIES FOR MENTAL RETARDATION
Birth asphyxia	
Intraventricular hemorrhage	
Head trauma	
Meningitis	
Encephalitis	
Heavy metal exposure (lead)	
Near drowning	
Psychosocial deprivation	
Malnutrition (severe)	

SELECTED DEVELOPMENTAL DISORDERS

LANGUAGE DELAY (DELAYED SPEECH)

The development of communication and language ability depends on the child's capacity to understand, process, and express his emotions or desires. Therefore, the evaluation of a child with delayed speech should include differentiation of defects in understanding (reception) versus expression. Hearing loss is an important cause of language delay, and its evaluation should include an audiologic assessment. Children with a defect in language reception have an increased incidence of other developmental deficiencies. Speech delay is present in approximately 10% of the general population.

TABLE 2-4	CAUSES OF LANGUAGE DELAY

A short frenulum does not contribute to speech delay.

Idiopathic
Hearing loss
Mental retardation
Pervasive developmental disorder
Landau-Kleffner syndrome
Rett syndrome
Dysarthria
Child abuse/neglect

HEARING LOSS

Competent hearing ability allows for cognitive brain and receptive language development. The normal pathway of hearing can be divided into two stages: conduction and processing. Normal sound waves travel from the air, to the external ear canal, and eventually to the tympanic membrane. Vibrations are sensed on the membrane by the hair cells of the organ of Corti and transmitted by the eighth cranial nerve to the auditory cortex for processing. The etiology of hearing loss can therefore be classified as conductive (abnormal function of the auditory canal or tympanic membrane) versus sensorineural (abnormal function of the neural pathway). Conductive hearing loss is usually acquired in the postnatal period. The most common etiologies include fluid in the middle ear (otitis media) or wax or a foreign body in the ear canal. Deformations of the tympanic membrane (i.e., scarring causing stiffness, or perforation) can also cause conduction problems. Sensorineural hearing loss is usually acquired perinatally. Risk factors include TORCH infections, genetic syndromes, prematurity, kernicterus, meningitis and ototoxic medications. Hearing disabilities affect nearly 21 million Americans (including approximately 5% to 7% of the children in the United States).

TABLE 2-5.	CAUSES OF HEARING DISABILITIES

TABLE 2-5	*COMMON CAUSES OF HEARING DISABILITIES*

CONDUCTIVE HEARING LOSS	SENSORINEURAL HEARING LOSS
• Otitis media (most common)	• TORCH infections (congenital rubella most common)
• Meningitis	• Prematurity
• Cholesteatoma	• Ototoxic medications
• Perforation of the tympanic membrane	• Kernicterus
• Foreign body	• Alport syndrome
• Craniofacial deformity (secondary otitis)	• Waardenburg syndrome
	• Mucopolysaccharidosis

TORCH, **t**oxoplasmosis, **o**ther viruses, **r**ubella, **c**ytomegalovirus, **h**erpes simplex.

ATTENTION DEFICIT HYPERACTIVITY DISORDER (ADHD)

DEFINITION: The presence of a combination of inattention, impulsivity, and /or hyperactivity (usually assessed by standardized scales), to a degree that is maladaptive and inconsistent with developmental level. In addition, the diagnostic criteria require that symptoms are chronic, have persisted for more than 6 months, and are present in two or more settings (i.e., school and home). Symptoms should be present before age 7.

ETIOLOGY: There is a strong genetic predisposition. Affects males more than females. Incidence decreases with increasing age.

CLINICAL PRESENTATION: Children frequently present before the age of 7 years with learning difficulty, inattention, and anxiety. Patients whose major symptom is inattentiveness with few behavior problems may not present until the adolescent period. Often children will show minimal symptoms in novel situations (i.e., the doctor's office), and increased symptomatology in situations that are "boring" or require sustained attention (i.e., reading a book). Poor self-esteem and comorbid depression are also common.

DIAGNOSIS: A detailed history with a comprehensive school report that outlines performance and behavior is helpful. The evaluation for diagnosis in many communities involves a multidisciplinary approach and includes a neurologist. There is no one specific test used for diagnosis. All children who are evaluated for ADHD should also be evaluated for anxiety and depression, which mimic the symptoms of inattention and hyperactivity. Routine lab tests including lead levels and thyroid panels are not indicated unless the history suggests a specific etiology.

TREATMENT: Once a diagnosis is confirmed, first-line therapy should include behavioral modification. Pharmacologic therapy with stimulant medications and antidepressants has been successful. Although the mechanism of action of stimulant medications in the treatment of ADHD is not completely understood, they are generally well tolerated. Side effects include appetite suppression, insomnia, mood disorders, and hypertension. Occasionally, children with ADHD have undiagnosed Tourette syndrome as well. These patients may have tics unmasked while on stimulant medications, leading to the additional diagnosis. If tics are observed, the medication should be discontinued and a nonstimulant medication substituted.

GILLES DE LA TOURETTE SYNDROME

DEFINITION: Presence of multiple motor and one or more vocal tics, occurring nearly every day for more than 1 year, with no more than 3 consecutive months without tics. The motor and vocal tics are not required to occur at the same time.

ETIOLOGY: Dopamine dysregulation is strongly suspected. There is a genetic predisposition.

CLINICAL PRESENTATION: Children will present by early school age with simple motor or verbal tics. Tics are usually involuntary and repetitive and may be exacerbated by stress or anxiety. Throat clearing, sniffing, and unusual vocal sounds are common. Symptoms wax, wane, and may last into adolescence and adulthood. The syndrome is most common in white males. There is no association with developmental or language delay. There is an increased risk for developing ADHD (50%) and obsessive-compulsive disorder (OCD).

DIAGNOSIS: The diagnosis is suspected if the child meets the criteria in the definition above. Additionally, the onset must be before age 18 years, and cause distress and impairment in daily activities. Other possible conditions should be ruled out (e.g., encephalitis).

TREATMENT: Dopamine blockade with haloperidol or pimozide. Treatment of associated ADHD or OCD should take precedence, as these disorders cause more disability.

PERVASIVE DEVELOPMENTAL DISORDERS (PDD)

DEFINITION: PDD are best characterized as continued disorders of language and social interaction that prevent the child from maturing as his/her peers do. They encompass a spectrum of impaired social interactions, language development and abnormal behavior. These disorders have developmental sequelae, predominately affecting speech. The two most common disorders are autism and Asperger syndrome. The overall incidence is approximately 2-4 per 1000 children in the United States.

ETIOLOGY: Unknown. There has been no proven association with the measles-mumps-rubella (MMR) vaccine. PDD are more common in males. There is a genetic predisposition.

CLINICAL PRESENTATION: Children often present by the age of 3 years with language delay. There are usually associated social and behavioral abnormalities.

Anxiety, hyperactivity, and depression may also be present. There is a progressive divergence from the norm. There is usually no significant past medical history.

TREATMENT: Aggressive multi-disciplinary behavior modification, speech and occupational therapy. Although there is no successful pharmacologic treatment available, medications may be used to help alleviate comorbid symptoms such as hyperactivity and depression. The prognoses of PDD are generally poor, with the exception of Asperger syndrome, which yields a good prognosis if intervention is early and consistent.

TABLE 2-6. *SIGNS/SYMPTOMS OF AUTISM*

TABLE 2-7. *PERVASIVE DEVELOPMENTAL DISORDERS*

TABLE 2-6	*SIGNS/SYMPTOMS OF AUTISM*
	Poor social interactions
	Does not seek comfort when distressed
	Impaired imagination
	Lack of desire to make friends
	Impaired language
	Preoccupation with objects
	Routines are common
	Avoids changes in environment
	Avoids eye contact
	Seizures (15%-35%)
	Mental retardation common (75%)

TABLE 2-7   *PERVASIVE DEVELOPMENTAL DISORDERS*

MILD: ASPERGER SYNDROME	SEVERE: AUTISM
Affects:	Affects:
• Social interaction	• Social interaction
• Restricted interests	• Language
• Development normal	• Imagination
	• Behavior
	• Play
	• Developmental delay present

RETT SYNDROME

DEFINITION: A neurodegenerative disorder characterized by microcephaly, language regression, and developmental delay.

ETIOLOGY: X-linked dominant inheritance. Affects females only.

CLINICAL PRESENTATION: Female children present at age 6 to 18 months with regression of language, loss of milestones, and associated poor head growth (acquired microcephaly). Ataxia, pervasive developmental symptoms, and characteristic flapping hand movements are common.

DIAGNOSIS: Clinical history and presentation. Genetic testing is now available.

TREATMENT: Supportive therapy. There is no known treatment available. There is a poor prognosis with mortality in the third decade of life.

LANDAU-KLEFFNER SYNDROME

DEFINITION: Epileptic aphasia.

ETIOLOGY: Epileptic discharges in temporal lobes result in the selected loss of language skills.

CLINICAL PRESENTATION: Children present by the age of 5 years with regression of previously acquired speech ability, onset of seizure disorder, and autistic behavior. Affects boys more frequently than girls.

DIAGNOSIS: Clinical history and EEG including sleep studies are often helpful. Seizure disorder and autism do not need to be present for diagnosis.

TREATMENT: Aggressive speech therapy and seizure control with anticonvulsants yield a good prognosis.

Primary Care Development

ENURESIS

DEFINITION: Involuntary and regular discharge of urine after toilet training is underway. There are two types: primary (child was never fully toilet trained), and secondary (child had been previously toilet trained for 3 months or longer). Enuresis can be further divided into nocturnal (nighttime) and diurnal (daytime).

ETIOLOGY: A genetic predisposition has been noted. Children with nocturnal enuresis are unable to recognize that the bladder is full, and do not wake from sleep in response. Children with diurnal enuresis exhibit dysfunctional voiding habits (bowel and bladder sphincter dysfunction) that are thought to be a major factor.

CLINICAL PRESENTATION: Nocturnal bedwetting is much more common than diurnal accidents. Affects males more than females. Nocturnal enuresis affects up to 25% of all 4-year-olds and decreases with increasing age to approximately 1% at age 15 years. The incidence of daytime enuresis is 10% at 4 years.

DIAGNOSIS: Clinical history and presentation. Urinalysis and urine cultures are adequate screening tests. Daytime enuresis should always be evaluated for an organic etiology. The differential diagnosis includes urinary tract infection, ectopic urethra, spinal cord disease, diabetes mellitus, diabetes insipidus, sickle cell disease, and sexual abuse.

TREATMENT: Parental understanding that the child is not voiding purposely is important. Bedwetting alarms are often adequate first-line therapy and are associated with high success rates and ease of use. Pharmacologic treatment with imiprimine or intranasal DDAVP may be useful in severe cases. DDAVP may also be used as short-term treatment in situations where bedwetting would be particularly undesirable, such as at sleep-away camp.

ENCOPRESIS

DEFINITION: Repeated, involuntary passage of stool into clothing by a child older than 4 years of age, for more than 1 month. Similar to enuresis, encopresis may be primary (bowel continence had never been achieved) or secondary (child had previously been continent of stool).

ETIOLOGY: Genetic predisposition. Chronic constipation with overflow incontinence is the most common cause. Affects males more frequently than females.

CLINICAL PRESENTATION: Children present with daytime and nighttime accidents. These accidents may occur in school and cause significant embarrassment to the child. Abdominal pain and avoiding the toilet are common. Children often deny the accident even when asked directly, or confronted with soiled clothing. Approximately 25% of affected children have associated enuresis. Late onset Hirschsprung disease is occasionally diagnosed during evaluation of encopresis.

DIAGNOSIS: Clinical history and presentation. An abdominal radiograph is helpful in evaluating overflow incontinence. Physical exam should include an assessment of the lumbosacral area, as well as an evaluation of lower limb sensory and motor function. Suspected cases of Hirschsprung disease should undergo rectal biopsy to visualize microscopic ganglion cells.

TREATMENT: In cases of chronic constipation, bowel evacuation with short-term use of enemas and laxatives may be necessary. Dietary adjustments to high-fiber, low-fat meals are important. Toilet retraining may be necessary. A behavioral modification program, which includes positive reinforcement, is the gold standard. All efforts should be made to avoid embarrassing the child.

TOILET TRAINING

Most children are fully toilet trained by 4 years of age. Communication of the desire to toilet train and developmental readiness are the keys to success. Daytime continence is usually achieved a few months before nighttime continence. Bowel control is usually obtained before bladder control. Girls often achieve successful training before boys. Children should not be forced to toilet train; they should be encouraged.

NIGHTMARES

Repeated episodes of frightening dreams that occur during REM sleep (i.e., several hours after the patient has fallen asleep). These dreams often awaken the patient from sleep in the late night/early morning hours. The dreams are usually recalled. This condition affects boys and girls equally. Spontaneous resolution by adolescence is common.

NIGHT TERRORS

Repeated episodes of violent, frightening (to observer), sudden screaming events with the eyes wide open. The child may appear awake, but does not respond to stimulation. Night terrors occur soon after falling asleep while in transition from stage 3 or 4 sleep to REM sleep. The episode is not remembered by the patient. Parents should not attempt to wake the patient during the episode. Spontaneous resolution by adolescence is common. Avoidance of stress and excessive fatigue is helpful, as is parental reassurance. There is usually a positive family history for parasomnias (sleepwalking, sleep talking).

TEMPER TANTRUMS

A normal component of development. Defined as outbursts of inappropriate behavior, screaming or stubbornness due to frustration or anger. A careful approach as to the possible cause of tantrums should be performed. Reassurance of the parent by the physician is useful. The "time-out" technique is also a useful disciplinary tool. A social history to rule out parental neglect or abuse should be obtained.

BREATH HOLDING SPELLS

Characterized as involuntary breath holding episodes often in response to pain, frustration or noxious stimuli. There are two main types of breath holding spells: cyanotic and pallid. Cyanotic spells are usually more severe and are often associated with crying, cyanosis and loss of consciousness. Pallid spells are not associated with crying. Children with pallid spells frequently lose consciousness and become limp. Anoxic seizures may be present with either category. Breath holding affects males and females equally, and occurs predominantly from infancy to 6 years of age. The episodes are often frightening to the parent. The main goals of therapy are to avoid situations of secondary gain by breath holding and to keep the child in a safe environment during an episode.

CHAPTER 3

NUTRITION

CALORIC REQUIREMENTS

Caloric requirements per kilogram of body weight:

- The premature neonate: approximately 120 kcal/kg/day
- The full-term neonate to 2 years: approximately 100 kcal/kg/day
- Age 2-10 years: approximately 90 kcal/kg/day
- Age 11-14 years: approximately 55 kcal/kg/day

Daily caloric requirements can be estimated by the following formula:

- First 10 kg: 1000 kcal/day
- Second 10 kg: 500 kcal/day
- Each kg after 20 kg: 1 kcal/day

Example: a 14-kg infant requires 1200 kcal/day; 1000 kcal for the first 10 kg + 200 kcal (500 × .40) for the next 4 kg.

PHYSICAL GROWTH

The normal full-term newborn:

- May lose up to 5% to10% of its birth weight during the first week of life mainly due to extracellular water loss. The infant should recover the lost weight by 2 weeks of age.
- Should gain approximately 30 grams (1 ounce) per day.
- Should double his birth weight by 6 months of age.
- Should triple his birth weight by 1 year of age.
- Should double his height by 4 years of age.

BREAST MILK VS. WHOLE COW'S MILK

- Colostrum (initial breast milk) is the most valuable form of breast milk. It is rich in macrophages and secretory IgA that help enhance early immunity and protect against infection.
- The relative water content of breast and cow's milks are equal.
- The caloric values of both milks are approximately 20 kcal/oz or 0.67 kcal/mL.
- Human milk contains more carbohydrate (predominately lactose).
- Human milk has less quantitative fat and iron than cow's milk; however, both substances are more readily absorbed from human milk.

TABLE 3-1.	*COMPARISON BETWEEN BREAST MILK AND WHOLE COW'S MILK*
TABLE 3-2.	*CONTRAINDICATIONS FOR BREAST-FEEDING*
TABLE 3-3.	*ACCEPTABLE CONDITIONS FOR BREAST-FEEDING*

TABLE 3-1   *COMPARISONS BETWEEN BREAST MILK AND WHOLE COW'S MILK*

	BREAST MILK	WHOLE COW'S MILK
Calories	=	=
Water content	=	=
Fat content	↓	↑
Protein	↓	↑
Carbohydrate	↑	↓
Iron	↓	↑
Sodium	↓	↑
Minerals	↓	↑
Vitamin C	↑	↓
Vitamin D	↓	↑
Vitamin K	↓	↑
Immunity	↑	↓

TABLE 3-2	*CONTRAINDICATIONS FOR BREAST-FEEDING*

HIV infection
Active tuberculosis
Breast cancer
Substance abuse
Maternal medications category D or X
Active herpetic lesions on the breast
Acute systemic herpes disease
Herpes zoster
Septicemia
Cytomegalovirus infection (premature neonate)
Postpartum psychosis

TABLE 3-3	*ACCEPTABLE CONDITIONS FOR BREAST-FEEDING*

Viral syndrome
History of tuberculosis
Mastitis
Hepatitis B
Hepatitis C
Rubella
Cytomegalovirus infection (full-term neonate)

VITAMIN AND MINERAL SUPPLEMENTATION

- Iron supplementation in the breast-fed infant should begin at age 4 to 6 months.
- Vitamin D supplementation in the breast-fed infant should begin at age 6 months.
- Formula-fed infants should receive iron-fortified formula from birth.
- Premature infants should receive multivitamin supplementation including vitamins A, C, E, and the B vitamins from birth.
- Fluoride supplementation depends on the local community water supply and should begin at 6 months of age in children who receive only fluoride-free tap or bottled water.

- Solid foods should be introduced at 6 months of age with careful observation for potential food allergies. One new food should be introduced each week as tolerated, beginning with cereal first, vegetable, and fruit later. Protein-containing foods should be introduced last.

COMMON MILK DEFICIENCIES

- Infants of vegetarian or vegan mothers are susceptible to vitamin B_{12} deficiency.
- Infants fed exclusively goat's milk are prone to folate-deficient megaloblastic anemia.
- Infants fed large amounts of evaporated milk are at risk for hypernatremia and dehydration if the milk is improperly prepared.
- Infants fed large amounts of cow's milk are at risk for iron deficiency anemia.

VITAMINS AND MINERALS

TABLE 3-4.   *VITAMINS*

TABLE 3-5.   *MINERALS*

TABLE 3-4 *VITAMINS*

VITAMIN	FUNCTION	EXCESS	DEFICIENCY
A **Retinol**	• Retinal pigmentation • Vision • Epithelial development • Tooth and bone structure	• Hyperostosis • Pseudotumor cerebri • Bulging fontanelle • Carotenemia • Anorexia • Skin desquamation	• Night blindness • Poor bone formation • Recurrent infection • Keratomalacia • Xerosis • Growth failure
B$_1$ **Thiamine**	• Oxidative decarboxylation of alpha keto acids and sugars	• None	• Beriberi • Cardiomegaly • Wernicke encephalopathy • Korsakoff psychosis • Radial nerve palsy • Fatigue • Irritability • Anorexia
B$_2$ **Riboflavin**	• Oxidative phosphorylation • Electron transfer reactions	• None	• Cheilosis • Greasy, scaly facial rash • Mucosal hyperemia

B$_3$
Niacin
	• NAD, NADPH cofactors
	• Synthesized from tryptophan
		• Skin flushing
		• Skin rashes
		• Bile stasis
		• Pruritus
		• Hyperuricemia
			• Pellagra
			  - Dermatitis
			  - Diarrhea
			  - Dementia
			• Black tongue

B$_6$ **Pyridoxine**	• Heme synthesis • Neurotransmission	• Sensory neuropathy	• Seizures • Glossitis • Dermatitis • Peripheral neuropathy with INH treatment

(Continued)

TABLE 3-4   *VITAMINS (CONTINUED)*

VITAMIN	FUNCTION	EXCESS	DEFICIENCY
B$_{12}$ **Cyanocobalamin**	• Methylation of homocysteine to methionine • Absorbed in ileum • Only found in animal products	• None	• Pernicious anemia • Macrocytic anemia • Common in small bowel disease, celiac disease, irritable bowel disease, fish tapeworm
Folate	• Synthesis of purines, pyrimidines, nucleoproteins	• Masks B$_{12}$ deficiency • Malaise • Irritability • Insomnia	• Megaloblastic anemia (macrocytic) • Glossitis
C **Ascorbic acid**	• Collagen stability • Aids iron absorption • Antioxidant	• Oxaluria • Renal stones • Diarrhea	• Scurvy • Poor wound healing • Bleeding gums • Infection • Anorexia
D **Ergosterol** **Ergocalciferol** **Cholecalciferol**	• Regulates calcium, phosphorus, bone development, and mineralization	• Hypercalcemia • Renal stones • Polyuria • Nausea • Diarrhea • Hypertension • Failure to thrive	• Rickets • Craniotabes • Rachitic rosary • Harrison grooves • Tetany
E	• Antioxidant	• None	• Hemolytic anemia in neonates • Neuropathies • Myopathies • Ataxia
K	• Procoagulant • Factors II, VII, IX, X • Produced by intestinal bacteria	• Hyperbilirubinemia • Hemolytic anemia • Kernicterus	• Hemorrhagic disease of the newborn • Vitamin A, D, E, and K deficiencies are common in cystic fibrosis, pancreatic disease, and cholestatic disease

INH, isoniazid; NAD, nicotinamide-adenine dinucleotide; NADPH, nicotinamide-adenine nucleotide, reduced.

TABLE 3-5   *MINERALS*

MINERAL	ROLE	EXCESS	DEFICIENCY
Calcium	• Structure of bones/teeth • Cardiac contractility • Muscle contraction • Nerve conduction • Blood coagulation • Breast milk production	• Shortened QT interval • Cardiac dysrhythmias • Renal stones • Calcification of soft tissues	• Increased QT interval • Tetany • Rickets • Scurvy • Parathyroid hyperplasia • Laryngospasm
Phosphorus	• Regulate pH • Structure of bones/teeth • ATP precursor • Vitamin D + PTH aid absorption	• Abdominal pain • Vomiting • Renal impairment • Neuromuscular impairment	• Muscle weakness • Rickets in premature infants • Anorexia
Fluoride	• Structure of bones/teeth	• Mottling of teeth	• Cavities
Iron	• Structure of hemoglobin • Structure of myoglobin • Absorption aided by vitamin C	• Fatigue • Abdominal pain • Vomiting • Hemachromatosis	• Hypochromic, microcytic anemia • Recurrent infection • Angular stomatitis
Potassium	• Muscle contraction • Nerve conduction • Major intracellular ion • Heart rhythm	• Fatal cardiac dysrhythmias • Peaked T waves	• Nausea • Muscle weakness • U waves on ECG • ACTH excess • Bone fragility • Adrenal hypertrophy • Failure to thrive
Sodium	• Major osmotic force • Major extracellular ion • Nerve conduction • Muscle contraction	• Seizures • Fluid shifts • Neurologic changes	• Anorexia • Nausea • Seizures • Increased intracranial pressure • Neurologic changes • Fluid shifts • Muscle atrophy

(Continued)

TABLE 3-5   *MINERALS (CONTINUED)*

MINERAL	ROLE	EXCESS	DEFICIENCY
Magnesium	• Muscle contraction • Nerve conduction • Protein synthesis • Calcium antagonist	• Hypotonia • Hyporeflexia	• Tetany • Muscle spasms • Depression
Copper	• Collagen stability	• None	• Microcytic anemia • Menke kinky hair syndrome
Zinc	• Collagen stability	• None	• Dwarfism • Acrodermatitis enteropathica • Poor wound healing • Scaling of the skin • Common in patients dependent on chronic total parenteral nutrition

ACTH, adrenocorticotrophic hormone; ATP, adenine triphosphate; PTH, parathyroid hormone.

DEFICIENCY SYNDROMES

TABLE 3-6.   *COMPARISON OF MARASMUS AND KWASHIORKOR*
FIGURE 3-1.   *MARASMUS VS. KWASHIORKOR.*

FAILURE TO THRIVE (FTT)

Failure to thrive is more of a descriptive term than a diagnosis, referring to a decrease in height and/or weight for age documented over a period of time. A growth chart will often reveal failure to maintain growth potential by crossing over 2 growth percentiles or by persistently maintaining less than the 3rd percentile for age. This will require more than one plot on a growth curve over time for diagnosis. A careful history is the most important evaluation and will help determine if the cause of FTT is organic (medical cause), nonorganic (nonmedical cause), or a combination of both. Children with FTT are clinically recognized by weight loss, reduced muscle mass, signs of vitamin deficiencies, hair loss, neurodevelopmental delay, and recurrent infection.

TABLE 3-6	COMPARISON OF MARASMUS AND KWASHIORKOR			
	DEFINITION	CLINICAL PRESENTATION	DIAGNOSIS	TREATMENT
Marasmus	• Calorie insufficiency	• Alert • Hungry • Dramatic weight loss • Emaciation • Loss of fat • Muscle atrophy	• Clinical history and presentation	• Caloric modification
Kwashiorkor	• Protein-calorie insufficiency	• Lethargic • Dramatic weight loss • Emaciation • Loss of fat • Muscle atrophy • Pitting edema • Neurologic changes • Recurrent infections • Striped red hair	• Low albumin • Low glucose	• *Slow* advancement of calories and nutrition • Antibiotic prophylaxis

Organic FTT

1. Decreased nutrient intake
   a. Cleft lip or palate
   b. Gastroesophageal reflux
   c. Lack of appetite (chronic infection, CNS pathology)
   d. Inability to swallow (CNS pathology)
2. Malabsorption, impaired utilization, and/or increased excretion of nutrients
   a. Insulin-dependent diabetes mellitus (IDDM)
   b. Cystic fibrosis
   c. Renal tubular acidosis
   d. Celiac disease
   e. Inborn errors of metabolism

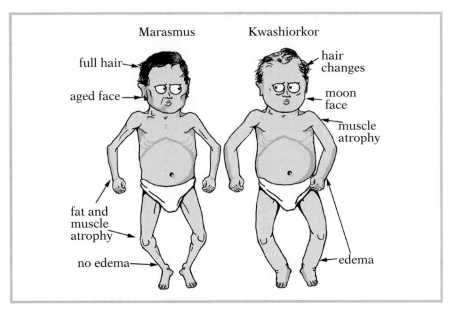

— **FIGURE 3-1** — Marasmus vs. kwashiorkor.

3. Increased energy requirement
   a. Congenital heart disease
   b. Malignancy
   c. Hyperthyroidism
   d. Chronic illness
   e. Bronchopulmonary dysplasia
4. Prenatal causes of FTT
   a. Trisomies
   b. Russell-Silver syndrome
   c. Achondroplasia
   d. Intrauterine growth retardation
   e. Maternal malnutrition
   f. Toxic exposure in utero

Nonorganic FTT

The most common causes of FTT associated with environmental and psychosocial factors:

1. Inexperienced parents
2. Poor feeding technique
3. Poverty
4. Child neglect
5. Dysfunctional family interactions

Combined Organic and Nonorganic FTT

When environmental and psychosocial factors contribute to FTT of organic etiology (example: psychosocial impact of chronic illnesses on family interactions).

OBESITY

Obesity is an increasing childhood epidemic in the United States. Inadequate physical activity is the greatest contributing factor. In addition, many children and adolescents eat poor diets deficient in key nutrients and high in fat. There are two forms of obesity: endogenous (medical causes) and exogenous (environmental influences). The endogenous causes of obesity, all of which are associated with delayed bone age, include: Prader-Willi, Laurence Moon-Biedl, and Cushing syndromes, and hypothyroidism.

Children with exogenous obesity are typically tall for age and have advanced bone development, although the final adult height may eventually be compromised. Approximately 75% of obese children become obese adults. Body mass index (BMI) is the most useful index for screening children and adolescents. A BMI greater than 30 or more than 85th percentile for age should be referred for further evaluation.

Childhood obesity contributes to early morbidity and mortality in adulthood due to:

- Hypercholesterolemia
- Hypertension
- Atherosclerosis
- Type II diabetes

Pediatric complications of obesity include:

- Poor psychosocial interactions
- Poor self-esteem
- Blount disease
- Polycystic ovarian syndrome (PCOS)
- Slipped capital femoral epiphysis (SCFE)
- Hyperestrogenism
- Primary menarche
- Hypertension
- Pseudotumor cerebri
- Obstructive sleep apnea (OSA)
- Mature-onset diabetes of youth (MODY)

Treatment options include exercise programs, nutritional counseling and family support. Caloric goals for weight reduction are based upon the desired weight.

[handwritten margin note: endogenous causes of obesity — Prader-Willi, Laurence Moon-Biedl, Cushing syndrome, hypothyroidism]

CHAPTER 4

GASTROENTEROLOGY

GASTROINTESTINAL SIGNS AND SYMPTOMS

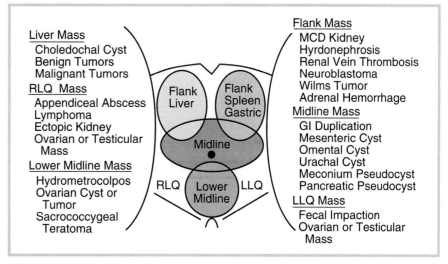

– FIGURE 4-1 – Causes of an abdominal mass based upon location.

Source: Rychman FC, Evaluation of abdominal masses in infants and children. In: Rudolph CD, Rudolph AM, Hostetter MK, Lister G, Siegel NJ, eds. Rudolph's Pediatrics. 21st ed. New York: McGraw-Hill, 2002, p. 1375.

TABLE 4-1	*CAUSES OF ABDOMINAL PAIN*

INFANTS	CHILDREN/ADOLESCENTS
• Colic	• Acute gastroenteritis
• Gastroesophageal reflux	• Gastritis
• Formula intolerance/allergy	• Gastroesophageal reflux
• Acute gastroenteritis	• Meckel diverticulum
• Meckel diverticulum	• Appendicitis
• Intussusception	• Diabetic ketoacidosis
• Volvulus	• Pneumonia
• Trauma	• Urinary tract infection/pyelonephritis
• Neuroblastoma	• Kidney stone
	• Trauma
	• Crohn disease
	• Ulcerative colitis
	• Mesenteric adenitis
	• Diskitis
	• Pancreatitis
	• Cholecystitis
	• Cholelithiasis
	• Lead poisoning
	• Black widow spider bite
	• Pelvic inflammatory disease
	• Pregnancy
	• Wilms tumor

TABLE 4-2	*CAUSES OF ASCITES*

Congestive heart failure
Tricuspid regurgitation
Malignancy
Cirrhosis
Budd-Chiari syndrome (hepatic vein obstruction)
Inferior vena cava obstruction
Lymphatic obstruction
Pancreatitis

Peritonitis
Severe malnutrition
Hypoalbuminemia
Nephrotic syndrome
Protein-losing enteropathy
Parasites

TABLE 4-3	*CAUSES OF UPPER GASTROINTESTINAL TRACT BLEEDING*

INFANTS	CHILDREN/ADOLESCENTS
• Swallowed maternal blood	• Gastritis
• Gastritis	• Peptic ulcer disease
• Necrotizing enterocolitis	• Foreign body
• Foreign body	• Epistaxis
• Trauma	• Mallory-Weiss tear
• Peptic ulcer disease	• Esophageal varices
• Food allergy	• Caustic ingestion
• Allergic enterocolitis	• Coagulopathy
• Volvulus	• Trauma
• Vascular malformation	

TABLE 4-4   *CAUSES OF LOWER GASTROINTESTINAL TRACT BLEEDING*

INFANTS	CHILDREN/ADOLESCENTS
• Necrotizing enterocolitis	• Hemorrhoids
• Allergic enterocolitis	• Infectious colitis
• Anal fissure	• Meckel diverticulum
• Intussusception	• Polyps
• Volvulus	• Crohn disease
• Hirschsprung disease	• Ulcerative colitis
• Hemolytic uremic syndrome	• Henoch-Schönlein purpura
• Meckel diverticulum	• Hemolytic uremic syndrome
• Infectious colitis	

DISORDERS OF THE ESOPHAGUS

GASTROESOPHAGEAL REFLUX DISEASE (GERD)

DEFINITION: The passage of gastric contents into the esophagus. It is the most common gastrointestinal disorder in children, and is very common in premature infants.

ETIOLOGY: The most common cause is transient lower esophageal sphincter relaxation. Additional contributing factors include delayed gastric emptying, impaired esophageal motility, and hiatal hernia.

CLINICAL PRESENTATION: In infants, the only presenting symptom may be subtle "spit-ups" that can occur anytime after feeding. Vomiting, gagging, and choking may be present in more severe cases. Reflux that passes to the laryngeal airway and irritates the glottis may result in a vagal reflex with subsequent apnea, bradycardia, limpness, cyanosis, and/or pallor. Arching can be a sign of reflux esophagitis. Extraesophageal signs of reflux include cough, wheezing, hoarse cry, stridor, and frequent pneumonias. Adolescents may present with halitosis or chest pain.

DIAGNOSIS: The diagnosis of GERD is made clinically. A pH probe is helpful in quantifying diagnosis and evaluating the response to treatment. In cases in which the diagnosis is unclear, an upper gastrointestinal series (UGIS) should be performed to rule out anatomical causes of vomiting (i.e., malrotation, obstruction, congenital webs, pyloric stenosis).

TABLE 4-5.   *TREATMENT OF GASTROESOPHAGEAL REFLUX DISEASE*

TABLE 4-6.   *COMPLICATIONS OF GASTROESOPHAGEAL REFLUX DISEASE*

TABLE 4-5	*TREATMENT OF GASTROESOPHAGEAL REFLUX DISEASE*

TREATMENT MODALITY	EXAMPLES/NOTES
Reflux precautions	• Head of bed at 30° for 30 min after feeds (infants)
Dietary modification	• Avoidance of fatty foods, caffeine, alcohol (adolescents)
Antacids	• Magnesium/aluminum salts • Histamine blockers (ranitidine) • Proton-pump inhibitors (omeprazole, pantoprazole)
Barriers	• Sucralfate
Prokinetics	• Metoclopramide • Erythromycin
Surgical intervention	• Nissen fundoplication • Gastrostomy feeding tube (often reserved for severe cases with recurrent aspiration)

TABLE 4-6	*COMPLICATIONS OF GASTROESOPHAGEAL REFLUX DISEASE*

Weight loss
Failure to thrive
Food aversion
Esophageal strictures
Barrett esophagus
Bronchospasm
Aspiration pneumonia
Obstructive apnea

ACHALASIA

DEFINITION: A neuromuscular disorder of the esophagus resulting in lack of normal peristaltic waves with an associated hypertonic lower esophageal sphincter.

ETIOLOGY: Loss of esophageal ganglion cells and subsequent degeneration of neuromuscular fibers result in loss of the natural rhythmic movement of the esophagus. This disorder is analogous to Hirschsprung disease in the colon and rectum.

CLINICAL PRESENTATION: The age of onset is usually after 5 years. The child presents with dysphagia, regurgitation, weight loss, nighttime cough, and chest pain.

DIAGNOSIS: A barium swallow reveals a classic tapered "bird beak" distal esophagus, and a dilated and tortuous proximal esophagus.

TREATMENT: Pharmacologic treatment with calcium-channel blockers and botulinum toxin injections provides transient symptomatic relief. Surgical correction or balloon dilation to relieve the lower obstruction is a more definitive cure.

TRACHEOESOPHAGEAL FISTULA

DEFINITION: A disorder of embryologic foregut development that results in abnormal communication between the trachea and esophagus.

ETIOLOGY: In normal embryologic development, the primitive gut tube is divided into the foregut (pharynx, trachea, esophagus), midgut (small intestines), and hindgut (colon, anus). The foregut is further divided into the esophagus dorsally and the trachea ventrally and separated by the tracheoesophageal septum. A defective septum allows an abnormal communication between the two structures, resulting in a fistula.

CLINICAL PRESENTATION: There are five types of tracheoesophageal fistulas (A through E); type A is most common (90%). This type is characterized by a blind esophageal pouch, and a fistula from the distal esophageal remnant to the trachea. Signs and symptoms include excessive accumulation of saliva and mucus, gagging, choking, vomiting, cyanosis, and aspiration pneumonias. Polyhydramnios is variably present on perinatal history.

DIAGNOSIS: The inability to pass a gastric tube into the stomach with the tube coiled into the blind esophageal pouch on radiograph is classic for type A disease. Contrast studies of the upper anatomy are often useful to determine the complete anatomy before surgical correction is attempted. Children with type C fistulas, where both the esophagus and trachea are patent and connected (often described as an H-type fistula), are difficult to diagnose due to the subtle anatomical defect and otherwise normal anatomy.

TREATMENT: An oral catheter placed into the blind pouch prevents aspiration of secretions pending evaluation. Surgical correction is definitive and leads to an excellent prognosis.

FIGURE 4-2. *TRACHEOESOPHAGEAL FISTULAS.*

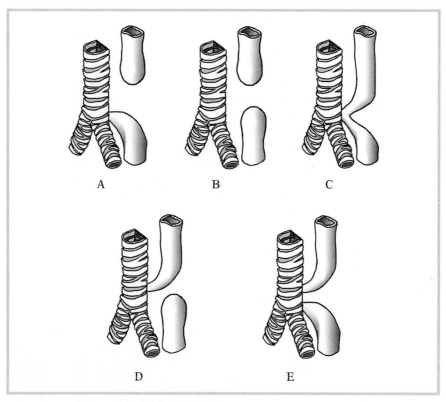

— **FIGURE 4-2** — Tracheoesophageal fistulas.

DISORDERS OF THE STOMACH

HYPERTROPHIC PYLORIC STENOSIS

DEFINITION: Idiopathic muscular hypertrophy that results in gastric outlet obstruction during the newborn period.

ETIOLOGY: There is a genetic predisposition. The disorder is most common in first-born male Caucasians.

CLINICAL PRESENTATION: Usually presents between 3 weeks and 3 months of age. The infant appears irritable and hungry, with nonbilious projectile vomiting after feeding. Prolonged vomiting results in a hypochloremic, hypokalemic metabolic alkalosis that is classic for the disease. During the physical examination, the hypertrophied pylorus may be palpated in the right upper quadrant (often described as "an olive"), and peristaltic waves may be visible.

TABLE 4-7. *PEPTIC ULCER DISEASE VS. GASTRITIS*

TABLE 4-7 *PEPTIC ULCER DISEASE VS. GASTRITIS*

Although these orders are interrelated, they are two distinct entities.

	PEPTIC ULCER DISEASE	GASTRITIS
Definition	• Ulceration of the gastric or duodenal mucosa	• Inflammation of the gastric mucosa
Etiology	• Duodenal more common than gastric in children • *H. pylori* infection is most common cause • Chronic gastritis • Burns (Curling ulcer) • Head trauma/surgery (Cushing ulcer) • Zollinger-Ellison syndrome (hypergastrinemia)	• *H. pylori* infection is the most common cause • Stress • Nonsteroidal anti-inflammatories • Alcohol • Aspirin • Spicy food • Celiac disease • Crohn disease

Clinical presentation	• Burning epigastric pain
	  - Gastric ulcers cause pain after eating
	  - Duodenal ulcers cause pain before eating
	• Duodenal ulcer pain can radiate to the back
	• Nausea
		• Burning epigastric pain after eating
		• Nausea
		• Halitosis

Diagnosis	• Esophagogastroduodenoscopy with biopsy
	• Histologic diagnosis
	• *H. pylori* diagnosis:
	  - Breath urea test
	  - Stool antigens
	  - Serum serology	

Treatment	• Histamine receptor blockers • Proton-pump inhibitors (PPI) • Antibiotics *and* PPI for confirmed *H. pylori* infection (clarithromycin, amoxicillin)	

DIAGNOSIS: The diagnosis is usually made clinically. An UGIS is not necessary, but is useful to confirm the obstruction and rule out other anatomical abnormalities prior to surgery. On the UGIS, the narrowed pyloric opening lets a thin stream of contrast through to the intestine, described as the "string sign." An abdominal ultrasound is frequently helpful in confirming the diagnosis.

TREATMENT: Pyloromyotomy.

DISORDERS OF THE INTESTINE

DUODENAL ATRESIA

DEFINITION: An abnormal development of the embryologic midgut resulting in absence of the lower duodenum.

ETIOLOGY: Multifactorial. There is a strong association with Down syndrome.

CLINICAL PRESENTATION: The newborn infant presents with abdominal distention and bilious emesis. There is often a perinatal history of polyhydramnios.

DIAGNOSIS: An abdominal radiograph shows the classic "double bubble" sign. An UGIS reveals the obstruction.

TREATMENT: Surgical repair.

MECKEL DIVERTICULUM

DEFINITION: A remnant of the fetal omphalomesenteric duct. (In utero, this duct connects the embryologic yolk sac to the primitive gut.)

ETIOLOGY: Persistence of the duct results in a true diverticulum, typically along the ileum. This diverticulum often contains ectopic gastric mucosa.

CLINICAL PRESENTATION: Painless rectal bleeding in a toddler is the most common presentation. The bleeding is secondary to intestinal ulceration caused by acid secretion from the ectopic gastric mucosa.

TABLE 4-8	RULE OF 2's FOR MECKEL DIVERTICULUM

2% of the population
Presents before age 2 y
Located 2 ft from the cecum
2 in. in length

DIAGNOSIS: A radionuclide scan using technetium 99m pertechnetate (Meckel scan) is used. This isotope locates and binds to the ectopic gastric mucosa.

TREATMENT: Surgical resection of the lesion.

INTUSSUSCEPTION

DEFINITION: A telescoping of adjacent intestinal segments, causing obstruction.

ETIOLOGY: Most cases of intussusception are idiopathic. Certain anatomical precipitating factors are associated with the disease. These "lead points" include lymph nodes, polyps and masses. The most common location for the prolapse is proximal to the ileocolic valve. It is most common in males and in children aged 3 months to 6 years, but can occur at any age.

CLINICAL PRESENTATION: The patient often presents with paroxysmal colicky pain, drawing up of the legs, vomiting, and bloody stools. Early in the disease, the child may appear well in between periods of pain. There is a classic description of "currant jelly" stools, although this is a late finding. If unrecognized, the child may progress to a state of shock, with lethargy, hypotension, fever, and respiratory compromise.

DIAGNOSIS: Plain radiographs of the abdomen may show a soft tissue mass outlined with air. Diagnostic and therapeutic air enema results in a reduction of the intussusception. Water-soluble contrast (i.e., barium) may also be used, but carries a higher risk of complication if perforation occurs. Failed reduction usually requires surgery.

CELIAC DISEASE

DEFINITION: Gluten-sensitive enteropathy.

ETIOLOGY: Gluten allergy and hypersensitivity cause intestinal mucosal damage and villous atrophy. Dietary history includes exposure to gluten-containing foods (wheat, oats, barley, and/or rye). There is a genetic predisposition with human leukocyte antigen (HLA) DQ2/DQ8.

CLINICAL PRESENTATION: The disease can present at any age. Failure to thrive, diarrhea, poor weight gain, abdominal distention, muscle wasting, and irritability are common.

DIAGNOSIS: Small bowel biopsy is the gold standard. Serum anti-gliadin, anti-endomysial and anti-reticulin antibodies are used as screening tests. Tissue-transglutaminase (TTG) antibody is the newest and most specific test. Patients with IgA deficiency do not produce the antibodies to gliadin, endomysium or reticulin, but may still have celiac disease.

TREATMENT: The intolerance to gluten is permanent. A gluten-free diet is the rule, although some patients may tolerate oats.

DISORDERS OF THE COLON AND RECTUM

FAMILIAL POLYPOSIS SYNDROMES

TABLE 4-9   *FAMILIAL POLYPOSIS SYNDROMES*

SYNDROME	ETIOLOGY	CLINICAL PRESENTATION
Familial polyposis coli	• APC gene mutation • The gene is located on chromosome 5 • Autosomal dominant inheritance	• Presents in second decade of life • Numerous intestinal polyps • Malignant transformation
Gardner syndrome		• Intestinal and extraintestinal polyps • Osteomas of the skull, maxilla and mandible • Subcutaneous fibromas • Desmoid tumors of abdomen • Extra teeth • Malignant transformation of polyps
Turcot syndrome		• Intestinal polyps • Central nervous system malignancy
Peutz-Jegher syndrome	• Autosomal dominant inheritance • No specific gene has been found	• Brown/black freckles of the lips and buccal mucosa • Hamartomatous polyps in the small intestine, colon, and stomach • Malignant transformation; however, less commonly than APC gene mutation

APC, adenomatous polyposis.

INFLAMMATORY BOWEL DISEASE (IBD)

While IBD classically presents with abdominal pain and bloody stool, it may also present with only fever, weight loss, or any of the extraintestinal manifestations listed in Table 4-10. It usually presents in adolescence and young adulthood. The underlying cause is unknown, although there is a genetic predilection.

TABLE 4-10	*INFLAMMATORY BOWEL DISEASE*	
	CROHN DISEASE	**ULCERATIVE COLITIS**
Location	• Mouth to anus	• Colon and rectum
Involvement	• Skip lesions	• Continuous lesions
	• Transmural inflammation	• Mucosal inflammation
Histology	• Granulomas	• Crypt abscesses
	• Fissures	
	• Fistulas	
	• Strictures	
	• Aphthous ulcers	
Clinical features	• Fever	• Fever
	• Weight loss	• Weight loss
	• Crampy abdominal pain	• Rectal bleeding
	• Diarrhea	• Tenesmus
	• Abscess formation	• Abscess formation
Extraintestinal manifestations (more common in Crohn disease)	• Erythema nodosum	• Erythema nodosum
	• Arthritis	• Arthritis
	• Anal skin tags	• Pyoderma gangrenosum
	• Oral ulcers	• Sclerosing cholangitis
	• Digital clubbing	• Ankylosing spondylitis
	• Gallstones	• Chronic active hepatitis
Cancer risk	• Low	• High

TABLE 4-10 *INFLAMMATORY BOWEL DISEASE (CONTINUED)*

	CROHN DISEASE	ULCERATIVE COLITIS

Diagnosis	• EGD/colonoscopy with biopsy
	• UGIS reveals:
	  • Thumbprint sign
	  • String sign
	• Serum ASCA
		• Colonoscopy with biopsy
		• Serum ANCA

Treatment	• Corticosteroids • Sulfasalazine • 6-mercaptopurine • Cyclosporin • Methotrexate • Antibiotics for suspected abscess • Surveillance for malignancy • Surgery is useful for complications only	• Corticosteroids • Sulfasalazine • 6-mercaptopurine • Cyclosporin • Methotrexate • Antibiotics for suspected abscess • Surveillance for malignancy • Surgery is useful, colectomy can be curative

ANCA, antineutrophil cytoplasmic antibody; ASCA, anti-*Saccharomyces cerevisiae* antibody; EGD, esophagogastroduodenoscopy.

HIRSCHSPRUNG DISEASE

DEFINITION: The absence of enteric ganglion cells in the anus, rectum, and/or sigmoid colon.

ETIOLOGY: Failure of migration of neural crest cells, which form enteric ganglion cells, during early embryologic development.

CLINICAL PRESENTATION: Premature infants may present with Hirschsprung-associated enterocolitis. This diagnosis must be distinguished from necrotizing enterocolitis. Newborn infants present with bilious vomiting, abdominal distention, absent passage of meconium, and enterocolitis. (The normal newborn should pass the first meconium within 48 hours). Some children present many years later with a history of constipation and encopresis. Any child evaluated for encopresis should have a careful history and physical exam to rule out Hirschsprung disease.

DIAGNOSIS: A rectal biopsy reveals an absence of ganglion cells. A barium enema demonstrates the narrow affected segment, a dilated proximal segment, and a funnel-shaped transition zone in between.

TREATMENT: Surgical reanastomosis of the proximal healthy sections of bowel.

DISORDERS OF THE PANCREAS AND LIVER

CHOLELITHIASIS

DEFINITION: Gallstones in the gallbladder.

ETIOLOGY: There are many conditions associated with the predisposition for developing gallstones. The most common conditions include hemoglobinopathies, hereditary spherocytosis, pregnancy, obesity, and chronic total parenteral nutrition. There is a genetic predisposition.

CLINICAL PRESENTATION: The majority of children with gallstones are asymptomatic. Older children and adolescents often present with right upper quadrant abdominal pain and vomiting, especially after eating a high-fat meal. Murphy's sign describes pain with palpation of the right upper quadrant during inspiration (inspiration displaces the gallbladder downward to the examiner's hand). Complications of gallstones include obstruction of the common bile duct resulting in acute pancreatitis, and inflammation of the gallbladder (cholecystitis).

DIAGNOSIS: The diagnosis is usually suspected by clinical history and presentation. The best screening test is an abdominal ultrasound to evaluate the anatomy of the liver and gallbladder and locate the gallstones. Patients with suspected gallstone pancreatitis benefit from endoscopic retrograde cholangiopancreatography (ERCP) to both diagnose the gallstone and relieve the obstruction.

TREATMENT: Mild cases of gallstones usually warrant symptomatic treatment with antipyretics and analgesics. Children who present with more severe symptoms and those with hemoglobinopathies benefit from cholecystectomy to prevent further recurrence. Lithotripsy is occasionally used in older children and adolescents.

CHOLECYSTITIS

DEFINITION: An acute inflammatory disease of the gallbladder.

ETIOLOGY: The most common cause of cholecystitis in children is gallstone formation and bile flow stasis. Viral and bacterial infections are important sources of the onset of the inflammatory process as well.

CLINICAL PRESENTATION: Most patients present with right upper quadrant pain, tenderness, and fever. Jaundice may also be present.

DIAGNOSIS: As with gallstones, clinical history and presentation are most important in suspecting the diagnosis. A complete blood count may reveal a leukocytosis with a left shift indicating an acute inflammatory process. Abdominal ultrasound is a useful screening test to evaluate the anatomy of the liver and gallbladder. A thickened gallbladder wall is a common finding with the disease. Complications include local abscess formation, and perforation.

TREATMENT: A cholecystectomy is the treatment of choice to prevent progression of the disease. Antibiotics are indicated if an abscess is suspected or prior to surgery in the immunosuppressed patient.

HEPATITIS A VIRUS (HAV)

ETIOLOGY: Hepatitis A is an RNA virus (picornavirus), transmitted by the fecal-oral route.

CLINICAL PRESENTATION: Early symptoms include anorexia, fever, and headache. The course progresses to acute onset of abdominal pain, nausea, and vomiting. Clinical jaundice in an adult who cares for the child will often lead to the diagnosis. Young children usually do not become jaundiced. The severity of the disease is variable.

DIAGNOSIS: Serum anti-HAV IgM. There is a mild elevation in serum transaminases.

TREATMENT: Supportive. Hepatitis A vaccine is available for those traveling to endemic areas. See pre/post-exposure prophylaxis/treatment in Table 11-20.

HEPATITIS B VIRUS (HBV)

ETIOLOGY: Hepatitis B is a DNA virus (hepadnavirus), transmitted by blood and body secretions. There is an increased risk in persons with multiple sex partners and in intravenous drug abusers.

CLINICAL PRESENTATION: There is often a slow onset of nonspecific symptoms: malaise, diffuse abdominal pain, anorexia, nausea, and vomiting. The development of arthritis and skin rashes is common. Jaundice may also be present. There are three possible courses of the disease: complete resolution, chronic disease, and fulminant hepatitis. Chronic disease is the most common outcome, and is associated with an increased risk of hepatocellular carcinoma. Maternal transplacental transmission is possible if the mother has active or chronic disease.

DIAGNOSIS: The diagnosis is made by demonstration of serologic markers. These include:

- HBV antigens
    - Surface antigen (HBsAg) = early sign of acute infection
    - Core antigen (HBcAg) = history of infection
    - Be antigen (HBeAg) = active infection, associated with high risk of transmission of disease
- HBV antibodies
    - IgG/IgM antibody to surface antigen (anti-HBAb) = prior infection or immunized (IgG), or acute/recent infection (IgM)
    - Antibody to core antigen IgM (anti-HBcAb) = acute infection

TREATMENT: Supportive. See pre/post-exposure prophylaxis/treatment (Table 11-20). Patients with chronic disease may be treated with interferon and lamivudine therapy.

HEPATITIS C VIRUS (HCV)

ETIOLOGY: Hepatitis C virus is an RNA virus transmitted by blood and body secretions.

CLINICAL PRESENTATION: Although acute HCV infection is often asymptomatic, it causes significant liver injury in over 30% of patients. Symptomatic patients present with malaise, anorexia, myalgias, and abdominal pain. The progression to chronic hepatitis occurs in 30% to 50%, and those patients have an increased risk of hepatocellular carcinoma.

DIAGNOSIS: The diagnosis is made by demonstration of serum anti-HCV antibodies. HCV polymerase chain reaction (PCR) is used to confirm the presence of the disease and diagnose infants born to seropositive mothers.

TREATMENT: Supportive. A combination of interferon and ribavirin has shown promise.

HEPATITIS D VIRUS (HDV)

ETIOLOGY: Hepatitis D virus is a defective RNA virus requiring HBV for replication. It is also transmitted by blood and body fluids

CLINICAL PRESENTATION: HDV infection can only occur in persons infected with HBV. Patients with HBV infection who acquire HDV have an increased risk of developing fulminant liver disease. Therefore, patients with a history of HBV who experience acute changes in liver function should be tested for HDV.

DIAGNOSIS: The diagnosis is made by demonstration of anti-HDV antibody in the serum.

TREATMENT: Supportive. The best therapy is currently prevention and treatment of HBV.

HEPATITIS E VIRUS (HEV)

ETIOLOGY: Hepatitis E virus is an RNA virus transmitted by the fecal-oral route, usually via contaminated water supplies.

CLINICAL PRESENTATION: The symptoms of HEV are similar to the other forms of hepatitis. There is a variable severity of disease. Young adults and pregnant women have an increased risk of progression to fulminant liver disease.

DIAGNOSIS: The diagnosis is made by the demonstration of anti-HEV antibody in the serum.

TREATMENT: Supportive. There is no specific therapy currently available.

DISORDERS OF LIVER METABOLISM

TABLE 4-11.   *DISORDERS CAUSING INDIRECT HYPERBILIRUBINEMIA*

TABLE 4-12.   *DISORDERS CAUSING DIRECT HYPERBILIRUBINEMIA*

TABLE 4-13.   *DISORDERS OF LIVER METABOLISM*

TABLE 4-11   *DISORDERS CAUSING INDIRECT HYPERBILIRUBINEMIA*

CONDITION	ETIOLOGY	CLINICAL PRESENTATION	DIAGNOSIS	TREATMENT
Physiologic jaundice	•Immature liver enzymes (deficient glucuronyl transferase) • ↑ Breakdown of RBCs releasing bilirubin • ↓ Bilirubin uptake by the liver • ↓ Life span of fetal hemoglobin	• Presents 24-72 h postdelivery • Mild jaundice • Bilirubin levels usually <15 mg/dL • No kernicterus	• History and clinical presentation	• Supportive • Reassurance • Phototherapy if severe
Breast-feeding jaundice	• Inadequate breast-feeding • Dehydration	• Mild jaundice • Onset 2+ d postdelivery	• History and clinical presentation	• Increase frequency of feedings • Fluid supplementation
Breast milk jaundice	• UDP-glucuronyl (UDPG) transferase inhibition by breast milk	• Mild jaundice • Onset 5+ d postdelivery	• History and clinical presentation	• Supportive • Temporary cessation of feeds
G6PD deficiency	• X- linked • Exposure to oxidant ingestants: sulfa drugs, antibiotics, fava beans	• Jaundice • Hemolytic anemia	• Measurement of G6PD enzyme activity	• Supportive • Phototherapy
Pyruvate kinase deficiency	• Autosomal recessive • Enzyme deficiency	• Jaundice • Hemolytic anemia • Splenomegaly	• Measurement of pyruvate kinase activity	• Supportive • Splenectomy
Glucuronyl transferase deficiency (Crigler-Najjar)	**Type I:** • Autosomal recessive • Absence of UDPG transferase • No formation of bilirubin glucuronide	• Jaundice • Kernicterus • Pale stool • No hemolytic anemia	• Marked elevated unconjugated bilirubin • Liver biopsy • Indirect bilirubin >20 mg/dL	• Poor prognosis • Phototherapy • Exchange transfusion

(Continued)

TABLE 4-11	DISORDERS CAUSING INDIRECT HYPERBILIRUBINEMIA (CONTINUED)			
CONDITION	**ETIOLOGY**	**CLINICAL PRESENTATION**	**DIAGNOSIS**	**TREATMENT**
	Type II: • Autosomal dominant • ↓ UDPG transferase	• Less severe form • Jaundice • No kernicterus • Pale stool	• ↓ Levels of bilirubin (<10 mg/dL) • Liver biopsy	• Responds well to phenobarbital • Phototherapy • Exchange transfusion

Gilbert syndrome	• Glucuronyl transferase enzyme deficiency
	• Genetic predisposition
		• Mild jaundice during:
		  - Illness
		  - Fasting
		• Neonatal jaundice
		• Presents at any age
			• Family history is helpful
			• Normal transaminases
			• Interventional studies of limited use
				• Supportive
				• Avoid fasting

Dubin-Johnson syndrome	• Deficiency of bilirubin transport	• Mild jaundice • Presents at any age • Persistent throughout life	• Clinical diagnosis • Normal transaminases	• Supportive

TABLE 4-12	DISORDERS CAUSING DIRECT HYPERBILIRUBINEMIA			
CONDITION	**ETIOLOGY**	**CLINICAL PRESENTATION**	**DIAGNOSIS**	**TREATMENT**
Alpha-1-anti-trypsin deficiency	• Enzyme deficiency • A serum protease inhibitor • Incidence 1:2000 • PiZZ allele most common	• Jaundice • Hepatomegaly • Acholic stools • Cirrhosis	• Alpha 1 anti-trypsin phenotype • Liver biopsy	• Liver transplantation

TABLE 4-12	DISORDERS CAUSING DIRECT HYPERBILIRUBINEMIA (CONTINUED)			
CONDITION	**ETIOLOGY**	**CLINICAL PRESENTATION**	**DIAGNOSIS**	**TREATMENT**
Hepatitis B and C	• Liver cell injury	• Jaundice • Hepatosplenomegaly • Acholic stools • Hypoglycemia	• Elevated transaminases • Hepatitis antibody panel • Maternal history of disease • Liver biopsy	• IVIG • Interferon
Neonatal hepatitis	• Diffuse intra-hepatic injury • Total parenteral nutrition • TORCH infection • Metabolic disorders • ↑ Incidence with premature infants	• Cholestatic jaundice • Acholic stools • Dark urine (urobilinogen)	• Elevated transaminases • Liver biopsy reveals "giant cells"	• Supportive • Fat-soluble vitamin supplementation
Biliary atresia	• Progressive obliteration of the biliary tree • Incidence 1:10,000	• Jaundice • Acholic stools	• Choliangiography • Liver biopsy	• Kasai procedure (anastomosis of porta hepatis to bowel) • High failure rate after age 3 mo associated with the need for transplantation
Alagille syndrome	• Paucity of intrahepatic ducts • Incidence 1:100,000 • Autosomal dominant	• Triangular face • Congenital heart disease • Cholestatic jaundice • "Butterfly" vertebrae • Ocular disease (posterior embryotoxin)	• Liver biopsy	• Supportive • Most children have poor prognosis, requiring liver transplant

IVIG, intravenous immunoglobulin; TORCH, **t**oxoplasmosis, **o**ther viruses, **r**ubella, **c**ytomegalovirus, **h**erpes simplex.

TABLE 4-13   *DISORDERS OF LIVER METABOLISM*

CONDITION	ETIOLOGY	CLINICAL PRESENTATION	DIAGNOSIS	TREATMENT
Wilson disease	• Hepatolenticular degeneration • Autosomal recessive • Deficiency of copper metabolism • ↑ Deposition of copper in liver, kidney, brain, eyes	• Behavioral changes • Learning disability • Psychiatric illness • Hepatic insufficiency • Cirrhosis • Esophageal varices • Upper GI bleed	• ↓ Serum ceruloplasmin • ↑ Urine copper • Liver biopsy shows ↑ hepatic copper • Ophthalmic exam demonstrates Kayser-Fleisher rings	• Chelation with D-penicillamine • Low-copper diet • Zinc supplementation
Reye syndrome	• Acute encephalopathy and fatty degeneration of the liver • Associated with salicylate administration during viral illness (influenza and varicella) • Incidence has decreased with decrease in pediatric aspirin use	• Vomiting • Encephalopathy • Mental status changes ranging from lethargy to coma • Seizures (infants) • Consider with children who are on chronic aspirin therapy (Kawasaki syndrome, thrombotic disease, rheumatologic disease)	• Markedly elevated AST, ALT • Fatty infiltration of the liver and kidney • Increased serum ammonia	• IV glucose administration • Control of intracranial pressure • The degree of encephalopathy determines prognosis

AST, aspartate aminotransferase; ALT, alanine aminotransferase.

PANCREATITIS

DEFINITION: An acute or chronic inflammatory disease of the pancreas.

ETIOLOGY: There are numerous precipitating factors including trauma, viral illness, bile duct obstruction, toxins, medications, congenital malformations of the pancreas, and metabolic abnormalities. Most cases of pancreatitis in children are idiopathic. The precipitating injury or illness triggers an enzymatic cascade of events resulting in pancreatic autodestruction.

CLINICAL PRESENTATION: Nausea, vomiting, anorexia, and abdominal pain are common. The abdominal pain is often epigastric and frequently radiates to the lower back. Metabolic abnormalities include hypocalcemia and hyperglycemia. Complications include ascites, pleural effusions, shock, and renal failure.

DIAGNOSIS: Clinical suspicion is most important in the expeditious diagnosis of pancreatitis. The pancreatic enzymes, amylase and lipase, measured in the serum, are good screening tests. Lipase is more specific, as amylase is also produced by the parotid glands. A normal pancreatic enzyme level does NOT rule out pancreatitis. An elevated serum bilirubin level may indicate gallstone pancreatitis. Abdominal ultrasonography is useful to rule out the formation of a pancreatic pseudocyst and evaluate the biliary anatomy. ERCP is often used in older children and adults with suspected gallstone pancreatitis to identify congenital abnormalities and relieve obstruction.

TREATMENT: Intravenous hydration is most important. Serum calcium and glucose should be followed carefully. Bowel rest and gastric decompression are indicated in symptomatic patients with moderate to severe disease. Analgesia may be helpful in moderate to severe cases. Some authorities believe morphine sulfate should be avoided, as it may exacerbate constriction of the sphincter of Oddi. Spontaneous resolution is common.

Ca^{2+}
glucose

DISORDERS OF CARBOHYDRATE METABOLISM

TABLE 4-14	DISORDERS OF CARBOHYDRATE METABOLISM			
CONDITION	**ETIOLOGY**	**CLINICAL**	**DIAGNOSIS**	**TREATMENT**
Galactosemia	• Deficiency of: 1. Galactose 1 phosphate uridylyl-transferase 2. Galactokinase • Incidence 1: 60,000	• Jaundice • Hepatosplenomegaly • Cataracts • Hypoglycemia • Seizures • Failure to thrive • Gram-negative sepsis	• Reducing substance in urine • Measurement of enzyme levels in red blood cells • Serum galactose levels	• Lactose-free diet • Lactose = glucose + galactose

(Continued)

lactose = glucose + galactose
sucrose = glucose + fructose

TABLE 4-14	DISORDERS OF CARBOHYDRATE METABOLISM (CONTINUED)			
CONDITION	**ETIOLOGY**	**CLINICAL**	**DIAGNOSIS**	**TREATMENT**
Hereditary fructose intolerance	• Deficiency of fructose 1,6 biphosphate aldolase • Accumulation of fructose 1-phosphate • Autosomal recessive	• Often presents after initiation of fruit juice to infant • Vomiting • Hypoglycemia • Jaundice • Hepatosplenomegaly	• Serum aldolase B activity • Genetic testing is available	• Avoidance of fructose, sorbitol, and sucrose • Sucrose is broken down to fructose and glucose
Hereditary tyrosinemia	• Deficiency of fumarylacetoacetate hydrolase • Autosomal recessive	• Jaundice • Hypoglycemia • Hepatosplenomegaly • Failure to thrive • Coagulopathy	• Increased serum alpha-fetoprotein • Liver biopsy	• Supportive • Liver transplantation • Poor prognosis

CHRONIC (NONINFECTIOUS) DIARRHEA

CHRONIC NONSPECIFIC DIARRHEA (TODDLER'S DIARRHEA)

DEFINITION: Three to six large watery bowel movements (often containing mucus and food particles) per day in a child aged 6 to 36 months. Diarrhea that is present for more than 3 weeks is termed "chronic." The patient has normal growth and development, and no evidence of infection or malabsorption.

ETIOLOGY: Excess fluid intake (especially fruit juice), increased intestinal motility, and low fat intake all contribute to the diarrhea.

CLINICAL PRESENTATION: The diarrhea is usually most prominent in the morning. There is no associated abdominal pain, nausea, vomiting, fever, or weight loss. The diet history usually reveals high carbohydrate intake. Parents may fear the patient will become dehydrated, and supplement with large amounts of fruit juice. The office evaluation reveals normal growth and development, with no sign of malnutrition.

DIAGNOSIS: History and physical are usually sufficient. A stool specimen may be evaluated for fecal fat, occult blood, and *Giardia* antigen if the diagnosis is unclear.

TREATMENT: Increase fiber and fat, and decrease juice in diet. Parental reassurance is important.

CHAPTER 5

PULMONOLOGY

The pathophysiology of lung disease can be divided into two main categories:

1. *Obstructive lung disease*: Obstruction of small airways resulting in increased resistance to airflow.
2. *Restrictive lung disease*: Decreased lung volumes due to parenchymal, pleural or chest wall disease.

TABLE 5-1.	*CAUSES OF OBSTRUCTIVE LUNG DISEASE*
TABLE 5-2.	*CAUSES OF RESTRICTIVE LUNG DISEASE*
TABLE 5-3.	*OBSTRUCTIVE VS. RESTRICTIVE LUNG DISEASE*

TABLE 5-1	*CAUSES OF OBSTRUCTIVE LUNG DISEASE*
Asthma	
Bronchiolitis	
Pneumonia (viral, mycoplasma)	
Cystic fibrosis	
Emphysema	
Foreign body	
Tumors	
Chronic lung disease	

TABLE 5-2	*CAUSES OF RESTRICTIVE LUNG DISEASE*

Respiratory distress syndrome
Acute respiratory distress syndrome
Pneumonia (lobar, bacterial)
Pulmonary fibrosis
Interstitial lung disease
Scoliosis
Pleural effusion
Pulmonary edema

TABLE 5-3	*OBSTRUCTIVE VS. RESTRICTIVE LUNG DISEASE*

	OBSTRUCTIVE	RESTRICTIVE
Tidal volume	↓	↓
Residual volume	↑	↓
Total lung capacity	↔ ↑	↔↓
Functional residual capacity	↑	↓
Vital capacity	↔↓	↓
FEV1	↓	↔↓
FEV1/FVC ratio	↓	↔↑
Forced vital capacity	↓	↔↓
FEF 25%-75%	↓	↔↓

FEF, forced expiratory flow; FEV1, forced expiratory volume in 1 sec; FVC, forced vital capacity.

PULMONARY FUNCTION TESTS (PFTS)

Pulmonary function tests are often used to aid in the diagnosis and management of lung disease. PFTs can help differentiate between obstructive and restrictive physiologies. They are reported in both absolute values and as a predicted percentage of normal. Bronchodilators are used to evaluate reversible airway disease. The most common modalities used are:

• **Spirometry**: Measures the volume and flow of air exhaled from a maximally inflated lung. Used to assess the physiologic performance of the lung using a volume-time curve.

* **Lung Volumes**: Measured by body plethysmography or helium dilution. Provides information independent of airflow velocity.

Definitions for the terms used in PFTs are:

* **Functional Residual Capacity (FRC)**: The volume in the lung following normal exhalation.
* **Vital Capacity (VC)**: The total amount of air that can be exhaled with no time limit following a deep breath, i.e., the volume change that occurs between maximal inhalation and maximal exhalation.
* **Total Lung Capacity (TLC)**: The total volume the lungs can hold at maximal inhalation. This value is often very diminished in restrictive lung disease.
* **Tidal Volume (TV)**: The volume inhaled or exhaled during each respiratory cycle.
* **Forced Vital Capacity (FVC)**: The total amount of air that can be exhaled as fast as possible following a deep breath.
* **Forced Expiratory Volume in 1 Second (FEV1)**: The volume exhaled during the first second of forced exhalation.
* **FEV1/FVC ratio:** Expressed as a percentage of the FVC. A useful index to evaluate airflow limitation. The FEV1 ratio may remain normal in restrictive lung disease due to reduction of both the FEV1 and FVC.
* **Residual Volume (RV):** A calculated volume (RV = TLC − VC). The amount of air remaining in the lungs after maximal exhalation. This volume is not exhaled and therefore is not measured by spirometry. Helium diffusion or body plethysmography is commonly used to make this calculation. RV is often increased during asthma exacerbations and obstructive lung disease due to air trapping.
* **Forced Expiratory Flow 25%-75% (FEF 25%-75%)**: The flow of forced air during mid-exhalation. This flow is often decreased in obstructive lung disease.

FIGURE 5-1. *SPIROMETRY.*

* **Flow-Volume Loops**: Flow-volume loops measure the volume dynamics of the respiratory cycle. The characteristic shape of a flow-volume loop can be a useful aid in diagnosis. Note the characteristic downward scooping of the expiratory flow-volume curve in obstructive lung disease, as shown in Figure 5-2.

FIGURE 5-2. *FLOW-VOLUME LOOPS.*

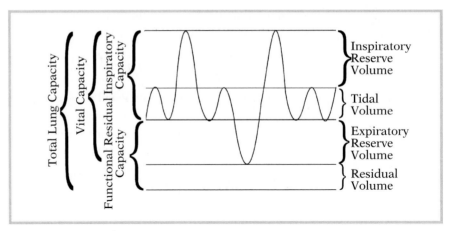

— FIGURE 5-1 — Spirometry.

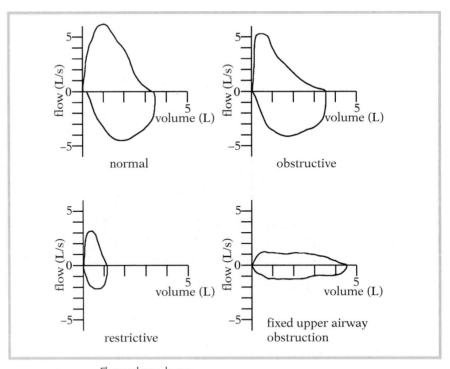

— FIGURE 5-2 — Flow-volume loops.

PULMONARY GAS EXCHANGE

Pulse Oximetry

A noninvasive method of measuring arterial oxygen saturation. Measures a percentage of hemoglobin heme sites bound by available oxygen. Factors limiting the accuracy of pulse oximetry include:

- Carboxyhemoglobin
- Methemoglobin
- Sickle cell anemia
- Hypothermia
- Diminished peripheral perfusion
- Jaundice

Oxyhemoglobin Dissociation Curve

The relationship of oxygen saturation to the partial pressure of oxygen. The "force" that either attracts or releases oxygen from hemoglobin. It is depicted as an S-shaped curve that can shift left or right.

- Forces that attract oxygen to hemoglobin (shift to the left):
    - Fetal hemoglobin
    - Increased pH
    - Decreased temperature
    - Decreased 2-3 diphosphoglycerate (DPG)
    - Decreased P_{CO_2}
    - Decreased hemoglobin
- Forces that release oxygen readily to the tissues (shift to the right):
    - Decreased pH
    - Increased temperature
    - Increased 2-3 diphosphoglycerate (DPG)
    - Increased P_{CO_2}
    - Cyanotic heart disease
    - Polycythemia

FIGURE 5-3.   *OXYHEMOGLOBIN DISSOCIATION CURVE.*

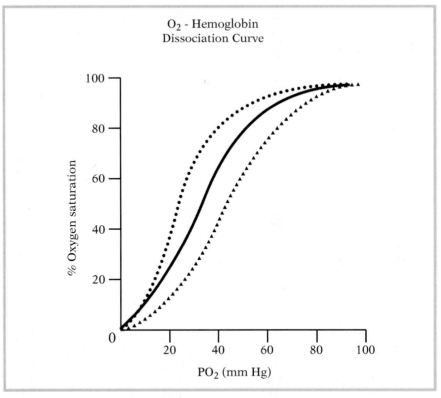

O$_2$ - Hemoglobin
Dissociation Curve

– FIGURE 5-3 – Oxyhemoglobin dissociation curve.

Acid-Base Disorders

The role of acid-base equilibrium is to maintain an optimal environment for human physiology. There are two systems involved:

- Metabolic: controlled by serum bicarbonate (HCO_3)
- Respiratory: controlled by carbon dioxide tension (PCO_2)

A primary process producing a change of one system leads to compensation by the other system to achieve a normal pH. Recognize that a compensated single disorder does not reach a normal pH. Mixed disorders can have a normal pH. (Example: metabolic alkalosis + respiratory acidosis.)

TABLE 5-4.   *COMPENSATED ACID-BASE DISORDERS*

TABLE 5-4   *COMPENSATED ACID-BASE DISORDERS*

PRIMARY DISORDER	PROCESS	COMPENSATION	PH	EXAMPLES
Metabolic alkalosis	↑ HCO_3	↑ P_{CO_2}	↑	• Diuretics • Vomiting
Metabolic acidosis	↓ HCO_3	↓ P_{CO_2}	↓	• Sepsis • DKA • Toxins
Respiratory alkalosis	↓ P_{CO_2}	↓ HCO_3	↑	• Asthma exacerbation (early) • Aspirin toxicity (early) • Pain • Fever
Respiratory acidosis	↑ P_{CO_2}	↑ HCO_3	↓	• CNS injury • Respiratory failure • Obstructive sleep apnea • Barbiturate toxicity • Chronic lung disease

SIGNS AND SYMPTOMS OF RESPIRATORY DISEASE

TABLE 5-5	CAUSES OF CHRONIC COUGH IN CHILDREN

Foreign body

Sinusitis

Asthma

Cystic fibrosis

Gastroesophageal reflux

Chronic aspiration pneumonia

Allergic rhinitis

Tracheoesophageal fistula

Vascular ring/sling

Mediastinal mass

Pulmonary hemosiderosis

Croup

Pertussis

Tuberculosis

Psychogenic (tics)

Vocal cord dysfunction

TABLE 5-6	CAUSES OF INFANTILE AND PEDIATRIC STRIDOR

INFANTS	CHILDREN
• Laryngomalacia	• Foreign body
• Tracheomalacia (extrathoracic)	• Croup
• Subglottic stenosis	• Epiglottitis
• Hemangioma	• Tracheitis
• Papilloma	• Gastroesophageal reflux
• Gastroesophageal reflux	• Papilloma
• Foreign body	• Retropharyngeal abscess
• Vascular rings/slings	• Peritonsillar abscess
• Vocal cord paralysis	• Vascular rings
	• Vocal cord dysfunction
	• Mediastinal mass
	• Angioedema
	• Psychogenic vocal cord dysfunction

TABLE 5-7	*CAUSES OF CHRONIC WHEEZING*

Asthma
Cystic fibrosis
Bronchopulmonary dysplasia
Foreign body
Gastroesophageal reflux
Tracheomalacia (intrathoracic)
Bronchomalacia
Pulmonary hemosiderosis

Congenital heart disease
Congestive heart failure
Mediastinal mass
Chronic bronchiolitis
Bronchogenic cyst
Congenital lobar emphysema

TABLE 5-8	*CAUSES OF HEMOPTYSIS IN CHILDREN*

Epistaxis
Foreign body
Bronchiectasis (cystic fibrosis)
Esophagitis
Mallory-Weiss tear
Congenital heart disease
Arteriovenous malformation
Pulmonary abscess
Pulmonary embolus
Wegener granulomatosis
Pulmonary hemosiderosis
Tuberculosis
Vitamin A deficiency
Trauma (pulmonary contusion)

DISORDERS OF THE RESPIRATORY SYSTEM

ASTHMA

DEFINITION: Airway hyperresponsiveness and chronic inflammation in the presence of inflammatory mediators. It is also defined as an obstructive airway disease that is fully or partially reversible using a bronchodilator. Recognize that the incidence, morbidity, and mortality are all increasing in the United States.

TABLE 5-9	*CLASSIFICATION OF ASTHMA*		
CLASSIFICATION	**CLINICAL SYMPTOMS**	**PEAK EXPIRATORY FLOW (PEF) OR FORCED EXPIRATORY VOLUME IN 1 SEC (FEV1)***	**PEF VARIABILITY**
Mild intermittent	• Daytime symptoms 2 times/wk or less • Infrequent nighttime symptoms	• ≥80%	• <20%
Mild persistent	• Daytime symptoms more than 2 times/wk • Nighttime symptoms 3-4 times/mo	• ≥80%	• 20%-30%
Moderate persistent	• Daily daytime symptoms • Weekly nighttime symptoms (≥5 times/mo)	• >60% to <80%	• >30%
Severe persistent	• Daily daytime symptoms • Frequent nighttime symptoms	• ≤60%	• >30%

*FEV1 and PEF are only relevant for patients age 6 years and older who can use these devices.

Modified from National Institutes of Health: Practical Guide for the Diagnosis and Management of Asthma. NIH Publication number 97-4053, October 1997.

TABLE 5-10	RISK FACTORS FOR ASTHMA

Family history

Atopy

Nasal polyps

Smoke exposure (passive)

Chronic lung disease

History of an RSV infection as a neonate

TABLE 5-11	COMMON TRIGGERS OF ASTHMA

Allergens	• Dust mites
	• Molds
	• Pollens
	• Cockroaches
	• Animal dander
Irritants	• Air pollution
	• Tobacco smoke
	• Cold air
	• Perfumes
	• Household cleaners
Infections	• Rhinitis
	• Sinusitis
	• Otitis
	• Viral respiratory infections
Others	• Aspirin
	• Beta blockers
	• Exercise
	• Gastroesophageal reflux
	• Emotional stress

TABLE 5-12   *SIGNS AND SYMPTOMS OF ASTHMA*

Nighttime cough

Exercise-induced cough

Wheezing

Nasal flaring

Intercostal retractions

Subcostal retractions

Suprasternal retractions

Decreased peak expiratory flow rates

Hyperinflation

Hypoxemia

Cyanosis

TABLE 5-13   *SIGNS OF SEVERE DISTRESS IN ASTHMA*

Cyanosis

Hypoxemia

Grunting

Lethargy

Pulsus paradoxicus

Hypotension

Metabolic acidosis (lactic acid)

Silent chest (no air movement)

Pulmonary edema

CLINICAL PRESENTATION: Children will often have a history of reactive airway disease as infants. Exercise-induced exacerbations will occur in a large percentage of patients with asthma due to environmental activation of bronchial hyperreactivity. Cough-variant asthma is characterized by nighttime and early morning cough, cough with exercise, and prolonged cough with viral syndromes.

DIAGNOSIS: History and physical examination are often enough to diagnose reactive airway disease. Recognize that all wheezing is not necessarily secondary to asthma. First-time "wheezers" should receive a baseline chest X-ray to look for foreign bodies and congenital malformations. Pulmonary function tests may be performed in a cooperative patient (starting at around age 5 years) using a bronchodilator to evaluate the reversibility of airway disease. Dust mites and other environmental allergens have become an important controllable etiology of asthma.

TREATMENT: The main principle of therapy is the regulation of chronic airway inflammation. Therapeutic interventions should be evaluated frequently. It is important to consider environmental control, drug delivery systems, and compliance in all patients who fail appropriate therapy. Antibiotics are generally not indicated. PFTs are helpful to monitor disease control and progress.

TABLE 5-14	*ASTHMA TREATMENT*
TYPE	**TREATMENT/NOTES**
Exercise-induced cough variant; mild intermittent	• Short-acting B-2 agonist 30 min before sports activity or: • Inhaled cromolyn sodium 30 min before sports activity and: • Histamine antagonist if allergic symptoms are present • Consider daily leukotriene modification during sports season
Mild persistent	• Daily inhaled anti-inflammatories (steroids, cromolyn) • Short-acting B-2 agonists as needed for exacerbations • Oral steroids for acute exacerbations • Consider trial of daily leukotriene modification
Moderate persistent	• Daily inhaled anti-inflammatories (steroids, cromolyn) • Long-acting B-2 agonist • Short-acting B-2 agonists as needed for exacerbations • Oral steroids for acute exacerbations • Consider trial of daily leukotriene modification
Severe persistent	• Daily inhaled anti-inflammatories (steroids, cromolyn) • Long-acting B-2 agonists • Frequent short-acting B-2 agonists as needed to control symptoms • Frequent oral steroids as needed for exacerbations • Consider trial of daily leukotriene modification

(Continued)

TABLE 5-14	*ASTHMA TREATMENT (CONTINUED)*
TYPE	**TREATMENT/NOTES**
Status asthmaticus	• Oxygen supplementation • Intravenous hydration • Intravenous steroids • Continuous inhaled or intravenous beta agonists (terbutaline) • Magnesium sulfate • Aminophylline/theophylline

CHRONIC LUNG DISEASE (OF INFANCY) (CLD)/BRONCHOPULMONARY DYSPLASIA (BPD)

DEFINITION: A persistent oxygen requirement and respiratory insufficiency in a premature infant after term postconceptual age.

ETIOLOGY: The treatment of respiratory failure in a premature infant. This includes therapies such as oxygen and high-inspiratory ventilator pressure resulting in airway damage, alveolar hypoplasia, interstitial fibrosis, and cystic changes. Other factors such as infection may play a role.

RISK FACTORS :
• Extreme prematurity
• Prolonged oxygen therapy
• High concentration of oxygen required during therapy

COMPLICATIONS:
• Bronchoconstriction
• Bronchomalacia
• Tracheomalacia
• Pulmonary fibrosis
• Pulmonary hypertension
• Cor pulmonale
• Chronic atelectasis
• Ventilation-perfusion mismatches (hypoxemia)
• Organic failure to thrive
• Congestive heart failure
• Increased resting energy expenditure (REE)

TABLE 5-15	SIGNS AND SYMPTOMS OF CHRONIC LUNG DISEASE/BRONCHOPULMONARY DYSPLASIA

Chronic wheezing or crackles

Tachypnea

Retractions

Chronic hypoxemia

Failure to thrive

DIAGNOSIS: History and physical presentation are often sufficient. Chest radiography reveals hyperinflated lungs with diffuse interstitial infiltrates and cystic changes.

TREATMENT: Prevention by the aggressive delay of extreme premature delivery is the best therapy. Prenatal steroids aid surfactant maturation. Once the patient is born, oxygen therapy should be administered at a minimal concentration for a minimal time both in the nursery and after discharge home. Once lung disease has occurred, oxygen, bronchodilators, and diuretic therapy are the mainstays of treatment. Aggressive nutritional support and vitamin A supplementation aid the growing lung. Respiratory syncytial virus prophylaxis is indicated.

CYSTIC FIBROSIS (CF)

DEFINITION: Deficient chloride transport regulation results in a clinical spectrum of pancreatic insufficiency, frequent pneumonias, infertility, and decreased life span. CF affects approximately 30,000 children and adults in the United States.

ETIOLOGY: Cystic fibrosis is inherited as an autosomal recessive disorder on the long arm of chromosome 7. It is most common in Caucasians and approximately 1/25 of them carry the mutation for the disease. There are over 1000 gene mutations that can cause the defect. The incidence ranges from 1/2500 to 1/3500 live births of Caucasians in the United States. The most common mutation is the DF508, cystic fibrosis transmembrane conductance regulator (CFTR), resulting in a lack of the CFTR protein. This mutation is expressed as a deficient chloride transport mechanism in epithelial cells, predominantly of the lungs and exocrine pancreas, which results in abnormal mucus accumulation in these and other organs.

TABLE 5-16.	CLINICAL PRESENTATION OF CYSTIC FIBROSIS
TABLE 5-17.	COMMON ORGANISMS COMPLICATING CYSTIC FIBROSIS

TABLE 5-16	*CLINICAL PRESENTATION OF CYSTIC FIBROSIS*
Pulmonary	• Wheezing • Persistent coughing • Frequent pneumonias • Chronic atelectasis (upper lobe) • Chronic bronchiolitis • Bronchiectasis • Hemoptysis • Pneumothorax • Clubbing
Gastroesophageal	• Meconium ileus • Rectal prolapse • Steatorrhea • Failure to thrive • Gastroesophageal reflux • Chronic diarrhea • Vitamin ADEK deficiency
ENT	• Nasal polyps • Chronic sinusitis
Genitourinary	• Infertility in males • Decreased fertility in females
Integumentary	• "Salty-tasting" skin • Acrodermatitis
Endocrine	• Pancreatic insufficiency • Glucose intolerance • Hyponatremia
Infection	• Bacterial colonization with complicating organism

TABLE 5-17	COMMON ORGANISMS COMPLICATING CYSTIC FIBROSIS

Staphylococcus aureus
Pseudomonas aeruginosa
Stenotrophomonas maltophilia
Haemophilus influenzae
Burkholderia cepacia
Atypical mycobacterium
Aspergillus

[handwritten: gold standard → sweat testing]

DIAGNOSIS: Sweat testing remains the gold standard. A positive sweat test is defined as a sweat chloride concentration higher than 60 mEq/L after stimulation with pilocarpine. A false-positive test can be seen with an inadequate sample (most common), malnutrition, adrenal insufficiency, infants with nephrogenic diabetes, and hypothyroidism. A negative sweat test in a patient with high suspicion of CF is an indication for repeat testing. Genetic DNA testing is also available. It is important to note that commercially available genetic tests can only detect approximately 90 of the more than 1000 defects.

TABLE 5-18	TREATMENT GOALS FOR CYSTIC FIBROSIS

GOAL	EXAMPLES
1. Improve and maintain pulmonary function	• Chest physiotherapy • Bronchodilators
2. Improve and maintain mucociliary clearance	• Mucolytic agents
3. Control infection	• Nebulized antibiotics • Oral antibiotics • Intravenous antibiotics
4. Optimize nutrition	• High-calorie diet • Supplemental nutrition via nasogastric or gastric feeding tube • Fat-soluble vitamin supplementation
5. Optimize pancreatic function	• Pancreatic enzyme supplementation

[handwritten notes: sweat test: pilocarpine → sweat [Cl⁻] > 60 meq/L is (+)]

[handwritten: False (+): inadequate sample, malnutrition, adrenal insufficiency, nephrogenic DI, hypothyroidism]

PULMONARY HEMOSIDEROSIS

DEFINITION: Pulmonary interstitial iron accumulation and hemorrhage.

ETIOLOGY: Idiopathic in most cases. Rarely, cases are attributed to cow's milk hypersensitivity (Heiner syndrome).

CLINICAL PRESENTATION: Often presents with acute life-threatening hemoptysis. Fever, chronic cough, expiratory wheezing, and hypoxemia are common signs and symptoms.

DIAGNOSIS: Chest radiography will reveal a diffuse interstitial pattern consistent with pulmonary hemorrhage. Diagnosis is often difficult to make. Emergent bronchoscopy is helpful during a life-threatening episode. Bronchoscopy specimens will reveal hemosiderin-laden macrophages, which is diagnostic if other causes have been excluded. A hematology profile will reveal a hypochromic microcytic iron-deficient anemia.

TREATMENT: Admission to an intensive care unit followed by oxygen supplementation and intubation if necessary pending bronchoscopy. Blood transfusions are often required. Intravenous corticosteroids have been useful in the acute episode. Idiopathic cases should be evaluated for cow's milk allergy.

DISORDERS OF RESPIRATION

APNEA

TABLE 5-19.   *DEFINITIONS OF APNEA*

OBSTRUCTIVE SLEEP APNEA (OSA)

DEFINITION: Upper airway obstruction during sleep despite continued chest wall effort and subsequent apnea. Also known as "Pickwickian syndrome."

TABLE 5-19	*DEFINITIONS OF APNEA*	
OBSTRUCTIVE	**CENTRAL**	
• Presence of respiratory effort	• No respiratory effort	
• Absent air flow	• Absent air flow	
• Tonsillar hypertrophy	• Apnea of prematurity	

RISK FACTORS: There is a predisposition in obese patients, and in patients with small airway openings, craniofacial deformities, muscular dystrophies, and hypotonia. There is an increased incidence in Down syndrome, achondroplasia, and neuromuscular disease.

ETIOLOGY: Any anatomical obstruction to the upper airway can result in obstructive sleep apnea. Enlarged tonsils and adenoids are the most common cause in otherwise healthy children.

CLINICAL PRESENTATION: Nighttime snoring with episodic airway obstruction (silent periods) is the typical presentation. This results in abnormal sleep patterns, hypoventilation, and hypoxemia. Daytime hypersomnolence, behavioral changes, and hyperactivity are important daytime manifestations.

DIAGNOSIS: Clinical history and presentation are important. Polysomnography is the gold standard.

COMPLICATIONS:

- Polycythemia
- Right ventricular hypertrophy
- Pulmonary hypertension
- Chronic carbon dioxide retention
- Chronic hypoxemia
- Chronic sleep deprivation
- Short stature
- Poor school performance

TREATMENT: An ECG should be performed in children suspected of having moderate or severe exacerbations to rule out pulmonary hypertension. Continuous positive airway pressure (CPAP) or bilevel positive airway pressure (BiPAP) have been successful in cooperative patients for whom surgical removal of the enlarged tonsils and adenoids has failed to relieve symptoms.

CENTRAL APNEA

Respiratory pauses with lack of respiratory effort usually lasting 20 seconds or more. May be associated with cyanosis and/or bradycardia. The differential diagnosis includes apnea of prematurity, meningitis, narcotic administration, gastroesophageal reflux, seizures, head trauma, intraventricular hypertension, Arnold-Chiari malformation, and brain tumors. A careful history and physical examination often indicate an etiology. Apnea of prematurity resolves by term gestational age.

CONGENITAL MALFORMATIONS OF THE RESPIRATORY SYSTEM

CHOANAL ATRESIA

Defined as a bony or membranous obstruction of the nasal airway. The etiology is failure of the choanal plates to cannulate. It may be unilateral or bilateral. The infant will often present with cyanosis during feeding that is relieved by crying. Recognize that most neonates are obligatory nasal breathers. The diagnosis is usually made by the inability to pass a suction catheter through the nasal airway. Orogastric tube feeding pending surgical correction is often necessary.

LARYNGOMALACIA (INFANTILE LARYNX)

The most common cause of newborn inspiratory stridor. Occurs secondary to floppy epiglottal and arytenoid tissues that obstruct the airway on inspiration. The infant will present with inspiratory stridor shortly after birth. The stridor is usually exacerbated during crying and improved while sleeping. Diagnosis is made by direct layngoscopy or bronchoscopy. Laryngomalacia resolves with weight gain and growth. Reassurance is necessary. Tracheostomy is rarely required.

SUBGLOTTIC STENOSIS

Defined as a narrowing of the area just below the vocal cords. Often occurs secondary to a prolonged intubation causing inflammation and granulomas. The infant will present with inspiratory and expiratory stridor. The diagnosis is made by direct laryngoscopy or bronchoscopy. Subglottic stenosis often resolves with weight gain and growth. Tracheostomy is occasionally necessary.

CONGENITAL LOBAR EMPHYSEMA (CLE)

The most common congenital lung lesion. Defined as an overdistention and obstruction of bronchial small airways resulting in lobar hyperinflation. The etiology is unknown. The infant will present with respiratory distress shortly after birth. A chest X-ray, revealing a segmental hyperinflation of the lung, is diagnostic. The left upper lobe of the lung is most commonly affected. The treatment is surgical correction.

CONGENITAL CYSTIC ADENOMATOID MALFORMATION (CCAM)

A cystic abnormality in one lobe of the lung with secondary compression of the proximal healthy lung. The etiology is unknown. The infant may present with respiratory distress, hypotension, even possibly cyanosis, and shock. A chest X-ray revealing a cystic lesion in a single lobe of the lung is usual. Secondary mediastinal shift and ipsilateral pneumothorax are also possible. The treatment is surgical correction.

MISCELLANEOUS RESPIRATORY DISORDERS

FOREIGN BODY ASPIRATION

Most commonly aspirated to the right side. May present at almost any age, although it is most common in older infants and those of preschool age. Any history of chronic cough in this age group warrants a chest radiograph to rule out a foreign body aspiration. Multiple visits to a physician office or emergency room will result in chest radiographs that reveal frequent, similarly located pneumonias. The radiographs may also reveal unilateral hyperinflation on the affected side of aspiration. Unilateral expiratory wheezing may be heard on physical examination. The treatment is to remove the obstruction via direct laryngoscopy or rigid bronchoscopy.

VASCULAR MALFORMATIONS

These anatomical malformations compress the upper airway. The typical presentation is a young infant with a chronic cough, failure to thrive, and inspiratory stridor. A double aortic arch (vascular ring) and pulmonary artery slings are the most common causes. This diagnosis should be suspected in any child who presents with a disorder of the upper respiratory system. Diagnosis is made by barium esophagram.

PNEUMOTHORAX

Defined as an accumulation of air in the pleural space. May be traumatic (blunt or penetrating force), spontaneous (ruptured bleb, severe asthma exacerbation), or iatrogenic (mechanical ventilation, subclavian venous access placement). The patient will present with decreased breath sounds on the affected side, respiratory distress, hypoxemia, and possible cardiovascular collapse. Therapy depends upon the degree of lung collapse. All patients should be treated initially with 100% oxygen, which aids in shrinking the pneumothorax by nitrogen washout. A small pneumothorax (<10%) may resolve spontaneously. A larger pneumothorax or any sign of respiratory distress warrants emergent chest tube placement or needle decompression to remove the air from the pleural space. In recurrent episodes of spontaneous pneumothorax, patients may require surgical exploration to treat persistent blebs or air leaks.

CHAPTER 6

CARDIOLOGY

CARDIOVASCULAR EXAMINATION

The cardiovascular examination of the newborn infant begins with an inspection for color, comfort, and activity level. Peripheral perfusion is assessed by visualization of color and palpation of temperature, pulses, and capillary refill. The abdomen is palpated to evaluate for organomegaly, and the chest is palpated to determine the magnitude of precordial activity and point of maximal cardiac impulse. Finally, chest auscultation is employed to evaluate heart rate, rhythm, and heart sounds. The absence of a heart murmur does not rule out congenital heart disease.

Peripheral cyanosis (acrocyanosis) is a common normal condition encountered in newborns during a routine evaluation. It is characterized by cyanosis of the hands and feet, with normal color and perfusion of the mucous membranes and the rest of the body. The arterial oxygen saturation in this condition is normal. It is benign and self-limited; no further evaluation or treatment is necessary. The patient who presents with differential cyanosis (different oxygen saturations in different parts of the body) or central cyanosis (cyanosis of the entire body) and those with an abnormal murmur should receive a chest radiograph and electrocardiogram (ECG) as screening tests.

Cardiovascular evaluation of the older child and adolescent typically takes place in the setting of a preparticipation physical examination for sports activity. The evaluation of these patients should include assessment of the family history for cardiac disease (including sudden death) and a cardiac examination to assess for activity-limiting diseases (i.e., hypertrophic cardiomyopathy).

• **Innocent Murmurs**: Extra heart sounds that are not associated with cardiovascular disease.

TABLE 6-1.   *INNOCENT MURMURS*

TABLE 6-1 *INNOCENT MURMURS*

MURMUR	ETIOLOGY	DESCRIPTION	COMMON AGE OF PRESENTATION
Peripheral pulmonary stenosis	• Relative stenosis of the pulmonary artery branches	• Systolic ejection murmur; often unilateral and louder over the back	• Newborn, young infant • Resolves by 6 mo
Vibratory ("Still's")	• Probably due to movement of the chordae tendineae of the mitral valve	• Systolic over left lower sternal border; musical or groaning in quality; supine > sitting	• 3-6 y
Venous hum	• High-velocity blood flow in the internal jugular vein	• Continuous over right midclavicular area; diminishes with turning head, supine position	• 3-6 y
Pulmonary flow	• Audible flow across the pulmonary valve and/or pulmonary arteries	• Systolic over left upper sternal border; supine > sitting	• School age to adolescence • Pregnancy
Carotid bruit	• High-velocity blood flow in the carotid artery	• Short, harsh systolic murmur over the supra-clavicular fossa, right upper sternal border	• Adolescents

CONGENITAL HEART DISEASE

Congenital heart defects affect approximately 1% of all children. The etiology of most congenital heart disease is likely multifactorial, however, some defects can be inherited. Intrauterine risk factors include maternal ingestions, medications, and infections (see Chapter 1). A review of the common structural heart defects follows.

TABLE 6-2. *ASSESSMENT OF THE INFANT WITH SUSPECTED CONGENITAL HEART DISEASE*

TABLE 6-3. *CHEST RADIOGRAPH FINDINGS IN INFANTS WITH CONGENITAL HEART DISEASE*

TABLE 6-2   *ASSESSMENT OF THE INFANT WITH SUSPECTED CONGENITAL HEART DISEASE*

TOOL	PURPOSE	PEARLS
Physical exam, including: • 4 limb blood pressures • Upper- and lower-extremity oxygen saturations	• Evaluates for differential blood pressure and oxygen saturations between the upper and lower extremities	• Differential blood pressure: coarctation of the aorta • Differential oxygen saturations: persistent pulmonary hypertension, transposition of the great arteries, coarctation of the aorta
Hyperoxia test: • Compares the arterial oxygen tension (PaO_2) in room air with the PaO_2 obtained during inspiration of 100% oxygen • Normal room air PaO_2 is ~70-80 mm Hg • Maximal PaO_2 during 100% O_2 is ~500-600 mm Hg	• Differentiates cardiac causes of cyanosis (i.e., a right-to-left shunt from CHD or persistent pulmonary hypertension) from pulmonary causes of cyanosis (i.e., pneumonia or respiratory distress syndrome)	• A PaO_2 of ≤70 mm Hg after hyperoxia challenge suggests congenital heart disease as a cause of cyanosis • A PaO_2 of ≥200 mm Hg after hyperoxia challenge rules out cyanotic heart disease as a cause of the cyanosis

ECG	• Evaluates rate, rhythm, axis, and intervals	• Left axis deviation:
		  - In presence of cyanosis:
		    • Tricuspid atresia
		  - In absence of cyanosis:
		    • Atrioventricular canal defect
		• Right axis deviation
		  - In presence of cyanosis:
		    • Total anomalous pulmonary venous return
		  - In absence of cyanosis:
		    • Normal in newborns
		    • Atrial septal defect (older children and adults)

Echocardiogram	• Provides ultrasonic visualization of cardiac anatomy	• Most children with suspected CHD will require an echocardiogram
Catheterization	• Provides definition of anatomy and physiology • Therapeutic intervention (balloon atrial septostomy, aortic/pulmonary valvuloplasty)	• Infrequently used for diagnostic purposes in the neonate due to ease and precision of echocardiography

CHD, congenital heart disease.

| TABLE 6-3 | *CHEST RADIOGRAPH FINDINGS IN INFANTS WITH CONGENITAL HEART DISEASE* |

Chest radiographs should be obtained in all infants in whom congenital heart disease is suspected, to evaluate heart size and position, and lung vasculature. You should be familiar with the classic patterns. These descriptions should be studied with an atlas.

CHEST RADIOGRAPH FINDING	DISEASE
"Boot-shaped heart"	• Classic tetralogy of Fallot
"Egg on a string," narrow mediastinum	• Transposition of the great arteries
"Figure 8" or "snowman"	• Total anomalous pulmonary venous return
Increased pulmonary blood flow in a patient with cyanosis	• Transposition of the great arteries • Total anomalous venous return • Truncus arteriosus
Decreased pulmonary blood flow in a patient with cyanosis	• Tricuspid atresia • Pulmonary atresia

The Fetal Circulation

In the fetus, high fetal pulmonary vascular resistance causes most circulating blood to bypass the fetal lungs. Blood entering the fetal right heart passes through the foramen ovale (an atrial-septal communication) to the left atrium and ventricle, or traverses the right ventricle and then passes from the pulmonary artery to the aorta through the ductus arteriosus. This allows oxygenated blood from the placenta to gain access to the fetal systemic circulation. At the time of delivery, with the first breath, pulmonary vascular resistance decreases; this allows increased pulmonary blood flow to the lungs for gas exchange. The foramen ovale and ductus arteriosus functionally close in the first days of life.

A *patent ductus arteriosis* (PDA) occurs when the ductus fails to close properly. PDA is frequently found in premature infants as well as normal infants without other associated congenital heart disease (isolated patent ductus arteriosus), and in infants with congenital heart disease that depend on the PDA for survival (ductal-dependent lesions). Premature infants and those without associated congenital heart disease may be observed carefully for possible spontaneous closure of the ductus. If the spontaneous closure does not occur in a symptomatic neonate, closure may be induced medically with indomethacin. If this fails, surgical ligation may be necessary. In the asymptomatic patient, the only clinical significance of a PDA is the risk for endocarditis. Elective closure by interventional catheterization is the treatment of choice.

Infants with ductal-dependent CHD require a PDA to provide either pulmonary blood flow (Table 6-3) or systemic blood flow (Table 6-4). These patients are often asymptomatic at birth, but may present in the first 1 to 2 weeks after delivery with cyanosis and shock, secondary to duct closure. These patients should be treated presumptively with prostaglandin infusion to keep the duct open until further evaluation and definitive interventions can be performed.

TABLE 6-4.   *LESIONS WITH DUCTAL-DEPENDENT PULMONARY BLOOD FLOW*

TABLE 6-5.   *LESIONS WITH DUCTAL-DEPENDENT SYSTEMIC BLOOD FLOW*

TABLE 6-6.   *NONCYANOTIC CONGENITAL HEART DISEASE*

Cyanotic Congenital Heart Disease

Cyanosis occurs when the deoxygenated blood returning from the systemic circulation mixes with oxygenated blood and reenters the systemic circulation. The peripheral arterial blood is not fully saturated with oxygen, and the baby appears dusky or blue. Table 6-7 summarizes the common lesions that result in cyanosis.

TABLE 6-7.   *COMMON CARDIAC LESIONS CAUSING CYANOSIS*

TABLE 6-4	*LESIONS WITH DUCTAL-DEPENDENT PULMONARY BLOOD FLOW*
	Pulmonary atresia (with or without intact interventricular septum)
	Pulmonary stenosis (severe)
	Tetralogy of Fallot (severe)
	Tricuspid atresia

TABLE 6-5	*LESIONS WITH DUCTAL-DEPENDENT SYSTEMIC BLOOD FLOW*
	Coarctation of the aorta
	Interrupted aortic arch
	Transposition of the great arteries
	Hypoplastic left heart syndrome

TABLE 6-6   NONCYANOTIC CONGENITAL HEART DISEASE

Patients should be monitored carefully for weight gain, feeding tolerance and breathing difficulty, which may be presenting signs of congestive heart failure (CHF). CHF can be treated with digoxin and diuretic therapy pending surgery.

LESION	PATHOPHYSIOLOGY	CLINICAL	DIAGNOSIS	TREATMENT/NOTES
Ventricular septal defect (VSD)	• A communication between the left and right ventricle • Left-to-right shunting across the defect • Right ventricular hypertrophy secondary to elevated pulmonary vascular resistance (large defect)	• Most common congenital heart defect • The patient is usually asymptomatic • A pansystolic murmur caused by shunting from the left ventricle (high pressure) to the right ventricle (low pressure) is auscultated over the left sternal border	• Diagnosed during routine physical exam • Echocardiogram is helpful to determine the location and size of the defect as well as the degree of shunting • Chest radiograph may be useful to determine cardiomegaly and increased pulmonary blood flow	• Small lesions require only observation, SBE prophylaxis • Large lesions result in continuous left-to-right shunting and pulmonary overcirculation that lead to congestive heart failure • Large lesions resulting in symptoms of congestive heart failure and/or failure to thrive require surgical correction • If uncorrected, development of Eisenmenger syndrome (reversal of left-to-right shunting) due to pulmonary hypertension results in a permanent right-to-left shunt, cyanosis, and congestive heart failure • Some patients qualify for minimally invasive device closure that seals the defect using interventional catheterization techniques

| Atrial septal defect (ASD) | • A communication between the left and right atrium
• Left-to-right shunting across the defect | • The patient is usually asymptomatic
• A systolic ejection murmur is caused by the increased blood flow into the pulmonary artery; the murmur is located at the upper left sternal border and radiates to the back
• The murmur is *not* caused by flow across the defect | • Diagnosed during a routine physical exam
• Echocardiogram is diagnostic to determine the location and size of the defect as well as the degree of shunting
• Chest radiograph is nonspecific
• ECG may reveal right axis deviation
• "Fixed splitting" of the second heart sound (S2) caused by delayed closure of the pulmonic valve is suggestive of an ASD | • Small lesions require only observation
• Large lesions result in continuous left-to-right shunting and right atrial enlargement that increase the risk for developing cardiac dysrhythmias
• Large lesions resulting in symptoms and/or failure to thrive require surgical correction
• Many patients qualify for "minimally invasive" device closure that seals the defect using interventional catheterization techniques
• A murmur over the back of a child aged >1 y should prompt suspicion of an ASD |

(Continued)

TABLE 6-6 NONCYANOTIC CONGENITAL HEART DISEASE (CONTINUED)

LESION	PATHOPHYSIOLOGY	CLINICAL	DIAGNOSIS	TREATMENT/NOTES
Isolated patent ductus arteriosus (PDA)	• The persistence of the embryologic ductus arteriosus (functions in utero to shunt blood from the pulmonary artery to the aorta, bypassing the fetal lungs) • Normally, the ductus arteriosus functionally closes in the first few days of life	• The presentation varies from an incidental heart murmur in an asymptomatic child to florid heart failure in a premature newborn with respiratory distress • The murmur is continuous (often described as "machinery-like") and is auscultated in the first and second left intercostal spaces in the left midclavicular line • A wide pulse pressure may also be present due to "pulmonary steal" through left-to-right shunting across the ductus	• When a ductus is present with other congenital heart lesions, it may be difficult to detect • Echocardiogram is helpful to determine the size of the lesion and degree of shunting • The ECG and chest radiograph in the uncomplicated ductus are nonspecific	• Therapy is dependent on the severity of the lesion • Medical closure is possible with indomethacin in premature infants • Surgical ligation of the PDA is definitive therapy and indicated for the symptomatic or complicated patient • In the older infant and child, the only clinical significance of a PDA is the risk of SBE; treatment is usually by coil embolization or device closure by catheterization

Coarctation of the aorta

(handwritten annotations: Turner's, DiGeorge)

- A narrowing of the aortic arch, most frequently adjacent to the origin of the left subclavian artery, proximal to the ductus arteriosus
- There is an increased incidence in males (2:1), Turner syndrome, and DiGeorge syndrome
- In critical coarctation, the patient is dependent on the patent ductus arteriosus for systemic perfusion

- The newborn infant may be asymptomatic
- At age 1-2 wk, the ductus closes, diminishing blood supply to the systemic circulation
- The infant presents with profound shock, metabolic acidosis, and multisystem organ failure mimicking septicemia
- Older children with isolated coarctation are asymptomatic and may be diagnosed incidentally with upper-extremity hypertension, pulse discrepancy, or claudication with exercise
- Blood pressure should always routinely be measured in the right arm so that precoarctation hypertension can be identified

- Four-extremity blood pressure reveals a striking differential between upper and lower extremities (right upper-extremity pressure will be higher)
- In older children, the heart size usually is normal on chest radiograph, but characteristic findings include:
  1. Dilatation of the ascending aorta above the site of stenosis (the "3" sign)
  2. Dilated pulmonary collaterals
  3. "Rib notching" from dilated collateral intercostal vessels
- Echocardiography is useful to determine degree of stenosis
- Cardiac catheterization or magnetic resonance imaging should be performed preoperatively to evaluate the extent of collaterals prior to surgery

- Newborns with critical coarctation require prostaglandin infusion
- Prostaglandin helps maintain the patency of the ductus arteriosus, and improves cardiac output, organ perfusion, and acidosis pending definitive surgery
- In older children, dilation and stent placement by catheterization may be useful
- An aortic ejection click and murmur indicate an associated bicuspid aortic valve, which is found in greater than 50% of patients with aortic coarctation

ECG, electrocardiogram; SBE, subacute bacterial endocarditis.

TABLE 6-7   COMMON CARDIAC LESIONS CAUSING CYANOSIS

These lesions are usually picked up because the child is cyanotic, NOT because a murmur is appreciated on examination.
A helpful hint: The 5 most frequently encountered cyanotic cardiac lesions begin with the letter "T".
Brain abscesses may occur in patients with right-to-left shunts because bacteria are not filtered in the lungs.

LESION	PATHOPHYSIOLOGY	NOTES
<u>T</u>ransposition of the great arteries	• Blood flows through the pulmonary and systemic circuits in parallel • Systemic deoxygenated blood is recirculated to the body (body → heart → body) • Pulmonary oxygenated blood is recirculated to the lungs (lung → heart → lung) • This anatomic abnormality is incompatible with life without a communication (ASD, VSD, PDA) to allow oxygenated pulmonary venous blood to enter the systemic circulation and systemic venous blood to enter the pulmonary circulation	• Presents within hours to days after birth • Alprostadil administration should be initiated to preserve pulmonary blood flow across the ductus arteriosus • Balloon atrial septostomy allows the oxygenated pulmonary blood to mix with the systemic blood flow and is life saving until a more definitive surgery can be performed • Arterial switch operation in the first week of life
Tetralogy of Fallot	• Consists of: (*IHOP*) 1. Interventricular septal defect 2. **H**ypertrophic right ventricle 3. **O**verriding aorta 4. **P**ulmonary stenosis/atresia • Right-to-left shunting across the VSD depends on the degree of right ventricular outflow tract obstruction (either pulmonary stenosis or atresia)	• Presents within days to months after birth • Signs and symptoms of hypercyanotic episodes; the classic "Tet spell" includes: 1. Agitation or irritability 2. Hyperpnea 3. Profound cyanosis 4. Syncope • Surgical correction is performed within the first year of life • Neonates with severe pulmonary stenosis or atresia require some type of arterial systemic–pulmonary shunt (Blalock-Taussig shunt)

Tricuspid atresia
- Functionally, acts as a single ventricle
- Agenesis of the tricuspid orifice with an absent connection between the right atrium and right ventricle
- Returning venous deoxygenated blood cannot pass to the right ventricle and continue to the lungs
- The blood from the right atrium is shunted across an ASD or PFO to the left atrium and ventricle

- Pulmonary blood flow may be ductal dependent in the absence of a VSD (Table 6-4)
- Presents within hours to days after birth when the ductus closes
- Alprostadil administration will preserve pulmonary blood flow across the ductus arteriosus and may be life saving
- Surgical palliation is performed as early as possible and may initially include an arterial systemic–pulmonary shunt (Blalock-Taussig shunt)

Truncus arteriosus
- One single outflow tract from the right and left ventricles
- A truncal valve (outflow tract) overriding a VSD is frequently present
- VSD facilitates blood flow to the lungs

- Presents within weeks to months after birth with severe CHF and mild cyanosis
- Surgical correction is performed before age 6 mo

Total anomalous pulmonary venous return
- There is an absence of any direct connection between the pulmonary veins and the left atrium
- Pulmonary venous blood returns to the right side of the heart, bypassing the systemic circulation: pulmonary veins → right heart → septal defect → left heart → aorta

- The age at presentation is variable and dependent on the degree of obstruction
- The degree of cyanosis may be minimal
- The patient frequently presents with either congestive heart failure or respiratory distress within the first year of life
- Surgical correction is performed shortly after diagnosis is made

(Continued)

TABLE 6-7   COMMON CARDIAC LESIONS CAUSING CYANOSIS (CONTINUED)

LESION	PATHOPHYSIOLOGY	NOTES

Persistent pulmonary hypertension of the newborn (PPHN) (persistent fetal circulation)
 	
• See Chapter 1
	• Blood shunts right to left through a PFO and a PDA secondary to high pulmonary vascular resistance	• Risk factors:
		  1. Fetal distress
		  2. Meconium aspiration
		  3. Group B streptococcal sepsis
		  4. Cesarean section
		  5. Congenital diaphragmatic hernia
		  6. Hyaline membrane disease
		• Respiratory distress and profound shock with significant hypoxemia are apparent within the first few hours of life
		• Most common in full-term infants
		• Pre- and postductal differential saturations are useful in diagnosis (higher in upper extremity)
		• Treatment consists of aggressive respiratory and hemodynamic support, inhaled nitric oxide, and ECMO if necessary

Pulmonary atresia	• Absence of the pulmonary outflow tract • Deoxygenated blood in the right ventricle cannot reach the lungs • The blood from the right side of the heart is shunted across a VSD, PFO, or ASD (right to left shunt)	• Pulmonary blood flow is ductal dependent (Table 6-4) • Presents within hours to days after birth when the ductus closes • Alprostadil administration will preserve pulmonary blood flow across the PDA and may be life saving

Pulmonary atresia	• Blood flow to the lungs is retrograde: aorta→PDA → pulmonary arteries	• Cardiac catheterization may be indicated for diagnosis and treatment • Pulmonary valvuloplasty during catheterization can improve blood flow to the lungs in select patients • Surgical correction is indicated if valvuloplasty is unsuccessful • Isolated pulmonary atresia functions like a single ventricle
Hypoplastic left heart syndrome	• A group of malformations characterized by marked underdevelopment of the entire left side of the heart • The right side of the heart supports both the pulmonary and systemic circulations • Pulmonary venous blood must shunt from the left atrium, across the PFO/ASD/right atrium → right ventricle → PDA → aorta	• Systemic blood flow is ductal dependent (Table 6-5) • Presents within hours to days after birth • Aprostadil administration will preserve systemic flow across the PDA and may be life saving • Surgical palliation usually includes a 3-stage approach and is initiated at the time of diagnosis: Stage 1 (arterial systemic–pulmonary shunt, aortic reconstruction); Stage 2 (SVC to pulmonary arterial anastomosis), performed at 4-6 months; and Stage 3 (IVC to pulmonary arterial anastomosis [Fontan]), performed in childhood.
Interrupted aortic arch/critical coarctation	• The descending aorta may be entirely supplied by deoxygenated blood via the PDA; baby may appear dusky or blue from the chest down	• Systemic blood flow is ductal dependent (Table 6-5) • Presents within hours to days after birth • Alprostadil administration will preserve systemic blood flow across the PDA and may be life saving

ASD, atrial septal defect; ECMO, extracorporeal membrane oxygenation; IVC, inferior vena cava; PDA, patent ductus arteriosus; PFO, patent foramen ovale; SVC, superior vena cava; VSD, ventricular septal defect.

Emergency Interventions for Congenital Heart Disease

TABLE 6-8	EMERGENCY INTERVENTIONS FOR CONGENITAL HEART DISEASE	
INTERVENTION	**PURPOSE**	**ANATOMY REQUIRING INTERVENTION**
Alprostadil* (prostaglandin PGE$_1$)	• Maintains patent ductus arteriosus	• Lesions with no (or dangerously little) blood flow from the heart to the pulmonary circulation (Table 6-4)
		• Lesions with no (or dangerously little) blood flow from the heart to the systemic circulation (Table 6-5)
		• Any patient who fails a hyperoxia test is likely to have a congenital heart disease with ductal-dependent pulmonary or systemic blood flow (Tables 6-4 and 6-5) and should receive alprostadil until anatomic diagnosis can be accomplished
Balloon atrial septostomy	• Enlarges the atrial communication	• Transposition of the great arteries
		• Hypoplastic left heart syndrome

*Alprostadil side effects include hypotension, apnea, fever, and seizures. Alprostadil administration is generally well tolerated and should be started immediately on all patients with presumed ductal-dependent anatomy.

Hypercyanotic Episodes

Hypercyanotic episodes, also know as "tet spells," are characterized as episodes of increased agitation, hyperpnea, cyanosis, and syncope in a patient with tetralogy of Fallot. The spell begins when the ratio of pulmonary to systemic vascular resistance increases and blood exits the right ventricle preferentially across the ventricular septal defect (VSD) to the aorta. The result is acute deoxygenation and cyanosis. This may be secondary to increased pulmonary vascular resistance or decreased systemic resistance (or both). Tet spells are infrequently seen in the modern era due to early surgical repair of tetralogy during infancy.

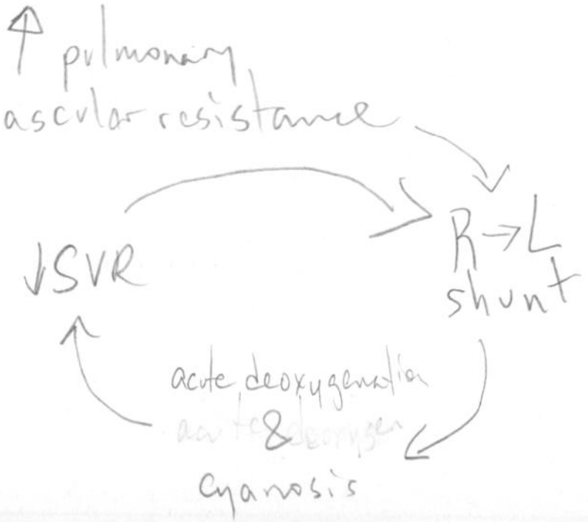

(handwritten annotations:)
↑ pulmonary vascular resistance

↓SVR → R→L shunt

acute deoxygenation & cyanosis

TABLE 6-9	TREATMENT OF A "TET SPELL"
METHOD	**PURPOSE**
Calm the patient; create a quiet environment	• Decreases physical activity and stress leading to reduced right-to-left shunting and increased pulmonary blood flow
Bring the knees to the chest	• Increases systemic vascular resistance, increases pulmonary blood flow, and reduces right-to-left shunting
Oxygen administration	• Oxygen is a direct pulmonary vasodilator and a peripheral vasoconstrictor, increasing pulmonary blood flow and reducing right-to-left shunting
Morphine sulfate	• The exact mechanism is unknown; the sedative effect decreases physical activity and stress causing a similar effect to calming the patient
Intravenous fluid	• Increases preload and cardiac output, presumably with a preferential increase in right-sided output and increased flow to the lungs
Bicarbonate	• Corrects acidosis; an increased serum pH promotes pulmonary arterial relaxation
Phenylephrine	• Increases systemic resistance, increases pulmonary blood flow and reduces right-to-left shunting
AVOID isoproterenol and epinephrine	• They may cause peripheral vasodilatation (dropping systemic resistance and increasing right-to-left shunting)

ACQUIRED HEART DISEASE

CARDIOMYOPATHIES

A cardiomyopathy is defined as a structural and/or functional abnormality of the ventricular myocardium that compromises cardiac output.

TABLE 6-10. *CARDIOMYOPATHIES*

INFECTIVE ENDOCARDITIS (IE)

In pediatric patients, IE is usually associated with congenital heart disease, valvular heart disease, a history of prolonged indwelling catheters (ICU admissions), or cancer therapy (Broviacs). Endocardial tissue or valves previously altered by surgery, trauma, or prior disease are exposed to turbulent blood flow and thrombin formation, predisposing the endocardium to infection. Although less common, IE can also affect the normal heart. The introduction of bacteria into the bloodstream is a necessary factor for precipitating IE.

TABLE 6-10   *CARDIOMYOPATHIES*

TYPE	PATHOPHYSIOLOGY	ASSOCIATIONS	TREATMENT
Restrictive	• Fibrosis of the heart muscle • Decreased ventricular compliance ("stiffening" of the myocardium) • Impaired diastolic filling • Poor ventricular diastolic function	• Idiopathic hypereosinophilic syndrome	• No specific treatment exists • Poor prognosis
Dilated	• Ventricular dilatation • Poor ventricular contraction • Cardiomegaly • Congestive heart failure	• Myocarditis (coxsackievirus) • Muscular dystrophies • Chemotherapy (doxorubicin)	• Fluid restriction • Diuretics • Digoxin • Vasodilators • Beta blockers
Hypertrophic	• Thick left atrium and ventricle • Poor ventricular relaxation • Congestive heart failure	• Sudden cardiac death • Hereditary tendency	• Beta blockers • Pacing

ETIOLOGY: Gram-positive cocci account for about 90% of overall infecting organisms in endocarditis. Gram-negative organisms and fungi are other important infectious causes, especially in immunocompromised hosts and in nosocomial infections. *Staphylococcus aureus* is the most common organism isolated in patients with fulminant, rapid-onset endocarditis. Many of these patients have no history of prior heart disease. More indolent cases of endocarditis, such as those acquired after dental cleaning, are usually caused by *Streptococcus viridans* and occur in patients with anatomical risk factors (see below). Coagulase-negative staphylococci and *S. aureus* are encountered more frequently in patients with prolonged indwelling catheters. Enterococci are also commonly seen in intravenous drug users. (The terms "acute" and "subacute" are often utilized to describe endocarditis, but these are mainly terms of historical interest used to describe the patient's expectant time until death: acute bacterial endocarditis victims died in less than 3 weeks, while those with subacute bacterial endocarditis died after 3 or more weeks of illness.)

CLINICAL PRESENTATION: Fever, fatigue, and splenomegaly are the most common clinical manifestations of IE. Children with a history of congenital heart disease, valvular heart disease, or indwelling catheters require a high level of suspicion if these symptoms are present. Less frequent manifestations include weight loss, abdominal pain, petechiae, new or changing murmur, and arthritis. Osler nodes (tender lesions found most commonly on the pads of the fingers and toes), Roth spots (small, hemorrhagic retinal lesions with pale centers), Janeway lesions (nontender, hemorrhagic macules on the palms and soles), and splinter hemorrhages may also be present. Occasionally a patient presents in extremis due to acute destruction of a cardiac valve caused by IE.

DIAGNOSIS: Multiple blood cultures (typically 3-5) from different sites should be obtained. Echocardiography and magnetic resonance imaging are useful to detect valvular and intra-atrial thrombi (vegetations) as a possible source of infection and to document progression of disease. Erythrocyte sedimentation rate (ESR) is usually elevated.

TREATMENT: A 4- to 6-week course of parenteral antibiotics should be tailored to the identification and sensitivity of the infecting organism. Penicillin, cephalosporins, and vancomycin are frequently used. Rifampin and gentamicin are useful adjuncts that act synergistically. Surgical intervention may be required if there is valvular damage.

TABLE 6-11	*CONDITIONS THAT REQUIRE ENDOCARDITIS PROPHYLAXIS*

Prosthetic cardiac valves
Prior endocarditis
Cyanotic congenital heart disease
Most congenital heart disease (except secundum atrial septal defect)
Acquired valvular heart disease (mitral regurgitation)
Hypertrophic cardiomyopathy
Mitral valve prolapse with regurgitation

PREVENTION: Endocarditis prophylaxis is recommended prior to dental, oral, respiratory tract, or esophageal procedures for the types of patients listed in Table 6-11.

Conditions that do *not* require prophylaxis include atrial septal defect (ASD), repaired ASD/VSD and PDA (at least 6 months past repair), innocent heart murmurs, or history of Kawasaki disease/rheumatic fever that did not induce valve dysfunction. Prophylaxis is not routinely recommended for bronchoscopy, endoscopy, or tympanostomy procedures.

ARRHYTHMIAS

TABLE 6-12.	*ARRHYTHMIAS*
FIGURE 6-1.	*SECOND-DEGREE ATRIOVENTRICULAR BLOCK*
FIGURE 6-2.	*COMPLETE ATRIOVENTRICULAR BLOCK*

TABLE 6-12   *ARRHYTHMIAS*

Questions regarding treatment of arrhythmias generally involve conditions that present acutely or are life-threatening (i.e., supraventricular tachycardia). A rule of thumb is to treat the patient with medication if the patient is stable and treat with electrocardioversion if the patient is symptomatic or unstable.

ARRHYTHMIA	DESCRIPTION/ NOTES	TRACING
Atrioventricular block **• 1st degree**	• Long PR interval for age and heart rate • Usually secondary to medication (digoxin), trauma, or cardiac surgery	
• 2nd degree—Mobitz type I (Wenckebach)	• Progressively longer PR intervals, then a dropped QRS • Seen in sleep and those with increased vagal tone (↑intracranial pressure, Valsalva)	• Figure 6-1
• 2nd degree—Mobitz type II	• Stable PR interval, then a dropped QRS • Every other P wave is conducted in a 2:1 block • Seen most commonly after cardiac surgery • Of more concern than Mobitz type I	
• 3rd degree (complete)	• Total A-V dissociation with P-P interval shorter than R-R interval • The QRS complexes are regular • Seen with connective tissue disorders (SLE/Sjögren syndrome)	• Figure 6-2
Sinus arrhythmia	• Normal variation, sinus node rate is irregular, but every P is followed by a QRS	• Figure 6-3
Atrial flutter	• "Sawtooth" baseline on ECG with a stable R-R interval • Reentrant rhythm • Flutter rate is determined by reentrant rate, which may be 300-500 bpm	• Figure 6-4 A and B
Atrial fibrillation	• "Fuzzy" or "irregularly bumpy" baseline on ECG with irregularly occurring QRS complexes; no true P waves	
Premature atrial contraction	• Early P wave, each followed by a QRS • May be an incidental finding	• Figure 6-5

TABLE 6-12   *ARRHYTHMIAS (CONTINUED)*

ARRHYTHMIA	DESCRIPTION/ NOTES	TRACING
Premature ventricular contraction	• Early QRS with no preceding P wave; the early QRS is wider than the baseline QRS and is followed by an abnormal T wave	• Figure 6-6
Ventricular tachycardia	• Wide QRS complexes without discernable P waves • Rate usually less than 250/min • May represent a life-threatening arrhythmia • Often associated with absent pulse and cardiac arrest	• Figure 6-7
Ventricular fibrillation	• Coarse high-amplitude wave forms varying in size, shape and rhythm • No clear P, QRS, or T waves • Always electrocardiovert • Almost always associated with an absent pulse and cardiac arrest	
Supraventricular tachycardia (SVT)	• Abrupt onset and unwavering rate of tachycardia; terminates abruptly as well • Administration of adenosine may be both diagnostic and therapeutic • Vagal maneuvers may also be used if the patient is stable	• Figure 6-8
Wolff-Parkinson-White (WPW) syndrome	• Predisposes to SVT; ECG shows delta waves and a short PR interval	• Figure 6-9
Prolonged QT syndrome	• Risk for ventricular tachycardia/fibrillation • Multiple inherited forms, some associated with hearing loss • May present with syncope, seizures, and sudden death, especially in setting of strong emotion or activity	• Figure 6-10

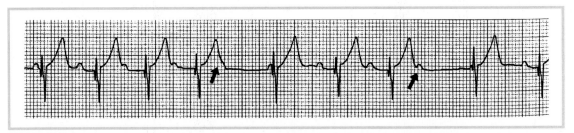

– FIGURE 6-1 – Second-degree atrioventricular block. Mobitz type 1 (Wenckebach block). Progressive lengthening of the P-R interval is present before the nonconducted or dropped beats occur. Arrow indicates dropped beat.

Source: Artman M, Mahoney L, Teitel D. Neonatal Cardiology. New York: McGraw-Hill, 2002, p. 164.

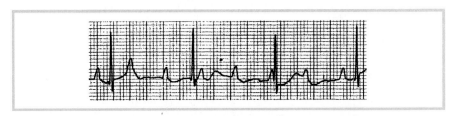

– FIGURE 6-2 – Complete atrioventricular block. Rhythm strip recorded in a neonate shows that P waves and QRS complexes are independent of each other. The atrial rate is 145 bpm and the ventricular rate is 62 bpm. The QRS complex is narrow.

Source: Artman M, Mahoney L, Teitel D. Neonatal Cardiology. New York: McGraw-Hill, 2002, p. 165.

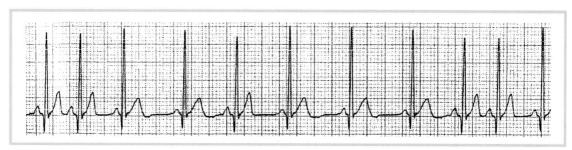

– FIGURE 6-3 – Sinus arrhythmia. The P-wave axis is normal and does not vary. The R-R interval varies from 400 to 700 milliseconds (86-150 bpm).

Source: Artman M, Mahoney L, Teitel D. Neonatal Cardiology. New York: McGraw-Hill, 2002, p. 163.

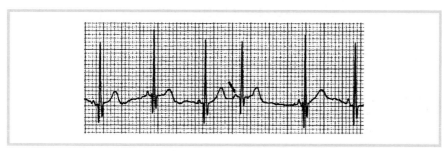

– FIGURE 6-4 – Premature atrial contraction (arrow).

Source: Artman M, Mahoney L, Teitel D. Neonatal Cardiology. New York: McGraw-Hill, 2002, p. 167.

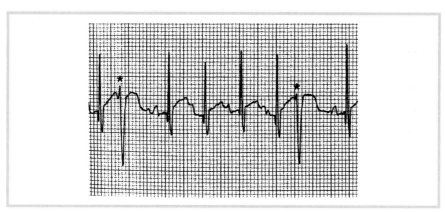

– FIGURE 6-5 – Premature ventricular contractions (*).

Source: Artman M, Mahoney L, Teitel D. Neonatal Cardiology. New York: McGraw-Hill, 2002, p. 175.

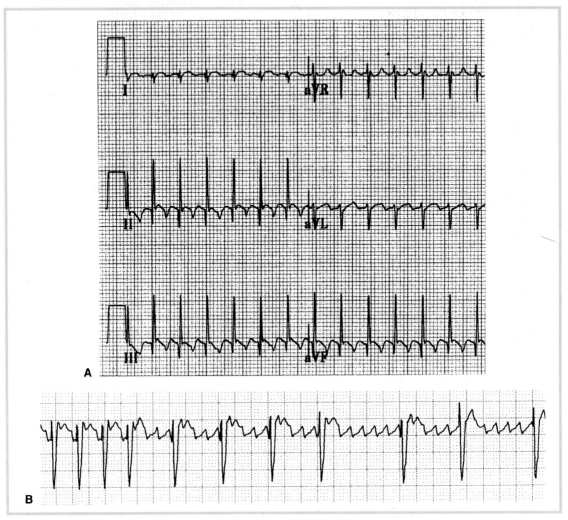

— FIGURE 6-6 — Atrial flutter. A: Negative flutter waves are present in lead II. The flutter rate is 400 bpm and there is 2:1 AV block. B: Administration of adenosine increases AV block and facilitates visualization of the flutter waves. The flutter rate in this patient is 460 bpm.

Source: Artman M, Mahoney L, Teitel D. Neonatal Cardiology. New York: McGraw-Hill, 2002, p. 174 .

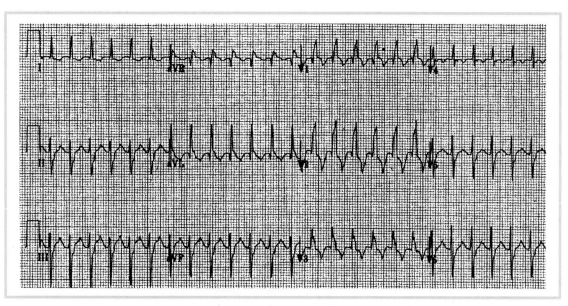

— **FIGURE 6-7** — Ventricular tachycardia. The heart rate is 195 bpm.

Source: Artman M, Mahoney L, Teitel D. Neonatal Cardiology. New York: McGraw-Hill, 2002, p. 176.

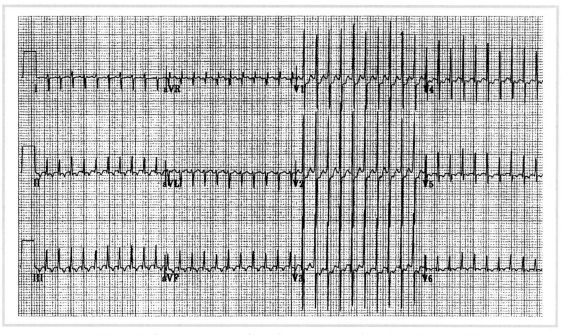

— **FIGURE 6-8** — Atrioventricular reciprocating tachycardia (supraventricular tachycardia). The QRS complex is normal. The heart rate is 325 bpm.

Source: Artman M, Mahoney L, Teitel D. Neonatal Cardiology. New York: McGraw-Hill, 2002, p. 171.

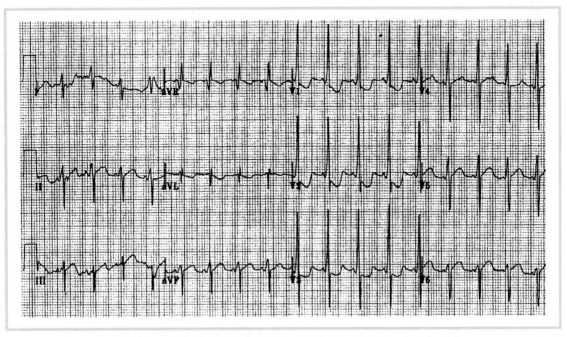

– FIGURE 6-9 – Wolff-Parkinson-White syndrome. The short P-R interval (80 ms) and a delta wave are present in multiple leads, which is consistent with preexcitation.

Source: Artman M, Mahoney L, Teitel D. Neonatal Cardiology. New York: McGraw-Hill, 2002, p. 168.

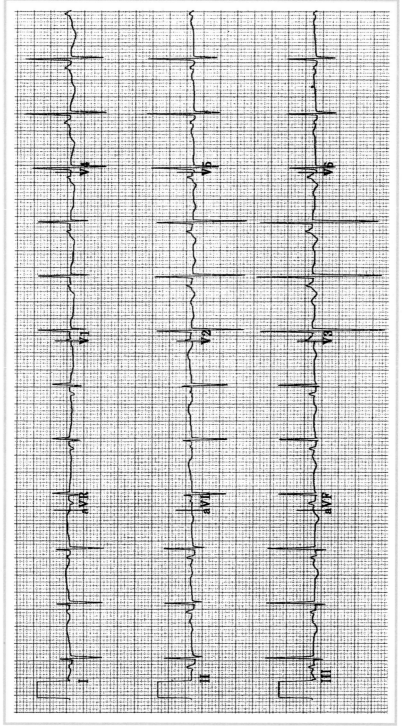

– FIGURE 6-10 – Long QT syndrome. Electrocardiogram from 1-day-old infant with congenital long QT syndrome shows markedly prolonged QT interval (460/670$^{1/2}$ 562 ms) measured in lead III and a heart rate of 90 bpm.

Source: Artman M, Mahoney L, Teitel D. Neonatal Cardiology. New York: McGraw-Hill, 2002, p. 180.

TABLE 6-13   *GENETIC SYNDROMES AND ASSOCIATED HEART ANOMALIES*

SYNDROME	HEART ANOMALY
Trisomy 21	• Atrioventricular septal defect • Ventricular septal defect • Patent ductus arteriosus
Turner	• Bicuspid aortic valve, coarctation, hypoplastic left heart
Noonan	• Valvular pulmonary stenosis • Hypertrophic cardiomyopathy
Williams	• Supravalvular aortic stenosis, peripheral pulmonary stenosis
Marfan	• Aortic aneurysm • Mitral valve prolapse
Tuberous sclerosis	• Rhabdomyoma
DiGeorge (del 22q11)	• Truncus arteriosus • Interrupted aortic arch
Infant of diabetic mother	• Myocardial hypertrophy • Transposition of the great arteries

Trisomy 21   AV canal defect
               VSD
               PDA

Turner — coarct   Noonan — valvular PS
         HLHS   hypertrophic
         bicuspid aortic valve   cardiomyopathy

CHAPTER 7

ACUTE/CRITICAL CARE

ALTERED MENTAL STATUS

Altered mental status is a term used to define central nervous system dysfunction. A child with altered mental status may present with a wide range of symptoms, ranging from irritability and stupor to lethargy and coma. The differential diagnosis of altered mental status in the pediatric age group is extensive. It is important that the practitioner complete an expeditious history and physical examination to narrow the differential and treat the underlying disorder.

TABLE 7-1. *CAUSES OF ALTERED MENTAL STATUS (AMS)*

SHOCK SYNDROMES

Shock is defined as the state in which oxygen and other nutrients/substrates are delivered at levels insufficient to meet the metabolic demands of the tissues. Presenting signs and symptoms of shock syndromes are variable, but usually include tachycardia, tachypnea, altered mental status, decreased urine output, and prolonged capillary refill. Shock may occur with a low, normal, or elevated blood pressure.

Functional Classification of Shock

- **Hypovolemic (bleeding, dehydration):** Inadequate volume to support appropriate cardiac output.
- **Distributive (early septic, anaphylactic, neurogenic):** Vasodilatation and shunting of blood from vital organs.
- **Cardiogenic (weak or stunned heart, late septic):** Inadequate cardiac output.
- **Obstructive (pneumothorax, tamponade):** Obstruction of cardiac output.

Phases of Shock

- **Compensated:** Vital organ function maintained; normal or elevated blood pressure.
- **Uncompensated:** Compromised blood pressure and altered perfusion.
- **Irreversible:** Severe and multiple end-organ damage.

121

TABLE 7-1	*CAUSES OF ALTERED MENTAL STATUS (AMS)*

T = Trauma, tumors

I = Ingestion, infection, intussusception, inborn errors of metabolism

P = Poisons

S = Sepsis, seizures

A = Abuse, arteriovenous malformations

E = Encephalopathy, electrolytes (glucose, sodium)

I = Insulin overdose

O = Opiates

U = Uremia

Formulas to Remember

- $\dot{D}O_2 = CO \times CaCO_2 \times 10$
- $CO = SV \times HR$
- $CaCO_2 = (1.34 \times Hgb \times SaO_2) + (0.003 \times PaO_2)$
  - $\dot{D}O_2$ = Oxygen delivery (LO_2/ min)
  - CO = Cardiac output (L/min)
  - SV = Stroke volume (L)
  - HR = Heart rate (beats/min)
  - Hgb = Hemoglobin (g/dL blood)
  - $CaCO_2$ = Arterial O_2 content (mLO_2/dL blood)
  - PaO_2 = Partial pressure of oxygen in the arterial blood (mm/hg)
  - SaO_2 = Arterial oxygen saturation (%)

Treatment of Shock

The treatment of all shock syndromes begins with the ABCs: control and maintenance of airway, breathing, and circulation. This is generally followed by oxygen supplementation, fluid resuscitation, and cardiorespiratory monitoring. Intravenous access should be obtained immediately to allow expeditious treatment with resuscitation fluids and medications. The subsequent specific treatment of shock disorders is dependent on the underlying cause. For example, a patient who presents with hemorrhagic shock after abdominal trauma requires swift blood replacement after the airway, breathing, and circulation are assured.

TABLE 7-2	SHOCK SYNDROMES		
CLASSIFICATION	**ETIOLOGY**	**PRESENTATION**	**TREATMENT/NOTES**
Hypovolemic	• Sudden decrease in intravascular volume • Profuse vomiting, diarrhea • Adrenal crisis • Diabetic ketoacidosis • Diabetes insipidus • Burns • Capillary leak syndromes	• Tachycardia • Tachypnea • ↓ CO • Hypotension • Oliguria • Cool extremities • Narrow pulse pressure • Lethargy	• Fluid resuscitation
Hemorrhagic	• Trauma (head, abdominal) • Fractures (pelvis, long bones) • Great vessel injury	• Tachycardia • Tachypnea • ↓ CO • Hypotension • Oliguria • Cool extremities • Narrow pulse pressure • Lethargy	• Blood replacement • Colloid administration • Surgical intervention
Distributive	• Anaphylaxis • Neurogenic (spinal cord trauma)	• Tachycardia • Tachypnea • Maldistribution of blood flow • Hypotension • Wide pulse pressure	• Fluid resuscitation • Epinephrine (for anaphylaxis) • Antihistamines (for anaphylaxis) • Dopamine • Norepinephrine • Corticosteroids (for spinal cord injury)
Septic	• Systemic inflammatory response syndrome (SIRS) • Capillary leak • Hypovolemia • Myocardial depression	Early: • Tachycardia • Tachypnea • Warm extremities • ↑ CO • Wide pulse pressure • Mild metabolic acidosis	• Fluid resuscitation • Dopamine • Norepinephrine (for early septic shock) • Epinephrine (for late septic shock) • Antibiotics

(Continued)

TABLE 7-2   *SHOCK SYNDROMES (CONTINUED)*

CLASSIFICATION	ETIOLOGY	PRESENTATION	TREATMENT/NOTES
Septic (*cont.*)		Late: • Tachycardia • Tachypnea • Cold extremities • ↓ CO • Severe metabolic acidosis	
Obstructive	• Mechanical obstruction of ventricular filling and/or cardiac output • Pneumothorax • Pericardial tamponade • Massive pulmonary embolus • Pulmonary hypertension • Congenital heart disease (coarctation)	• Tachycardia • Tachypnea • Cool extremities • Oliguria • Metabolic acidosis • ↓ CO	• Relief of obstruction
Cardiogenic	• Myocarditis • Cardiomyopathy	• Tachycardia • Tachypnea • Cool extremities • Oliguria • Metabolic acidosis	• Monitored fluid resuscitation • Dopamine • Dobutamine • Milrinone • Epinephrine

CO, cardiac output.

TABLE 7-3.   *HEMODYNAMIC VARIABLES OF SHOCK STATES*

TABLE 7-4.   *DIFFERENTIAL DIAGNOSIS OF SHOCK BY AGE*

TABLE 7-3   *HEMODYNAMIC VARIABLES OF SHOCK STATES*

	CO	SVR	MAP	PAOP	CVP
Hypovolemic	↓	↑	↔ or ↓	↓	↓
Distributive	↑	↓	↔ or ↓	↔ or ↓	↔ or ↓
Septic (early)	↑	↓	↔ or ↓	↓	↓
Septic (late)	↓	↓	↓	↑	↑ or ↔
Obstructive	↓	↑	↔ or ↓	↑	↑
Cardiogenic	↓	↑	↔ or ↓	↑	↑

CO, cardiac output; SVR, systemic vascular resistance; MAP, mean arterial blood pressure; PAOP, pulmonary artery occlusion pressure (wedge pressure); CVP, central venous pressure.

TABLE 7-4   *DIFFERENTIAL DIAGNOSIS OF SHOCK BY AGE*

NEWBORN	CHILD
• Sepsis	• Sepsis
• Trauma	• Trauma
• Congenital heart disease	• Ingestion
• Congenital adrenal hyperplasia	• Burns
• Bleeding	• Adrenal crisis
	• Diabetic ketoacidosis
	• Bleeding
	• Anaphylaxis
	• Dehydration

VASOACTIVE MEDICATIONS

Vasoactive medications are used to manipulate the cardiovascular responses to shock syndromes. A basic understanding of the actions of each of the frequently used medications is necessary.

TABLE 7-5.   *VASOACTIVE MEDICATIONS*

TABLE 7-5   *VASOACTIVE MEDICATIONS*

AGENT	RECEPTOR	DOSAGE (µG/KG/MIN)	EFFECT/NOTES	CONSIDER USE IN
Dopamine	Dopaminergic	Low dosage = 0-4	• Splanchnic and renal vasodilatation	• Renal dysfunction associated with multisystem organ failure
	$\beta_{1,2}$	Moderate dosage = 5-10	• ↑ Contractility • ↑ Heart rate • ↑ Conduction velocity	• Cardiogenic shock
	$\alpha_1 > \beta_{1,2}$	High dosage = 10-20	• Peripheral vasoconstriction	• Distributive and septic shock
Dobutamine	$\beta_{1,2}$	1-20	• ↑ Contractility • ↑ Heart rate • ↑ Conduction velocity • Peripheral vasodilatation • Pulmonary vasodilatation	• Cardiogenic shock • Postoperative myocardial dysfunction • May cause excessive tachycardia
Epinephrine	$\beta_{1,2}$	Low/moderate dosage = 0.05-0.50	• ↑ Contractility • ↑ Heart rate • ↑ Conduction velocity • Peripheral vasodilatation • Pulmonary vasodilatation	• Cardiogenic shock • Postoperative myocardial dysfunction • Myocardial dysfunction
	$\alpha_{1,2} > \beta_{1,2}$	High dosage = 0.5-2.0	• ↑ Contractility • ↑ Conduction velocity • Peripheral vasoconstriction • Pulmonary vasoconstriction	• Cardiogenic shock • Septic shock (late) • Cardiovascular collapse

(Continued)

TABLE 7-5   *VASOACTIVE MEDICATIONS (CONTINUED)*

AGENT	RECEPTOR	DOSAGE (µG/KG/MIN)	EFFECT/NOTES	CONSIDER USE IN
Norepinephrine	$\alpha_{1,2} > \beta_{1,2}$	0.05-2.0	• Peripheral vasoconstriction • Pulmonary vasoconstriction • ↑ Contractility (weak)	• Distributive and septic shock (early)
Sodium nitroprusside	Arterial > venous	0.5-10.0	• Rapid onset • Short duration • ↑ ICP • V/Q mismatch • Causes cyanide toxicity in patients with renal failure	• Hypertensive crisis • Afterload reduction in congestive heart failure
Nitroglycerin	Venous > arterial	1-20	• Peripheral vasodilatation • ↑ ICP	• Myocardial ischemia • Preload reduction in congestive heart failure
Alprostadil (PGE-1)		0.05-2	• Maintains patency of ductus arteriosus • Peripheral vasodilatation • Causes fever, apnea	• Ductal-dependent congenital heart disease
Milrinone	Phosphodiesterase inhibitor	0.5-1.0	• Afterload reduction • ↑ Contractility • ↑ Conduction velocity	• Myocardial dysfunction

ICP, intracranial pressure; PVR, peripheral vascular resistance; SVR, systemic vascular resistance; V/Q, ventilation/ perfusion.

RESPIRATORY DISTRESS AND FAILURE

Respiratory distress is defined as insufficient oxygenation and/or ventilation. Signs and symptoms of respiratory distress include tachypnea, tachycardia, grunting, head bobbing, abnormal breathing patterns, and abdominal retractions. Impaired gas exchange leads to hypoxemia, hypercarbia, and acidosis. Respiratory distress is the first sign of impending respiratory failure.

Acute respiratory failure can occur rapidly in children due to the high oxygen and metabolic demands of the tissues. Conditions that increase the metabolic and oxygen demands of tissues include fever, infection, and shock syndromes. Respiratory failure is best defined by standard blood gas criteria: PaO_2 <60 mm Hg, PCO_2 >60 mm Hg in patients without preexisting lung disease. Frequently encountered causes of respiratory failure include airway obstruction (foreign body), obstructive lung disease (RSV, bronchiolitis, asthma), restrictive lung disease (pneumonia), and neurologic disease (apnea, head trauma). Respiratory failure requires prompt management of the airway and control of breathing. In skilled hands, this is most efficiently accomplished by endotracheal intubation and mechanical ventilation. In emergency situations, the proper use of a bag, valve, and mask can be life saving. Acute respiratory failure that remains untreated or unrecognized is the most common cause of cardiac arrest in children.

Handwritten margin note: Respiratory failure $PaO_2 < 60 mmHg$ $PCO_2 > 60 mmHg$ in pts $\bar{s}$ preexisting lung dz

Ventilator Basic Principles

A basic understanding of ventilator mechanics is necessary for the board exam. Think of mechanical ventilation as two separate processes:

1. Control of oxygenation
2. Control of ventilation

Oxygenation is dependent upon the fractional concentration of inspired oxygen (FiO_2) and mean airway pressure. Ventilation is a function of tidal volume (TV) and breath rate (BR) and is quantified as minute ventilation.

- Minute ventilation (MV) = TV $\times$ BR

The effectiveness of ventilator management is monitored by arterial blood gases (ABG), pulse oximetry, and end-tidal carbon dioxide ($ETCO_2$) measurements. An arterial blood gas is the most accurate method of determining metabolic homeostasis (pH), ventilation, and oxygenation. If an arterial sample is not available, a capillary or venous sample may be substituted. The precision of a capillary blood gas is less than that of an arterial blood gas. The precision of a venous blood gas is less than that of a capillary blood gas and cannot be used to assess oxygenation. Pulse oximetry determines oxygenhemoglobin saturation by photoelectric measurements through the skin of the fingers, toes, ears, or forehead. $ETCO_2$ measures exhaled carbon dioxide and minute ventilation from a direct connection to the ventilator tubing or, with recent developments in technology, by a small probe that can be placed in the nose or mouth.

There are three basic ventilator modalities employed in the management of respiratory failure in children; volume-controlled, pressure-controlled, and high-frequency oscillatory ventilation (HFOV). Volume- and pressure-controlled ventilation are considered conventional modalities in mechanically ventilated children. During conventional ventilation, oxygenation is controlled by FiO_2, positive end-expiratory pressure (PEEP), and inspiratory time. Ventilation is controlled by tidal volume and respiratory rate.

High-frequency oscillatory ventilation is generally reserved for patients with acute hypoxemic respiratory failure (AHRF) due to neonatal and acute respiratory distress syndromes (RDS, ARDS). HFOV is a unique modality of support that utilizes a piston driven at 3 to 10 Hz to actively move small volumes of inhaled and exhaled gases. Oxygenation is controlled by FiO_2 and mean airway pressure (MAP). Ventilation is dependent on a continuous flow of gas to and from the alveoli and is controlled by the amplitude and frequency of the oscillations around the mean airway pressure. Fewer oscillations allows for greater volumes of exchanged gas leading to better ventilation.

TABLE 7-6.   *VENTILATOR TROUBLESHOOTING*

TABLE 7-7.   *CAUSES OF HYPOXEMIA/ DECOMPENSATION WHILE ON A VENTILATOR*

TABLE 7-6	*VENTILATOR TROUBLESHOOTING*	
	CONVENTIONAL	**HFOV**
To ↑ oxygenation	• ↑ PEEP • ↑ FiO_2 • ↑ Inspiratory time	• ↑ MAP • ↑ FiO_2
To ↓ oxygenation	• ↓ PEEP • ↓ FiO_2	• ↓ MAP • ↓ FiO_2
To ↑ ventilation	• ↑ Tidal volume • ↑ Respiratory rate • ↑ Expiratory time	• ↑ Amplitude • ↓ Frequency
To ↓ ventilation	• ↓ Tidal volume • ↓ Respiratory rate	• ↓ Amplitude • ↑ Frequency

FiO_2, fractional inspired oxygen; HFOV, high-frequency oscillatory ventilation; MAP, mean airway pressure; PEEP, positive end-expiratory pressure.

TABLE 7-7	CAUSES OF HYPOXEMIA/DECOMPENSATION WHILE ON A VENTILATOR

D = Disconnection

O = Tube obstruction

P = Pneumothorax

E = Equipment failure

CARDIAC ARREST (CARDIOPULMONARY ARREST)

Cardiac arrest is defined as the cessation of cardiac mechanical activity. The most frequent cause of cardiac arrest in children is respiratory failure. Signs and symptoms of cardiac arrest include unresponsiveness, absent pulse, and absent respirations. Treatment begins with expeditious protection and management of the airway, breathing, and circulation. Once the patient is stabilized, the underlying cause (if known) should be treated.

TABLE 7-8	COMMON CAUSES OF CARDIAC ARREST IN CHILDREN

Airway obstruction (most common cause)

Hypoxia (near drowning)

Uncompensated shock

Pulseless arrhythmia

Severe acidosis

Pneumothorax

Pulmonary embolus (massive)

Pericardial tamponade

TOXICOLOGY AND POISONINGS

The diagnosis of poisoning in children is often difficult. A child is often fearful of disclosing an ingestion and the parent is often unaware that an ingestion has taken place. Consideration of poisoning should be included in the differential diagnosis in any child who presents with an altered mental status, respiratory distress, seizures, lethargy, coma, unexplained acidosis, or unexplained bizarre symptoms.

Approach to the Poisoned Patient

ABCDE: **A**irway, **B**reathing, **C**irculation, **D**econtamination, **E**limination:

- Airway: Check protective reflexes, administer oxygen, and attach monitors.
- Breathing: Check rate, pattern, and oxygen saturation.
- Circulation: Check heart rate, blood pressure, rhythm, and ECG; establish IV access; draw labs.
- Decontamination: Remove toxin from the environment (skin, eyes, clothes) and GI tract (emesis, lavage, syrup of ipecac).
- Elimination: Administer charcoal and/or specific antidotes

The history and physical examination, done concurrently, should include quantity and time of ingestion, and possible toxins and medications in the environment. The exam should focus on vital signs, level of consciousness, skin, eyes, mouth (odors, secretions), heart rhythm, bowel sounds, and motor activity (fasciculations, hyperkinesias, weakness).

General Interventions

INDUCED EMESIS: SYRUP OF IPECAC

Ipecac can remove some toxins by gastrointestinal decontamination if administered within 30 minutes of the ingestion. The administration of ipecac may be at home, but should be performed in conjunction with a poison control consultation.

DOSAGE :

- <6 months: contraindicated
- 6-12 months: 10 mL with 8 oz water
- 1-5 years: 15 mL with 8 oz water
- >5 years: 30 mL with 8 oz water

CONTRAINDICATIONS :

- Benign ingestion
- Patient already vomited
- Expected or evident neurologic changes (resulting in inability to protect the airway; patient may aspirate vomitus)
- Bleeding
- Ingestion of caustic substances or sharp metals

LAVAGE

Gastric lavage can also remove some toxins by gastric decontamination if administered within 2 hours of the ingestion.

PROCEDURE: Ensure airway protection; intubate if necessary. Saline is administered several times to "wash out" the upper gastrointestinal tract, in most cases followed by administration of activated charcoal.

CONTRAINDICATIONS:

- Benign ingestion
- Ingestion of caustic substances
- Bleeding from oropharynx

ACTIVATED CHARCOAL

Activated charcoal is the most frequently employed and most effective method of gastric decontamination. It is most successful if administered within 4 hours of ingestion. However, even later administration is effective in eliminating many medications (barbiturates, theophylline) through so-called "gut dialysis" and/or as drugs return to the stomach vascular bed via the enterohepatic circulation. Multiple doses may be required.

ADMINISTRATION: The usual dose is 0.5 to 1 g/kg of activated charcoal. The solution is not very palatable, although most patients are able to drink it (add cherry syrup to improve taste). Infants and patients unable to protect their airway should have a nasogastric tube placed for administration. Always verify placement of nasogastric tube prior to starting charcoal because aspiration can cause severe pneumonitis.

CONTRAINDICATIONS:

- Caustics (obscure endoscopy, accumulate in burned areas)
- Ileus or bowel obstruction
- Aspiration risk (if not intubated)
- Charcoal prepackaged with sorbital should be avoided due to the risk of diarrhea and hypernatremic dehydration when multiple doses are administered.

time course

emesis   < 30 min
lavage   < 2 h
activated
charcoal   < 4 h
  → later for barbiturates, theophylline

	TABLE 7-9	*COMMON ACUTE POISONINGS*	
TOXIN	**PRESENTATION**	**DIAGNOSIS**	**ANTIDOTE/TREATMENT**
Acetaminophen	• Anorexia, nausea, and vomiting • Vital signs, mental status normal	• Abnormal liver function tests • Acetaminophen level 4 h after ingestion • Fulminant liver failure is a late finding	• *N*-acetylcysteine
Amphetamines (crank, ecstasy)	• Dilated pupils • Hypertension • Tachycardia • Tremors • Hyperthermia • Agitation	• Urine toxicology	• Supportive • Benzodiazepines for severe cases • Ecstasy is a slang name for 4-methylenedioxymethamphetamine (MDMA)
Anticholinergics (belladonna alkaloids)	• "Hot as a hare, mad as a hatter, dry as a bone, red as a beet, blind as a bat:" • Hyperthermia • Agitation • Dry skin and mucous membranes • Flushed skin • Dilated pupils	• History • Wide QRS complex	• Cholinesterase inhibitor (physostigmine) • Gastric lavage (if oral ingestion) • Remember, diphenhydramine overdose can be present in a similar manner
Beta blockers	• Bradycardia • Hypotension • Hypoglycemia • Bronchospasm	• History • ↑ PR interval • Atrioventricular block	• Supportive • Glucagon • Beta agonists • Dialysis
Botulism	• Constipation • Bulbar palsies (poor suck, weak cry, ptosis) • Weakness, hypotonia • Poor feeding • Respiratory compromise	• Mostly affects infants • History of honey ingestion • Isolation of *C. botulinum*, or toxin in the stool	• Supportive • Human-derived botulism immune globulin • Avoid aminoglycosides as they may further potentiate neuromuscular blockade

(Continued)

TABLE 7-9   *COMMON ACUTE POISONINGS (CONTINUED)*

TOXIN	PRESENTATION	DIAGNOSIS	ANTIDOTE/TREATMENT
Carbon monoxide	• Headache • Dizziness, confusion • Nausea, vomiting,	• Cherry red lips • Cutaneous pulse oxygen saturation measurements are falsely normal; patient may be hypoxemic • ↑ Carboxyhemoglobin • ↑ Lactate • Metabolic acidosis	• Oxygen • Hyperbaric oxygen therapy
Cocaine	• Tachycardia • Hypertension • Agitation • Mydriasis (dilated pupils) • Seizures	• ↑ CPK • Urine toxicology	• Supportive • Halperidol • Benzodiazepines • Antiarrhythmic • Antihypertensive
Digitalis	• Hypotension • Bradycardia • Nausea, vomiting, anorexia • Visual changes • Confusion	• Hyperkalemia • Digoxin level • T-wave depression • Prolonged PR interval	• Antidigoxin antibody • Digoxin levels are not reliable in neonates and infants due to endogenous digoxin-like substances
Ethylene glycol (antifreeze)/ methanol	• Tachypnea • Lethargy • Coma • Blindness (methanol)	• Anion gap acidosis • Hypocalcemia • Acute renal failure • Difference between calculated and measured serum osmolality (↑ serum osmolality)	• Ethanol • Bicarbonate • Hemodialysis • Fomepizole (antidote)

| TABLE 7-9 | COMMON ACUTE POISONINGS (CONTINUED) | | |

TOXIN	PRESENTATION	DIAGNOSIS	ANTIDOTE/TREATMENT
Iron	• Nausea, vomiting, abdominal pain • Hematemesis • Hypoglycemia • Hypotension • Coma	• Anion gap acidosis • Iron level • Heme-positive stools	• Induce vomiting if early ingestion • Deferoxamine chelation
Isoniazid (INH)	• *INH:* **I**njures **N**eurons and **H**epatocytes • Nausea, vomiting • Seizures	• Anion gap acidosis • Abnormal LFTs • Eosinophilia • Hyperglycemia	• Pyridoxine
Isopropyl alcohol (rubbing alcohol)	• Lethargy • Coma • Acetone odor • Hemorrhagic tracheobronchitis	• Absent acidosis • Normal glucose • Difference between calculated and measured serum osmolality (↑ serum osmolality)	• Supportive • Hemodialysis for severe cases
Lead	• Nausea, vomiting, abdominal pain • Constipation • Headache, lethargy, altered mental status • Wrist and foot drop	• Blood lead levels drawn by venipuncture • Increased heme precursors: FEP and ZPP	• EDTA • DMSA • BAL dimercaprol • Penicillamine • Children with blood lead levels >45 µg/dL should receive chelation therapy • BAL is administered as an intramuscular injection; it is generally suspended in peanut oil

(Continued)

TABLE 7-9   *COMMON ACUTE POISONINGS (CONTINUED)*

TOXIN	PRESENTATION	DIAGNOSIS	ANTIDOTE/TREATMENT
Lithium	• Altered mental status • Myoclonus, ataxia, seizures • Diabetes insipidus • Acute renal failure	• Lithium level • Hypernatremia • Sinus node dysfunction • Atrioventricular block	• Hydration • Hemodialysis for severe cases
Mercury	• Hypertension • Tachycardia • Sweating • Erythema of extremities • Swollen gums with a blue line around the teeth • Hypotonia • Photophobia • Nephrotic syndrome	• Sinus node dysfunction • Clinical history	• EDTA • BAL • Penicillamine
Opioids	• Hypotension • Miosis (constricted pupils) • Altered mental status • Ileus • Respiratory depression	• Urine toxicology • Respiratory acidosis • Hypoxemia	• Naloxone (repeat doses usually required due to short half-life)
Organophosphates (pesticides)	Cholinergic "DUMBELS" • Defecation • Urination • Miosis • Bronchospasm	• Clinical history • Abnormal plasma cholinesterase activity	• Decontamination • Atropine • Pralidoxime (restores cholinesterase activity at the neuromuscular junction)

TABLE 7-9   *COMMON ACUTE POISONINGS (CONTINUED)*

TOXIN	PRESENTATION	DIAGNOSIS	ANTIDOTE/TREATMENT
Organophosphates (pesticides) (*continued*)	• Emesis • Lacrimation • Salivation • Seizures		
Phencyclidine (PCP)	• Hyperthermia • Hypertension • Vertical nystagmus • Myoclonus • Hallucinations • Excessive salivation	• Myoglobinuria • ↑ Creatine phosphokinase • Toxicology screen	• Gastric lavage • Benzodiazepines
Salicylates	• Hyperthermia • Tachypnea • Tinnitus • Vomiting • Bleeding • Coma	• Mixed primary respiratory alkalosis and metabolic acidosis (anion gap) • Abnormal LFTs • Abnormal coagulation studies • Serum toxicology	• Urine alkalinization (bicarbonate) • Gut dialysis • Hemodialysis • Suspect overdose with patients who have rheumatologic disease, Kawasaki, or arthritis
Sedatives (barbiturates, benzodiazepines)	• Hypothermia • Hypotension • Respiratory depression	• Elevated P_{CO_2} • Urine toxicology	• Supportive care • Flumazenil (benzos) • Use care in those with seizure disorders as flumazenil may precipitate a seizure • Significant enough overdose can mimic brain death
Theophylline	• Hyperthermia • Tachypnea • Tachycardia • Hypotension • Tremor • Vomiting • Confusion, coma	• Hypokalemia • Hyperglycemia • Metabolic acidosis • Theophylline level	• Supportive care • Gut dialysis • Charcoal hemoperfusion for severe cases (charcoal rapidly binds to theophylline)

BAL, dimercaprol; DMSA, 2,3-dimercaptosuccinic acid; EDTA, edetate calcium-disodium; FEP, free erythrocyte protoporphyrin; LFT, liver function test; ZPP, zinc protoporphyrin.

POISONOUS BITES AND STINGS

TABLE 7-10   *POISONOUS BITES AND STINGS*

POISON	ETIOLOGY	PRESENTATION	TREATMENT/NOTES
• **Jellyfish** • **Portuguese man-of-war** • **Fire coral**	• Tropical environments • Nematocysts are used to inject toxin into the susceptible host	• Painful, erythematous rash • Headache, fever, myalgias, muscle spasms, nausea, vomiting • Paralysis and death are possible	• Supportive • Avoid irrigating the wound (releases more toxin from nematocysts) • Local reactions should be treated with topical vinegar, or baking soda (neutralizes toxin) • Systemic reactions may require antihistamines, epinephrine, and corticosteroids
• **Stingrays**	• Tropical environments • Large barbed tail is used to inject toxin and injure the susceptible host	• Laceration or puncture wound is often present • Nausea, vomiting, cramps, weakness • Shock and death in severe cases	• Supportive • Irrigation of the wound with sea water • Soak the wound in hot water
• **Black widow spider**	• Spider is shiny black with a red hourglass marking on abdomen (females)	• Local sharp pain at the site of injury • Mild local reaction • Muscle cramping, nausea, vomiting, abdominal muscle rigidity	• Supportive • Antivenin is available for severe reactions
• **Brown recluse spider**	• Spider has a brown violin-shaped mark on dorsum	• Large localized reaction, with erythema, ischemia, and necrosis at the site of injury • Fever, nausea, vomiting, weakness, hematuria	• Supportive

TABLE 7-10		POISONOUS BITES AND STINGS (CONTINUED)	
POISON	**ETIOLOGY**	**PRESENTATION**	**TREATMENT/NOTES**
• **Scorpions**	• Tail contains a cytotoxic venom • Located predominantly in the southwestern U.S.	• Local erythema and tenderness • Begins with throat spasms, muscle fasciculations, and abdominal cramps • Respiratory distress, convulsions, hypothermia, cyanosis, shock, pancreatitis	• ABCs • Supportive care • Antivenin is available in endemic areas • Benign course except for small children

• **Snakes**	Poisonous snakes include:
	• Pit vipers (Crotalidae):
	  - Rattlesnakes
	  - Diamondback
	  - Cottonmouth
	  - Copperhead
	• Non–pit vipers (Elapidae):
	  - Coral snakes
		• Local erythema, swelling, and edema
		• Fang marks may be present
		• Immediate numbness and paresthesias
		• Nausea, vomiting, weakness, chills
		• Respiratory failure, shock
		• Disseminated intravascular coagulation
			• Poisonous snakes have:
			  - Small triangular head
			  - Elliptical pupils
			  - Large frontal fangs
			  - Rattles
			• Coral snakes have red stripes on yellow stripes
			• ABCs
			• Supportive therapy (if mild)
			• Both the decision to use antivenin and the dosage required for the patient are dependent on the severity of symptoms
			• Antivenin should be administered to all confirmed cases of coral snake bites due to the possible delayed, sudden onset of severe symptoms
			• Antivenin is a horse serum product; skin testing should be performed prior to administration

(Continued)

TABLE 7-10	POISONOUS BITES AND STINGS (CONTINUED)		
POISON	**ETIOLOGY**	**PRESENTATION**	**TREATMENT/NOTES**
Hymenoptera (bee stings)	• Venom can induce any class of hyper-sensitivity reaction • Anaphylaxis is IgE-mediated	• Local erythema and tenderness • Nausea, vomiting, lethargy, shock	• ABCs • Remove the stinger • Supportive care • Severe reactions and anaphylaxis require antihistamines, corticosteroids, and epinephrine • Sensitive individuals should carry an emergency epinephrine kit

CHAPTER 8

NEPHROLOGY

Hematuria

Hematuria is defined as the presence of more than 5 to 10 red blood cells (RBCs) per high-power microscopic field from a centrifuged midstream-voided urine sample. Hematuria can be divided into two forms, gross and microscopic. Gross hematuria may originate from anywhere along the urinary tract and is most frequently associated with urinary tract infection, trauma, and exercise. Microscopic hematuria frequently originates from the kidney and may be associated with systemic or glomerular disease.

A urine dipstick is often employed as the first screening modality for the detection of hematuria. A positive dipstick for hemoglobin should be verified using microscopic analysis; false-positive results are possible in the presence of myoglobin, ascorbic acid, sulfonamides, and other medications.

TABLE 8-1.   *COMMON CAUSES OF HEMATURIA*

The most frequent causes of hematuria are listed in Table 8-1. Important clinical considerations include the presence of proteinuria, edema, and hypertension, which suggests glomerulonephritis; and abdominal pain and bloody diarrhea, which suggests Henoch-Schönlein purpura (HSP).

The evaluation of hematuria includes a complete urinalysis, urine culture, urine calcium/creatinine ratio, serum complement, and ASLO titers, as well as serum BUN and creatinine. A renal ultrasound should be considered in cases with suspected anatomic etiology (renal vein thrombosis).

Proteinuria

The presence of protein in the urine is most often discovered during routine urine dipstick screening. Protein excretion by the kidney may be found in the urine of healthy children and up to 0.15 grams per day is considered normal. Albumin derived from plasma makes up the largest percentage of protein excreted by the urine. Children with protein on dipstick require either a quantitative 24-hour urine collection for protein or

TABLE 8-1   *COMMON CAUSES OF HEMATURIA*

Urinary tract infection
Cystitis
Urethritis
Trauma
Strenuous exercise
Idiopathic hypercalciuria
Kidney stones
Acute glomerulonephritis
IgA nephropathy
Renal vein thrombosis
Systemic lupus erythematosus
Sickle-cell disease
Henoch-Schönlein purpura
Alport syndrome

a semiquantitative calculation of urinary protein-to-creatinine ratio with the first morning void. Generally, a ratio of 0.2 or higher suggests significant proteinuria. In children with alkaline urine, a dipstick may be falsely positive for protein.

TABLE 8-2.   *COMMON CAUSES OF PROTEINURIA*

Serum electrolytes, BUN, creatinine, and complement levels should be measured in patients with patients with suspected intrinsic disease.

Hypertension

Hypertension is defined as systolic or diastolic blood pressure greater than or equal to the 95th percentile for age, measured on three separate occasions, each measurement at least 3 weeks apart. Hypertension in an infant should invoke a lower threshold for further evaluation. Hypertension in children is associated with an increased risk for hypertension as an adult, associated cardiovascular disease, and early morbidity and mortality.

TABLE 8-3.   *COMMON CAUSES OF HYPERTENSION BY AGE GROUP*

Diagnostic evaluation should be tailored to the history, additional presenting symptoms, and physical examination. Screening modalities include vital signs, four-extremity blood pressure measurements, urinalysis, urine culture, and serum BUN and creatinine. Renal sonography and echocardiography are used to evaluate suspected underlying renal and cardiac disease. In obese patients with idiopathic hypertension, weight loss and exercise are cornerstones of therapy.

TABLE 8-2	COMMON CAUSES OF PROTEINURIA	

BENIGN CAUSES (MOST COMMON)	PATHOLOGIC CAUSES
• Orthostatic proteinuria • Fever • Exercise	• Idiopathic nephrotic syndrome • Minimal change disease • Acute/chronic glomerulonephritis • Focal segmental glomerulosclerosis • Mesangial proliferative glomerulonephritis • Membranoproliferative glomerulonephritis • Acute tubular necrosis • Interstitial nephritis

TABLE 8-3	COMMON CAUSES OF HYPERTENSION BY AGE GROUP	

INFANTS	CHILDREN/ADOLESCENTS
• Renal artery thrombosis • Renal artery stenosis • Parenchymal renal disease • Coarctation of the aorta • Reflux nephropathy • Renal failure	• Idiopathic (most common cause) • Obesity • Post–infectious glomerulonephritis • Pyelonephritis • Reflux nephropathy • Renal artery stenosis • Parenchymal renal disease • Corticosteroid use • Oral contraceptive use • Medications (decongestants) • Drug abuse (cocaine) • Renal trauma • Henoch-Schönlein purpura • Coarctation of the aorta • Connective tissue disorders • Pheochromocytoma • Renal failure • Intracranial tumor

CONGENITAL AND INHERITED KIDNEY DISORDERS

Renal masses (congenital and inherited) are the most frequently encountered abdominal masses in newborn infants. Many of these conditions are diagnosed prenatally during routine ultrasound. The most frequently encountered disorders are summarized in Table 8-4.

TABLE 8-4	*CONGENITAL/ INHERITED KIDNEY DISORDERS*		
CONDITION	**CLINICAL**	**DIAGNOSIS**	**TREATMENT/NOTES**

Congenital hydronephrosis	• Most frequently caused by fetal ureteropelvic junction obstruction
	• 80% of cases are unilateral
	• Consequences include:
	  - Vesicoureteral reflux
	  - Urinary tract infection
	  - Oliguria
	  - Hematuria
		• Renal ultrasound
		• VCUG
		• Nuclear imaging to assess renal function
		• Rising serum creatinine
			• Most common cause of abdominal mass in newborns
			• Poor prognosis
			• Most patients progress to renal failure
			• Transplantation often necessary

Polycystic kidney disease (autosomal recessive)	• Diagnosed in infancy
	• Prenatal oligohydramnios
	• Associated findings:
	  - Pulmonary hypoplasia
	  - Hepatic fibrosis
	  - Portal hypertension
	  - Hypertension
		• Family history
		• Renal ultrasound
		• Kidney biopsy
			• Variable clinical course
			• Most patients progress to renal failure
			• Transplantation often necessary

(autosomal dominant)	• Diagnosed later in life (adult form)
	• Hypertension
	• Hematuria
	• Associated findings:
	  - Berry aneurysms
	  - Hepatic cysts		

TABLE 8-4   *CONGENITAL/ INHERITED KIDNEY DISORDERS (CONTINUED)*

CONDITION	CLINICAL	DIAGNOSIS	TREATMENT/NOTES

Medullary cystic disease	• Hematuria
	• Enuresis
	• Associated findings:
	  - Growth retardation
	  - Hepatic fibrosis
	  - Ophthalmologic abnormalities
		• Renal ultrasound
		• Kidney biopsy
			• Poor prognosis
			• Transplantation often necessary

Alport syndrome	• Hereditary progressive nephritis • Asymptomatic hematuria • X-linked dominant (most common) • Associated with sensorineural hearing loss	• Renal ultrasound • Kidney biopsy • Diagnosis is aided by electron microscopy that reveals a thickened glomerular basement membrane	
Prune belly syndrome (Eagle-Barrett syndrome)	• Pulmonary and renal dysplasia • Abdominal wall muscle defect • Wrinkled loose abdominal skin • Dilated ureters • Oligohydramnios • Undescended testes • >90% are bilateral	• Renal ultrasound • Clinical diagnosis	

(Continued)

TABLE 8-4	CONGENITAL/ INHERITED KIDNEY DISORDERS (CONTINUED)		
CONDITION	**CLINICAL**	**DIAGNOSIS**	**TREATMENT/NOTES**
Cystinosis	• Proximal tubular dysfunction • Proximal tubular acidosis • Intralysosomal accumulation of cystine • Fanconi syndrome (cystinosis is the most common cause of Fanconi syndrome) • Retinopathy due to crystalline deposits (slit lamp exam) • Failure to thrive • Glucosuria	• Increased levels of cystine found in leukocytes	• Poor prognosis • Transplantation often necessary • Don't confuse cystinosis with cystinuria, a defect in the renal transport of the amino acids cystine, ornithine, arginine, and lysine (COAL); the only clinical consequence of cystinuria is renal stones

VCUG, voiding cystourethrogram.

GLOMERULAR DISORDERS

Glomerular disorders affect renal structure and function. The glomerular disorders can be classified by their clinical pathophysiology. Generally, there are three classes of disease: nephrotic syndrome, nephritic syndrome (glomerulonephritis), and hemolytic uremic syndrome.

NEPHROTIC SYNDROME

DEFINITION: Nephrotic syndrome is a glomerular disorder characterized by the presence of proteinuria, hypoproteinemia, and generalized edema. Albumin is wasted in the urine to a greater degree than globulin, although both are present in the urine. Nephrotic syndrome can occur as a primary kidney disorder, or secondary to an underlying condition.

ETIOLOGY: Minimal change disease is the most frequent overall cause of nephrotic syndrome and accounts for up to 90% of cases. Other important primary causes include focal segmental glomerulosclerosis, membranoproliferative glomerulonephritis, diffuse mesangial proliferation, and membranous nephropathy. Important secondary causes of nephrotic syndrome are poststreptococcal glomerulonephritis, hepatitis B and C, human immunodeficiency virus, systemic lupus erythematosus, and

Henoch-Schönlein purpura. The incidence of nephrotic syndrome is greatest in children from 1 to 6 years of age and is more common in boys than in girls.

CLINICAL PRESENTATION: Common presenting symptoms include periorbital edema, abdominal pain, and fatigue. As the disease progresses, generalized edema and an increased frequency of infections may occur.

TABLE 8-5. *DIAGNOSTIC CRITERIA FOR NEPHROTIC SYNDROME*

TABLE 8-6. *IMPORTANT CONDITIONS CAUSING NEPHROTIC SYNDROME*

COMPLICATIONS: Complications of nephrotic syndrome include severe anasarca, pleural effusions (from loss of oncotic pressure), severe infections (from loss of antibodies in urine), and hypercoagulability (from loss of anticlotting proteins in urine).

TREATMENT: The treatment of nephrotic syndrome consists of oral corticosteroids. Up to 95% of patients with minimal change disease respond within 4 weeks as evidenced by the absence of urine protein measured by dipstick. A sodium- and fat-restricted diet should also be initiated. Patients with anasarca require fluid restriction and albumin administration (followed by furosemide) to increase intravascular oncotic pressure. Patients with fever should be carefully evaluated for evidence of infection. Patients resistant to corticosteroids require a renal biopsy to confirm diagnosis and may respond to other immunomodulating agents (cyclosporin, tacrolimus).

TABLE 8-5	*DIAGNOSTIC CRITERIA FOR NEPHROTIC SYNDROME*
Generalized edema	
Hypoproteinemia (decreased albumin, complement, and immunoglobulins)	
Urine protein-to-creatinine ratio >2 in a first morning void	
24-h quantitative urine protein level greater than 50 mg/kg of body weight	
Hypercholesterolemia (>200 mg/dL)	

TABLE 8-6		*IMPORTANT CONDITIONS CAUSING NEPHROTIC SYNDROME*		
CONDITION	**ETIOLOGY/DEMOGRAPHICS**	**CLINICAL**	**EVALUATION**	**TREATMENT**
Minimal change nephrotic syndrome	• Peak incidence is age 2-6 y • The most common cause of nephrotic syndrome • Idiopathic	• Periorbital edema (may resemble an allergic reaction) • Ascites • Recurrent or severe infections	• The renal biopsy of children with minimal change disease demonstrates effacement of podocytes • Steroid-resistant cases frequently require a renal biopsy to confirm diagnosis	• Corticosteroids • 95% of patients respond to steroids within 4 wk • Excellent prognosis
Focal segmental glomerulosclerosis	• Peak incidence is age 2-6 y • Idiopathic	• Presentation identical to minimal change nephrotic syndrome • Characterized as steroid-resistant nephrotic syndrome	• Renal biopsy required for diagnosis	• Poor prognosis with eventual development of end-stage renal disease • There is a high recurrence rate after transplantation • Responsiveness to steroid therapy usually dictates the overall prognosis

NEPHRITIC SYNDROME (GLOMERULONEPHRITIS)

Glomerulonephritis occurs when glomerular injury leads to glomerular inflammation, disorder, and dysfunction. The clinical manifestations include hematuria, proteinuria, hypertension, and renal insufficiency. The most important causes of glomerulonephritis are summarized in Table 8-7.

TABLE 8-7. *IMPORTANT CONDITIONS CAUSING GLOMERULONEPHRITIS*

HEMOLYTIC UREMIC SYNDROME (HUS)

DEFINITION: HUS can best be defined as a triad of microangiopathic hemolytic anemia, thrombocytopenia, and renal insufficiency. It is the most frequent cause of acute renal failure in healthy children.

ETIOLOGY: The most common etiology of HUS is *E. coli* 0157:H7. This *E. coli* strain produces a shiga-like toxin that damages renal glomeruli and induces a systemic inflammatory response manifested by platelet and red blood cell destruction. The peak incidence is 9 months to 4 years of age. Risk factors include consumption of undercooked beef and inadequate washing of fruits and vegetables contaminated with manure. Thrombotic thrombocytopenic purpura (TTP) is an important differential diagnosis; many authorities suggest that HUS and TTP are different clinical manifestations of a single disorder.

CLINICAL PRESENTATION: Onset of disease is abrupt. Initial symptoms include abdominal pain, nausea, vomiting, and bloody diarrhea. Microangiopathic hemolytic anemia follows, with development of pallor, fatigue, and petechiae. Renal insufficiency is variable, and may be manifest with oliguria and hypertension. Neurologic manifestations are frequent and range from irritability to lethargy and seizures.

DIAGNOSIS: The diagnosis is principally made on clinical grounds. The triad of hemolytic anemia, thrombocytopenia, and renal insufficiency is pathognomonic. Stool cultures for *E. coli* O157:H7 should be obtained.

TREATMENT: Once a diagnosis of HUS is confirmed, supportive care is the most important therapy. Some authorities believe that antibiotic treatment of children with bloody gastroenteritis may increase the risk for developing HUS. Fluid management is important for renal insufficiency, as some patients ultimately develop acute renal failure requiring dialysis. Peritoneal dialysis, hemodialysis, and plasma exchange are potentially beneficial in removing the offending toxin. Platelet transfusions should be avoided if possible, as they may potentiate thrombotic episodes. The long-term prognosis is variable and largely dependent on the degree of renal insufficiency.

TABLE 8-7 IMPORTANT CONDITIONS CAUSING GLOMERULONEPHRITIS

CONDITION	ETIOLOGY/DEMOGRAPHICS	CLINICAL	EVALUATION	TREATMENT/NOTES
Acute poststreptococcal glomerulonephritis (APGN)	• The most frequent cause of glomerulonephritis • Peak incidence is age 5-15 y • Occurs after infection with group A β-hemolytic *Streptococcus* (usually skin infection) • Immune complex-mediated glomerular damage	• May occur many weeks after antecedent bacterial infection • Generalized edema • Gross hematuria (smoke or tea colored) • Hypertension is frequent	• Immunofluorescence reveals subepithelial deposits of IgG and C3 • Decreased serum C3 level • Normal C4 level • Azotemia • Increased urine osmolarity • Decreased urine sodium	• Supportive • Fluid restriction for renal insufficiency • Good prognosis
Membrano-proliferative glomerulonephritis	• Peak incidence is age 8-30 y • Idiopathic • Immune complex-mediated glomerular damage • May be associated with systemic diseases (SLE, hepatitis B and C, leukemia, lymphoma)	• Similar presentation to APGN • Generalized edema, proteinuria, hypoproteinemia (nephrotic syndrome) also present	• Immunofluorescence reveals subendothelial deposits of IgG and C3 • Decreased serum C3 and C4 levels • Renal biopsy is often necessary to confirm diagnosis	• Supportive therapy • Corticosteroids and immunosuppressive therapies are controversial • Poor prognosis with progression to ESRD likely
Lupus nephritis	• Peak incidence is in adolescence and adulthood • Immune complex-mediated glomerular damage • Nephritis is one of the 11 diagnostic criteria of SLE (see Chapter 17)	• Hematuria • Proteinuria • Acute renal failure	• The presence of renal disease with the diagnosis of SLE is generally sufficient for diagnosis	• Corticosteroids in combination with immunomodulating agents may be effective • Poor prognosis with progression to ESRD likely

IgA nephropathy

- Peak incidence is age 10-30 y
- Immune complex–mediated glomerular damage

- Gross hematuria
- May occur a few days after an antecedent URI
- Frequently, there are no other associated signs or symptoms

- Immunofluorescence reveals mesangial deposits of IgA, IgG, and C3
- Serum C3 and C4 levels are normal
- Children with additional associated symptoms (edema, hypertension) usually require a renal biopsy to confirm diagnosis

- Variable course
- Most patients with a mild course have a good prognosis
- Complicated disease often requires angiotensin-converting enzyme inhibitors and corticosteroid therapy to help prevent ESRD
- Do not confuse IgA nephropathy with nephritis due to HSP. A patient with HSP can have nephritis resulting in IgA nephropathy. A patient with IgA nephropathy does not necessarily have HSP. Histologically the diseases are identical.

ESRD, end-stage renal disease; HSP, Henoch-Schönlein purpura; SLE, systemic lupus erythematosus; URI, upper respiratory tract infection.

RENAL TUBULAR DISORDERS

Renal tubular acidification defects occur when the kidneys are unable to maintain a normal serum pH, due either to excessive excretion of bicarbonate or deficient secretion of acid into the urine. There are three major types of RTA: Type 1, Type 2, and Type 4. RTA may occur secondary to a systemic condition (SLE, sickle cell anemia), as a medication effect (amphotericin B, lithium, cyclosporin), or as a primary inherited disease. Patients with RTA usually have a hyperchloremic metabolic acidosis and a normal plasma anion gap. RTA is treated with bicarbonate administration.

TABLE 8-8	RENAL TUBULAR DISORDERS
RTA TYPE	**CHARACTERISTICS***
RTA type 1 (distal tubule)	• Decreased hydrogen ion (acid) secretion • Children present with failure to thrive, **hypokalemia,** and kidney stones • **Urine pH >5.5**
RTA type 2 (proximal tubule)	• Decreased bicarbonate reabsorption (decreased threshold for bicarbonate reabsorption) • The patient presents with failure to thrive, and a **hypokalemic,** hyperchloremic metabolic acidosis • Almost always seen as part of Fanconi syndrome • **Urine pH <5.5**
RTA type 4 (hyperkalemic),	• Decreased mineralocorticoid-dependent excretion of potassium • The patient presents with a **hyperkalemic**, hyperchloremic metabolic acidosis • **Urine pH <5.5** • Treatment consists of mineralocorticoid replacement in addition to bicarbonate administration
Fanconi syndrome	• Decreased proximal tubular transport of sodium, glucose, amino acids, and phosphorus • Most frequent cause is cystinosis (autosomal recessive) • Patient presents in infancy with polydipsia, polyuria, hypophosphatemic rickets, failure to thrive, and **hypokalemic**, hyperchloremic metabolic acidosis • Overall prognosis is poor, with high rate of progression to end-stage renal disease

*Important differences are in bold.

DISORDERS OF WATER BALANCE

POLYURIA

Polyuria occurs when a child who is not drinking excessive amounts of fluid experiences increased frequency and/or volume of urination. A urine dipstick for specific gravity (SG) is a good screening test to evaluate renal concentrating ability. A urine specific gravity of 1.020 or higher indicates the ability of the kidney to concentrate the urine and generally rules out pathologic disease. A urine specific gravity of 1.010 or lower is frequently seen with both nephrogenic and central diabetes insipidus.

Psychogenic polydipsia is common in children and often confused with DI (see below). Patients present with polydipsia polyuria, normal serum sodium and osmolarity, and low urine osmolarity.

TABLE 8-9	COMMON CAUSES OF POLYURIA
	Caffeine
	Diuretics
	Mannitol
	Glucosuria
	Diabetes mellitus
	Central diabetes insipidus
	Nephrogenic diabetes insipidus
	Chronic renal failure
	Psychogenic polydipsia
	Sickle-cell disease

DIABETES INSIPIDUS (DI)

Normally, antidiuretic hormone (ADH) acts at the level of the renal tubule collecting ducts to increase water reabsorption, resulting in concentrated urine. DI occurs when the renal tubule is unable to concentrate the urine, resulting in excessive free water loss and subsequent hypernatremia. DI can occur with either ADH deficiency (central DI) or ADH resistance (nephrogenic DI).

Central DI occurs in a variety of conditions, most frequently head trauma, intraventricular hemorrhage, meningitis, and craniopharyngioma. *Nephrogenic DI* can either be inherited (multiple modes of inheritance) or acquired. Disease states associated with nephrogenic DI include sickle cell disease, obstructive uropathy, electrolyte imbalance, and medications (lithium, amphotericin, general anesthesia).

Common presenting symptoms include polydipsia, polyuria, nocturia, dehydration, and headaches. Laboratory evaluation reveals elevated serum osmolarity, low urine osmolarity (SG <1.005), and hypernatremia. Response to DDAVP (ADH) as manifested by decreased urine output and correction of hypernatremia can differentiate between central and nephrogenic DI. Patients with central DI (absence of hormone) respond to intravenous vasopressin, while patients with nephrogenic DI (absence of receptors) do not. An additional finding in patients with nephrogenic DI is the presence of elevated vasopressin levels

Treatment of central DI consists of arginine vasopressin, titrated to clinical effect. Treatment of nephrogenic DI consists of a low-sodium diet, close monitoring of hydration status, and diuretics, specifically hydrochlorothiazide.

SYNDROME OF INAPPROPRIATE ANTIDIURETIC HORMONE (SIADH)

DEFINITION: This syndrome occurs when ADH is secreted in the absence of intravascular depletion or increased serum osmolarity.

TABLE 8-10	*CAUSES OF SYNDROME OF INAPPROPRIATE ANTIDIURETIC HORMONE (SIADH)*
Meningitis	
Encephalitis	
Brain abscess	
Brain tumors	
Pulmonary disease	
Paraneoplastic disease	
Head trauma	
Major surgery	
Drugs (cyclophosphamide, vincristine, etc)	
Glucocorticoid deficiency	

CLINICAL PRESENTATION: The severity of symptoms is dependent on both the serum sodium level and rate of fluctuation. Symptoms usually develop when serum sodium levels are below 120 mEq/L. Presenting signs and symptoms include decreased urine output, nausea, vomiting, irritability, headache, muscle cramps, and, when severe, ataxia, seizures, and coma.

DIAGNOSIS: Laboratory evaluation of affected patients reveals hyponatremia (<125 mEq/L), decreased BUN, serum uric acid, and serum hypoosmolality, as well as elevated urine sodium (>20 mEq/L), urine hyperosmolality, and urine specific gravity.

TREATMENT: Treatment of patients with SIADH is reliant on fluid restriction, sodium replacement, and treatment of the underlying cause. Hypertonic saline and diuretic use should be reserved for patients who develop seizures or profound changes in mental status.

DISORDERS OF ELECTROLYTE BALANCE

- **Hyponatremia**: Defined as a sodium concentration lower than 130 mEq/L. Hyponatremia can occur with increased, normal, or decreased total body sodium (TBNa).

TABLE 8-11	CAUSES OF HYPONATREMIA	
TOTAL BODY SODIUM (TBNA)	**MECHANISM**	**LABORATORY FINDINGS**
Decreased TBNa (usually occurs with hypovolemia)	Renal losses: • Adrenal dysfunction (Addison disease, congenital adrenal hyperplasia, adrenal hemorrhage, birth asphyxia) • Bartter syndrome • Intrinsic renal disease	• Increased urinary sodium excretion (>20 mEq/L) • Hyperkalemia • In Bartter syndrome, a renal transport defect decreases potassium absorption in the kidney; hyperkalemia is not present
	Extrarenal losses: • Gastrointestinal loss (diarrhea, vomiting) • Sweat • Pancreatitis • Burns • Effusions	• Decreased urinary sodium excretion (<20 mEq/L) • Hypokalemia
Increased TBNa (usually occurs with hypervolemia)	• Congestive heart failure • Nephrotic syndrome • Cirrhosis	• Decreased urinary sodium excretion (<20 mEq/L) • Hypokalemia
Normal TBNa (usually occurs with euvolemia)	• SIADH • Fluid overload • Acute renal failure with severe oliguria • Glucocorticoid deficiency	• Increased urinary sodium excretion (>20 mEq/L)

SIADH, syndrome of inappropriate antidiuretic hormone.

• **Hypernatremia**: Defined as a serum sodium concentration higher than 150 mEq/L. It can occur with increased, normal, or decreased total body sodium.

TABLE 8-12	CAUSES OF HYPERNATREMIA	
TOTAL BODY SODIUM (TBNA)	**MECHANISM**	**LABORATORY FINDINGS**
Decreased TBNa (usually occurs with hypovolemia)	• Gastrointestinal losses • Renal losses • Skin losses (perspiration)	• In all of these disorders except for hypernatremia due to renal losses, urinary sodium is <20 mEq/L
Increased TBNa (usually occurs with hypervolemia)	• Increased salt in formula • Iatrogenic (increased sodium bicarbonate administration, sodium chloride solutions) • Hyperaldosteronism	
Normal TBNa (usually occurs with euvolemia)	• Diabetes insipidus (central and nephrogenic)	

HYPOKALEMIA

Hypokalemia is defined as a potassium level lower than 4 mEq/L for infants younger than 10 days, and lower than 3.5 mEq/L for infants and children older than 10 days. The most frequent etiologies include gastrointestinal losses from diarrhea, diabetic ketoacidosis, diuretic or laxative abuse, and hyperhidrosis.

Inherited defects of electrolyte transport proteins in the kidney can also result in hypokalemia. Examples include RTA type I, Fanconi syndrome, and Bartter syndrome. In these disorders, urinary chloride is higher than 10 mEq/L, which differentiates them from hypokalemia due to GI losses or hyperhidrosis.

Additional etiologies include inherited impairments of sodium absorption in the distal tubule of the kidney. Examples include Cushing's disease, hyperaldosteronism, and some forms of congenital adrenal hyperplasia (CAH).

HYPERKALEMIA

Hyperkalemia is defined as a higher than normal serum potassium (generally greater than 5.5 mEq/L) due to either an increase in total body potassium or excessive release of potassium from the cells into the bloodstream. Excess potassium is normally excreted by the kidney. Any disorder that affects kidney function may reduce kidney's ability to excrete potassium.

TABLE 8-13	CAUSES OF HYPERKALEMIA

CAUSE	EXAMPLE
Renal	• Renal failure (acute and chronic) • Adrenal insufficiency • Salt-wasting congenital adrenal hyperplasia • Pseudohypoaldosteronism • Systemic lupus erythematosus • Drugs (i.e., spironolactone, ACE inhibitors)
Cellular breakdown	• Hemolysis • Severe burns • Crush injury • Tumor lysis after chemotherapy • Rhabdomyolysis
Metabolic acidosis	• Diabetic ketoacidosis (although total body potassium depleted) • Inborn errors of metabolism • Septic shock

UROLOGIC ABNORMALITIES

HYPOSPADIAS

Hypospadias is defined as incomplete development of the anterior urethra, resulting in an abnormal opening of the urethral meatus anywhere along the shaft of the penis. The prepuce is frequently malformed, with the ventral surface of the glans exposed. This preputial malformation is called a dorsal hood. Hypospadias is one of the most common congenital abnormalities, affecting as many as 1 in every 300 children. Newborn infants born with hypospadias should not be circumcised because the foreskin is used to repair the defect. Hypospadias associated with undescended or nonpalpable testes should raise the suspicion of an intersex disorder.

PHIMOSIS/PARAPHIMOSIS

Phimosis is defined as the inability to retract the foreskin. This is a normal finding in children less than 2 years of age. By age 3, 90% of foreskins should be retractable without force. Early forceful retraction of the foreskin should be avoided because of the risk of adhesion formation. In some children, the foreskin will not retract appropriately, resulting in balanoposthitis, or inflammation of the glans and foreskin. This may result in obstruction of the urethral meatus, discomfort, and urinary tract infection.

Paraphimosis is the entrapment of the prepuce proximal to the coronal margin, resulting in swelling and pain of the glans and foreskin. Prompt attention is required to prevent ischemic necrosis of the glans penis secondary to venous occlusion from the strangulated foreskin. The paraphimosis can be reduced in the office or emergency room with local anesthesia. Paraphimosis has a high rate of recurrence.

Scrotal Masses and Swelling

Acute scrotal masses and scrotal pain are a challenging dilemma for the pediatric practitioner. Signs and symptoms of an acute scrotum in children include abdominal pain, testicular pain, nausea, vomiting, fever, and a painful testicle. The differential diagnoses of acute scrotal pain in children include epididymitis, testicular torsion, torsion of a testicular appendage, incarcerated hernia, acute hydrocele, Henoch-Schönlein purpura, and testicular trauma. Selected disorders are discussed below.

EPIDIDYMITIS

DEFINITION: Epididymitis is an inflammation of the epididymis, a structure located on the posterior aspect of the testicle.

ETIOLOGY: In prepubertal boys, epididymitis may be secondary to an ectopic ureter, bladder outlet obstruction (secondary to posterior urethral valves), and congenital urethral abnormalities. In older children and adolescents, the most frequent cause of epididymitis is a bacterial infection or sexually transmitted disease. Other important causes of epididymitis include viral and fungal infections, sterile urine reflux, and amiodarone-induced chemical epididymitis.

CLINICAL PRESENTATION: The patient with epididymitis presents with fever, abdominal pain, nausea, and possibly a painful swollen testicle. This condition can be easily confused with testicular torsion in young children due to vague signs and symptoms.

DIAGNOSIS: The primary evaluation should include a thorough history and physical exam, urinalysis with Gram stain, urine culture, and white blood cell count. Adolescent patients, those with urethral discharge, or children suspected of being victims of sexual abuse should be evaluated for a possible sexually transmitted disease. A Doppler ultrasound or nuclear medicine testicular scan is valuable when trying to distinguish epididymitis from torsion of the testicle.

TREATMENT: Treatment of epididymitis includes antibiotics, analgesics, and scrotal elevation. If the diagnosis is unclear in a patient with an acute scrotum, emergent consultation with a pediatric urologist should be obtained.

VARICOCELE

DEFINITION: A varicocele is defined as an engorgement of the pampiniform plexus of veins within the spermatic cord, which coalesce to become the testicular vein at the internal inguinal ring.

ETIOLOGY: The etiology of varicoceles is unclear. Varicoceles most frequently occur on the left side (85% of cases) due to the perpendicular insertion of the left testicular vein into the left renal vein. The left renal vein has higher pressures compared to the vena cava, which receives the right testicular vein.

DIAGNOSIS: Large varicoceles may be visible on the initial inspection of the scrotum. On palpation, they are characterized as feeling like a "bag of worms." The presence of an acute or right-sided varicocele should raise suspicion of venous obstruction from a retroperitoneal mass. The differential diagnosis includes neuroblastoma, congenital mesoblastic nephroma, Wilms tumor lymphoma, and renal cell carcinoma.

TREATMENT: Varicoceles should be followed to ensure ipsilateral testicular development. If there is a discrepancy in testicular growth, surgical correction is warranted. Varicoceles are associated with decreased fertility in adulthood. As many as 40% of adult males have a varicocele, and it is the most common surgically correctable cause of male factor infertility.

HYDROCELE

A hydrocele is defined as a collection of fluid that accumulates between the parietal and visceral layers of the tunica vaginalis. The fluid collection is frequently the result of the failure of fusion and obliteration of the processus vaginalis and is typically associated with a hernia. The patient often presents with an asymptomatic scrotal mass. On physical exam, the mass can be transilluminated, revealing the fluid-filled sac. When the testicle cannot be examined due to a large hydrocele, scrotal ultrasound is warranted. Spontaneous resolution without treatment is frequent. In infants, parents should be warned about the signs and symptoms of an incarcerated hernia since most hydroceles in this age group are associated with hernias.

TESTICULAR TORSION

Testicular torsion is defined as twisting of the spermatic cord with strangulation of the blood supply to the affected testicle. Testicular torsion is a surgical emergency and prompt recognition of this condition with immediate surgical consultation is of paramount importance. Failure of timely diagnosis and delayed treatment is directly correlated to the potential viability of the affected testicle. The incidence of testicular torsion is 1 in 4000 males and is most frequent in children between the ages of 3 and 20 years. Testicular torsion is the most common cause of a scrotal mass in the newborn. When newborn testicular torsion occurs, the testicle is rarely viable. In rare cases, neonatal torsion may be confused with a yolk sac tumor of the testicle.

CLINICAL PRESENTATION: The patient with testicular torsion presents with the acute onset of scrotal pain, nausea, and vomiting. On physical exam the affected testicle may be elevated with an absent cremasteric reflex. The presence of an undescended testicle does not exclude the diagnosis of testicular torsion. Intra-abdominal testicles may also twist, presenting as acute abdominal pain.

DIAGNOSIS: Doppler ultrasonography or nuclear medicine studies reveal decreased flow to the affected testicle. If there is a strong suspicion of torsion, surgical consultation should not be delayed pending Doppler ultrasound results. During surgical exploration and correction of the torsion, the surgeon will often perform contralateral orchiopexy, although this practice is somewhat controversial.

TORSION OF THE TESTICULAR APPENDAGES

Torsion of a testicular appendage is the most common cause of acute scrotal pain in children and the most frequent condition confused with testicular torsion. The appendix testis, a remnant of the müllerian duct, is the usual appendage involved in torsion. The appendix of the epididymis or paradidymis is less frequently involved. Torsion of a testicular appendage presents with the same signs and symptoms as testicular torsion. In some patients, a "blue dot" sign may be visualized on inspection of the affected hemiscrotum. A Doppler ultrasound reveals either normal or increased flow to the affected testicle with a cold spot corresponding to the torsed appendage. Treatment consists of supportive therapy. The affected testicular appendage will usually autoamputate within a few days to 1 week, with resolution of symptoms in most cases.

CRYPTORCHIDISM (UNDESCENDED TESTES)

An undescended testicle is defined as the failure of testicular descent into the scrotum. The undescended testicle may be located in the abdominal cavity or in the inguinal canal. The presentation may be unilateral or bilateral. It occurs most frequently in premature infants. The undescended testicle should be differentiated from a retractile testicle on physical exam. Changing position from supine to standing or squatting often allows the practitioner to palpate the testicle in the distal inguinal canal.

An undescended testicle that cannot be located on physical exam (a nonpalpable testicle) frequently requires laparoscopy to confirm presence or absence of testicular tissue. Undescended testicles are associated with an increased risk for torsion, infertility, and malignancy. Patients may be treated with human chorionic gonadotropin (hCG) to facilitate migration of the undescended testicle into the scrotum. However, this practice is usually unsuccessful.

Children with failure of descent by 2 years of age should have an orchiopexy performed to bring the testicle into proper position. After 2 years of age, permanent histologic damage is evident. The risk of malignancy is unchanged by orchiopexy but it does allow for easier examination and follow-up. Whether fertility is affected by orchiopexy is controversial.

VESICOURETERAL REFLUX (VUR)

DEFINITION: Vesicoureteral reflux is defined as the retrograde flow of urine from the bladder into the ureter and kidney.

ETIOLOGY: Reflux is caused by an anatomical or functional abnormality of the ureterovesical junction and may be unilateral or bilateral. Reflux can also be due to bladder outlet obstruction, high voiding pressures (neurogenic bladder), and dysfunctional voiding. There is a genetic predisposition for developing VUR, as siblings and offspring of affected patients have an increased risk for the disease.

DIAGNOSIS: Children with VUR are usually diagnosed during the evaluation of a febrile urinary tract infection or hydronephrosis. The evaluation of a child with suspected VUR, hydronephrosis, or a febrile urinary tract infection includes a renal ultrasound and a voiding cystourethrogram (VCUG). The severity of VUR is graded based on the amount of reflux and associated anatomical pathology visualized on the study. There are five grades (I-V), grade I representing the most minimal amount of reflux visualized on a voiding study and grade V representing significant dilatation of the ureter, pelvis, and calyces.

COMPLICATIONS: Complications of VUR include frequent urinary tract infections, pyelonephritis, renal scarring, hydronephrosis, and renal failure.

TREATMENT: The goal of management is to prevent renal injury and scarring. Treatment options include antibiotic prophylaxis and serial imaging or operative repair via ureteric reimplant. Sterile reflux is not likely to cause renal damage in those patients with normal bladder function. Most patients with low-grade VUR (grades I-III) should be managed conservatively with antibiotic prophylaxis and annual voiding cystograms to evaluate for resolution. Serial renal ultrasounds or DMSA scans should be obtained to evaluate for renal scarring if a patient is being managed conservatively. Renal scarring can occur during follow-up in children who never present with a breakthrough infection. The majority of patients with low-grade reflux resolve spontaneously.

Although there is controversy regarding which patients require surgery, most authorities agree that patients with unilateral grade V reflux or bilateral grade IV reflux are good candidates for early surgical repair. Functional causes of reflux such as neurogenic bladder and dysfunctional voiding should always be addressed prior to surgical repair. Indications for operative repair include breakthrough infections, progressive renal scarring, poor compliance, the inability to tolerate antibiotic prophylaxis, and the development of complications from long-term antibiotic therapy. Screening of siblings with VUR may be performed with a nuclear medicine study, which has less radiation and improved sensitivity than the standard fluoroscopic study. The presence of reflux on the nuclear medicine study warrants a standard VCUG to grade the reflux and rule out bladder outlet obstruction.

CHAPTER 9

NEUROLOGY

ABNORMAL HEAD SIZE

Normal head growth is consistent with linear growth and weight gain. An abnormal head circumference in a child can indicate abnormal brain development. Head circumference and shape should be documented from the newborn period through late childhood. Children with abnormal head sizes (large or small) require further diagnostic evaluation for central nervous system abnormalities. Additionally, children who have a change in the pattern of head growth (i.e., rapid increase or arrest of growth) also require further evaluation.

MICROCEPHALY

Microcephaly is defined as a head circumference that is more than 3 standard deviations below the mean. Children with microcephaly have an increased incidence of mental retardation and developmental delay. Microcephaly can be congenital or acquired. *Congenital* disease results from abnormal brain development, as seen with chromosomal abnormalities, migration disorders, neural tube defects, toxin exposure, craniosynostosis, and intrauterine infections. *Acquired* microcephaly may result from perinatally acquired infection (i.e., meningitis), hypoxic-ischemic insults (i.e., perinatal asphyxia, intraventricular hemorrhage), metabolic derangements (i.e., hypothyroidism, aminoacidurias), and in Rett syndrome. Familial microcephaly occurs as well; the parent's head circumference should be measured when evaluating any child with microcephaly.

Affected infants should undergo evaluation as directed by clinical presentation. Serologic testing for toxoplasmosis, rubella, cytomegalovirus, HIV, and syphilis; radiologic imaging; metabolic screening; and /or chromosomal analysis can all provide clues to the underlying cause. Treatment options depend on the underlying cause.

TABLE 9-1. *COMMON CAUSES OF MICROCEPHALY*

MACROCEPHALY

Macrocephaly is defined as a large head size, greater than 3 standard deviations above the mean. Macrocephaly can be associated with increased brain mass and

163

TABLE 9-1   *COMMON CAUSES OF MICROCEPHALY*

CONGENITAL	ACQUIRED
• Trisomy 13 (Patau syndrome)	• Meningitis
• Trisomy 18 (Edwards syndrome)	• Perinatal asphyxia
• Trisomy 21(Down syndrome)	• Hypothyroidism
• Rett syndrome	
• Cornelia de Lange syndrome	
• Cri-du-chat syndrome (5p-syndrome)	
• Cytomegalovirus	
• Rubella	
• Toxoplasmosis	
• Familial—autosomal recessive	
• Familial—autosomal dominant	
• Maternal drug exposure (alcohol, phenytoin)	

size or increased ventricle size (hydrocephalus). Hydrocephalus is the most common cause of macrocephaly in children who have an underlying cause. Almost half of all cases of macrocephaly are familial in origin and are generally benign. The parent's head circumference should be measured when evaluating any child with macrocephaly.

TABLE 9-2   *COMMON CAUSES OF MACROCEPHALY*

Familial
Hydrocephalus
Megalencephaly
Neurocutaneous disorders (neurofibromatosis)
Achondroplasia
Metabolic (Alexander disease, Canavan disease)
Mucopolysaccharidosis

CRANIOSYNOSTOSIS

In normal infants, the cranial sutures remain open until the first year, and generally are completely closed by 2 years of age. Craniosynostosis is the inappropriate, premature fusion of one or more sutures. Premature closure results in asymmetric growth of the skull and/or abnormal skull shapes. Bony growth continues in the axis parallel to the fused suture, while growth perpendicular to the suture is arrested. For example, in isolated sagittal suture synostosis (the most common form of craniosynostosis), growth continues anterioposteriorly, with arrest in lateral growth. The result is an elongated, oval-shaped skull, termed dolichocephaly. Continued, unrepaired disease can lead to abnormal brain development, abnormal orbit and eye development, and facial distortion.

Craniosynostosis may occur due to a defect in the bone itself (primary craniosynostosis), or secondary to an underlying condition (secondary craniosynostosis). Primary craniosynostosis is most common in Caucasians and affects males more frequently than females. It may occur as an isolated defect, or in association with certain genetic syndromes (see below).

TABLE 9-3.   *COMMON ABNORMAL HEAD SHAPES*

TABLE 9-4.   *COMMON GENETIC SYNDROMES CAUSING CRANIOSYNOSTOSIS*

The most common underlying disorder in secondary craniosynostosis is abnormal development of the central nervous system. Patients with craniosynostosis secondary to abnormal brain development are usually microcephalic with some degree of mental retardation. Additionally, hyperthyroidism, mucopolysaccharidosis, malnutrition (chronic illnesses and/or congenital heart disease), and severe anemia can all result in craniosynostosis.

TABLE 9-3	*COMMON ABNORMAL HEAD SHAPES*	
CONDITION	**SHAPE**	**SUTURE INVOLVED**
Brachycephaly	• Broad head with recessed lower forehead	• Coronal suture
Dolichocephaly	• An elongated oval-shaped skull	• Sagittal suture
Occipital plagiocephaly	• Flattening on one side of the head	• Commonly seen in infants who are mainly positioned supine • May also be secondary to premature closure of the lambdoid suture
Trigonocephaly	• Triangular-shaped head with a vertical ridge in the mid-forehead	• Metopic suture

TABLE 9-4   *COMMON GENETIC SYNDROMES CAUSING CRANIOSYNOSTOSIS*

SYNDROME	ETIOLOGY/ DEMOGRAPHICS	CLINICAL	DIAGNOSIS	TREATMENT
Apert syndrome	• Autosomal dominant	• Craniosynostosis • Syndactyly of the hands and feet • Mental retardation • Mid-face hypoplasia • Frontal bossing • Hearing and vision loss	• Clinical	• Surgical correction of primary defect • Supportive care of secondary defects
Crouzon disease	• Autosomal dominant	• Craniosynostosis • Mid-face hypoplasia • Proptosis • Exotropia • Exophthalmos • Hypertelorism • Hearing and vision loss • Syndactyly of the hands and feet does *NOT* occur		

Children with craniosynostosis are initially evaluated with plain skull radiographs. If abnormalities are detected (either suture fusion or abnormal skull shape), then a magnetic resonance imaging scan or a computed tomographic scan with computerized three-dimensional reconstruction should be obtained. Secondary causes and genetic syndromes associated with craniosynostosis should be considered in the evaluation. Children with craniosynostosis should be referred to a surgeon capable of performing craniofacial reconstruction.

CENTRAL NERVOUS SYSTEM MALFORMATIONS

HYDROCEPHALUS

Hydrocephalus is characterized by dilated ventricles filled with cerebrospinal fluid (CSF), caused by an imbalance between CSF production and absorption. Hydrocephalus may be caused by blockage of CSF flow (obstructive hydrocephalus) or decreased CSF absorption (communicating hydrocephalus).

Obstructive hydrocephalus is the most frequently encountered form; causes include:

- Aqueductal stenosis (obstructing the fourth ventricle)
- Posterior fossa malformations (i.e., Dandy-Walker syndrome)
- Postinfectious inflammation (i.e., following TORCH infections or meningitis)
- Tumors directly obstructing flow
- Bleeding (causing inflammation)
- Arteriovenous malformation

Communicating (nonobstructive) hydrocephalus occurs when the subarachnoid cisterns or arachnoid villi do not absorb CSF in a normal fashion. The most common conditions resulting in communicating hydrocephalus include:

- Benign enlargement of the subarachnoid space (external hydrocephalus)
- Intraventricular hemorrhage
- Meningitis
- Meningeal spread of a malignancy
- Congenital toxoplasmosis

Accumulation of CSF can cause an increase in intracranial pressure. If the process is acute (i.e., trauma, bleeding), the patient may present with headache, vomiting, altered mental status, lethargy, coma, papilledema, and/or Cushing's triad (hypertension, bradycardia, and abnormal respirations). Most cases of chronic hydrocephalus manifest with subtle neurologic symptoms, including behavioral changes and developmental delay. Physical examination findings include macrocephaly, frontal bossing, dilated scalp veins, and paralysis of upward gaze (termed "sun-setting eyes"). Computed tomography is the initial diagnostic tool of choice. Surgical intervention and placement of a ventriculoperitoneal shunt system restores CSF flow patterns and relieves intracranial pressure.

CHIARI MALFORMATION

The Chiari malformation is characterized by the downward displacement of the cerebellum and brainstem through the foramen magnum. There are three classes of malformation, defined by the degree of displacement. Type I is defined by the presence of the cerebellar tonsils and vermis below the level of the foramen magnum. It is usually diagnosed in adolescents during evaluation for headaches, and is not associated with hydrocephalus. Type II is the most common, consists of displacement of the inferior vermis, pons, and medulla below the level of an elongated fourth ventricle, and is often associated with hydrocephalus and myelomeningocele. Type III is the most severe, defined by the presence of a herniated cerebellum through a defective cervical spinal canal. Magnetic resonance imaging is the preferred diagnostic modality. In many cases, the treatment will be surgical.

DANDY-WALKER MALFORMATION

Dandy-Walker malformation is characterized by:

- Partial or complete agenesis of the cerebellar vermis
- Cystic dilatation of the posterior fossa
- Hydrocephalus

This condition is usually diagnosed during the evaluation of hydrocephalus in an infant or young child. Ventricular shunt systems are generally required to relieve the obstruction and restore CSF flow.

NEURAL TUBE DEFECTS (NTDS)

The failure of the embryologic neural tube to completely close during early fetal development can result in NTDs. These defects occur extremely early in fetal development (2-3 weeks of gestational age), usually before the mother realizes she is pregnant. These conditions affect up to 5 in 1000 live births and have a genetic predisposition. There is an association between neural tube development and folic acid metabolism; administration of folic acid to women of childbearing age may prevent a substantial number of these defects from occurring. Other causes of neural tube defects include maternal radiation, maternal hyperthermia, vitamin A excess or deficiency, TORCH infections, and drugs such as pyrimethamine, trimethoprim/sulfasalazine, and certain anticonvulsants and chemotherapeutic agents. An elevated maternal serum alpha-fetoprotein level can indicate the presence of a neural tube defect, and is generally assessed around 18 to 20 weeks of gestation. There are many forms of neural tube defects; the most common are discussed below.

Anencephaly is the absence of the cranial vault and cerebral hemispheres. It is caused by a failure of the anterior neural tube to close during fetal development. This condition is usually diagnosed by routine prenatal ultrasound, and accounts for about 50% of all NTDs. Almost half of anencephalic infants are spontaneously aborted, and those who survive to term die in the neonatal period.

An *encephalocele* is the herniation of part of brain and meningeal tissue through a defect in the skull (cranium bifidum), resulting from a defective closure of the anterior portion of the neural tube. The patient usually presents with a sac-like structure protruding from the occipital portion of the skull. Surgical correction is necessary. Prognosis depends upon the extent of the defect and presence or absence of associated abnormalities.

Spinal dysraphisms are characterized as a group of disorders that result in the incomplete closure of the posterior portion of the neural tube. These defects are usually located in the lumbosacral area and have a variety of associated clinical manifestations. There is a wide spectrum of disease and clinical manifestations, depending on the location and severity of the defect.

A *meningomyelocele* results when a portion of the spinal cord and meninges herniate through a defect in the vertebral column. A sac with a thin layer of skin is present at birth. These patients have neurologic manifestations consistent with a spinal cord injury at the level of the defect. Frequent associated findings include bladder and bowel dysfunction, lower extremity weakness, and orthopedic problems (i.e., ankle and foot deformities). Most patients have an associated hydrocephalus or Chiari II malformation.

Patients with isolated meningomyelocele and hydrocephalus have low-average intelligence, although problems with memory and concentration are common. Children with lesions located higher on the spine and children who develop related infections, intracranial bleeding, or require shunting are at higher risk for mental retardation.

A *meningocele* is the herniation of meninges through the spinal and vertebral canal. The patient is often free of neurologic manifestations, and may present only with a fluctuant midline spinal mass. The incidence of hydrocephalus and associated central nervous system malformations is decreased relative to myelomeningocele.

Spina bifida occulta is a defect of the vertebral canal without herniation of meninges or spinal cord. The patient is asymptomatic and the diagnosis is generally made serendipitously. The presence of a dimple, hairy tuft, or birthmark on the lumbosacral spinal area should warrant suspicion. Infants and young children may present with recurrent urinary tract infections and/or meningitis.

SEIZURE DISORDERS

Seizure disorders are the most common neurologic diseases of childhood, affecting approximately 5% of all children prior to adolescence. The general pediatric practitioner encounters seizure disorders frequently, and should become familiar with the classifications, manifestations, etiologies, evaluation, prognosis, and treatment of these disorders.

A *seizure* is the result of excessive electrical discharge of cortical neurons, resulting in a disruption or alteration of brain function. *Epilepsy* is defined as two or more unprovoked seizures. The classification of seizures is determined by the origin of the electrical discharges and pattern of spread. A *partial seizure* occurs when the electrical discharges originate in a localized area of the brain. A *primary generalized* seizure occurs when the underlying electrical disorder originates in both hemispheres of the brain simultaneously. Additionally, seizures that are not associated with altered mental status are termed *simple* seizures; those associated with changes in mental status are termed *complex* seizures. Common etiologies of seizures include trauma, infection (i.e., meningitis, encephalitis), toxins (i.e., lead), arteriovenous malformations, hypoxia, and electrolyte disturbances (i.e., glucose, sodium). Frequent clinical manifestations of seizures include behavioral changes, loss of consciousness, visual disturbances, autonomic dysfunction, and motor dysfunction. These clinical manifestations may be representative of the specific region of the underlying electrical disturbance. For example, a seizure involving a localized region of the occipital lobe may be manifested as a visual disorder.

FEBRILE SEIZURES

Febrile seizures are the most frequently encountered seizures in children, affecting 2% to 5% of children under 5 years of age. They occur in children between 5 months and 5 years of age who have no associated neurologic disease (e.g., meningitis, encephalitis). A younger age at the time of the first febrile seizure is associated with a greater risk of recurrent febrile seizures. Common causes of febrile seizures include viral syndromes, otitis media, and roseola.

TABLE 9-5.   *SEIZURES*

TABLE 9-5   *SEIZURES*

SEIZURE TYPE	ETIOLOGY/DEMOGRAPHICS	CLINICAL	DIAGNOSIS	TREATMENT
Febrile seizures				
Simple febrile seizure	• Children with simple febrile seizures have an only slightly increased chance of developing epilepsy when compared to the rest of the population (2% vs. 1%)	• Age 5 mo to 5 y • Normal development • Generalized seizure • <15 min in duration • One seizure in 24 h	• The first simple febrile seizure in a child aged <12 mo should be evaluated with (strongly consider): • Lumbar puncture • Other diagnostic studies (CBC, electrolytes should be tailored to signs/symptoms of current illness) • EEG is not routinely recommended	• Antiepileptic medications are not routinely recommended for the first episode of a simple febrile seizure • Antipyretics and cold compresses are *not* useful in preventing a recurrent febrile seizure
Complex febrile seizure	• Up to a 10% chance of developing epilepsy when compared to the rest of the population	• Age 5 mo to 5 y • Normal development • Generalized or focal seizure • >15 min in duration • Two or more within 24 h	• Neurologic imaging is not routinely recommended • Children aged >12 mo should be evaluated with a lumbar puncture depending upon presenting signs/symptoms on a case-by-case basis • The evaluation of a complex febrile or second simple febrile seizure may require an EEG or neurologic imaging on a case-by-case basis	• For any recurrent febrile seizure, rectal diazepam may be given at the onset of a seizure • For any recurrent febrile seizure, phenobarbital may play a role

Partial seizures: The underlying electrical discharges originate in a localized area of the brain.

Simple partial seizure	• The most common cause of nonfebrile seizures in children • Can occur at any age	• Tonic and/or clonic movements • Auras uncommon • No loss of consciousness	• EEG is routinely performed • Video EEG is useful in cases where seizures are suspected but interictal EEGs are normal	• Antiepileptic medications are not routinely indicated following a single episode of an uncomplicated simple partial seizure or complex partial seizure
Complex partial seizure	• Can occur at any age	• Episodes may last 30 sec or more • Auras are common • Loss of consciousness • Tonic and/or clonic movements	• Magnetic resonance imaging may be indicated to rule out structural lesions • Severe, refractory epilepsy usually requires a focal cortical surgical resection targeted to the focus of electrical disturbance; this procedure has relatively good results in most centers	• Options for recurrent partial seizures include: - Phenobarbital - Phenytoin - Carbamazepine - Gabapentin - Oxcarbazepine - Levetiracetam - Zonisamide - Valproate

Generalized seizures: The underlying electrical discharges originate in both hemispheres of the brain simultaneously.

Absence seizure	• Onset around age 5-6 y	• Episodes last only a few seconds: - Staring - Eye blinking - Lip smacking • Many occur many times/day • Poor school performance is frequent	• EEG is routinely performed; a 3/sec generalized spike and wave pattern is pathognomonic of absence seizures • Video-assisted electroencephalography is useful in cases where seizures are suspected but interictal EEGs are normal • Magnetic resonance imaging is not routinely required	• Ethosuximide • Can be induced by hyperventilation

(Continued)

TABLE 9-5 SEIZURES (CONTINUED)

SEIZURE TYPE	ETIOLOGY/DEMOGRAPHICS	CLINICAL	DIAGNOSIS	TREATMENT
Myoclonic seizure	• Can occur at any age	• Brief, repetitive, synchronous muscle contractions • Auras uncommon • No loss of consciousness	• Clinical	• Valproate
Generalized tonic-clonic seizure	• Can occur at any age	• Repetitive, synchronous muscle contractions • Auras common • Loss of consciousness • Todd paralysis (postictal refractory period) is frequent	• Clinical • EEG	• Phenobarbital • Phenytoin • Lamotrigine • Gabapentin • Zonisamide • Valproate

CBC, complete blood count; EEG, electroencephalogram.

SELECTED EPILEPSY SYNDROMES

These syndromes include infantile spasms, Lennox-Gastaut syndrome, Landau-Kleffner syndrome, benign focal epilepsy of childhood, juvenile myoclonic epilepsy, and Rasmussen syndrome. Each disorder has a distinct constellation of symptoms, with seizures as the predominant one.

TABLE 9-6. *EPILEPSY SYNDROMES*

MUSCULAR DYSTROPHIES

Muscular dystrophies are a group of disorders characterized by the progressive degeneration of skeletal muscle function. These disorders are generally classified by the severity of muscle weakness and by pattern of inheritance. The overall incidence of muscular dystrophy is variable. The most common forms of muscular dystrophy are the Duchenne and Becker type.

TABLE 9-7. *MUSCULAR DYSTROPHIES*

NEUROMUSCULAR DISORDERS

Neuromuscular disorders are a group of disorders that affect the structure and function of the neuromuscular system. These conditions have similar clinical manifestations and require prompt diagnosis and treatment to prevent associated morbidity and mortality. The most frequently encountered disorders are summarized in Table 9-8.

TABLE 9-8. *NEUROMUSCULAR DISORDERS*

TABLE 9-6   EPILEPSY SYNDROMES

SYNDROME	ETIOLOGY/ DEMOGRAPHICS	CLINICAL	DIAGNOSIS	TREATMENT

Infantile spasms (West syndrome)	• Onset usually age 6 mo to 1 y
	• Characteristic seizure type associated with a variety of structural, metabolic or bio-chemical abnormalities of the central nervous system, including:
	  - Hypoxic ischemic encephalopathy
	  - Tuberous sclerosis
	  - Metabolic disorders
	• Many cases are cryptogenic
		• Convulsive episodes consist-ing of flexion of the head and trunk with sudden jerking of upper and lower extremities (Salaam movements)
		• May occur in clusters
		• Developmental delay occurs in most children with this type of seizure
			• EEG reveals classic abnor-mality: "hypsarrhythmia"	• ACTH
				• Prednisone
				• Vigabatrin
				• Up to 50% may resolve by age 2 y
				• Prognosis depends upon underlying disorder

Lennox-Gastaut syndrome (epileptic encephalopathy)	• Onset usually before age 3-4 y
	• Associated with:
	  - Perinatal asphyxia
	  - Traumatic brain injury
	  - Intraventricular hemorrhage
	• Many cases are idiopathic
		• Individual patients will have a variety of seizures, including generalized tonic-clonic, partial, atypical absence, and atonic
		• Status epilepticus is common
		• Developmental delay common
			• EEG reveals generalized, synchronous, sharp and slow wave complexes occurring at a rate of 2/sec	• Seizures are usually difficult to manage with AEDs
				• Poor prognosis

Landau-Kleffner syndrome (acquired epileptic aphasia)	• Epileptic discharges in the temporal lobes result in the selected loss of language skills • Onset usually before the age of 5 y • Affects boys more than girls	• Regression of previously acquired speech • Generalized seizures • Autistic behavior	• Clinical diagnosis • EEG reveals temporal lobe discharges that may only be present during sleep	• Speech therapy • Corticosteroids • AEDs may be helpful

	Etiology	Clinical Features	Diagnosis	Treatment/Prognosis
Benign focal epilepsy of childhood (Rolandic epilepsy)	• Idiopathic in most cases • Onset usually between ages 4 and 13 y	• Partial or generalized seizures	• EEG reveals spikes and sharp waves in the central and midtemporal regions	• AEDs include carbamazepine and gabapentin • Good prognosis with spontaneous resolution during adolescence
Juvenile myoclonic epilepsy (Janz syndrome)	• Idiopathic in most cases • Genetic predisposition • Onset usually between ages 12 and 16 y	• Myoclonic jerks in the morning shortly after awakening • Often described as "throwing objects across the room" • May develop generalized tonic-clonic seizure if left untreated	• EEG: 4-6 sec irregular spike and wave pattern • Enhanced by photostimulation	• Lifelong valproate results in dramatic improvement
Rasmussen syndrome (epilepsia partialis continua)	• Idiopathic in most cases • Postinfectious etiology suspected • Onset usually before age 10 y	• Partial and generalized seizures which progress in intensity over time • Developmental delay	• Clinical diagnosis	• Hemispherectomy • AEDs are of limited use • Poor prognosis

ACTH, adrenocorticotropic hormone; AEDs, antiepileptic drugs; EEG, electroencephalogram.

TABLE 9-7   *MUSCULAR DYSTROPHIES*

TYPE	ETIOLOGY/ DEMOGRAPHICS	CLINICAL	DIAGNOSIS	TREATMENT/NOTES
Duchenne muscular dystrophy (DMD)	• X-linked recessive inheritance • Defective DMD gene leads to absent dystrophin protein • Progressive onset, age at presentation is 4-5 y	• Progressive muscle weakness, initially presents with proximal weakness • Delayed, clumsy walking • Waddling gait • Inability to jump or climb stairs • Gower maneuver when pulling to a stand • Prominent calf muscles (pseudohypertrophy) • Scoliosis • Progressive disease with eventual loss of ambulation, restrictive lung disease, and cardiomyopathy	• Clinical diagnosis • DNA testing for DMD gene mutation is available • Increased serum CPK • EMG may be helpful • Muscle biopsy with special staining for dystrophin is negative (no dystrophin present)	• Supportive care • Corticosteroids may help transiently early in the disease • Patients are wheelchair-bound by adolescence • Poor prognosis, with eventual dependence on medical technology (ventilator, tracheostomy)
Becker muscular dystrophy	• Dystrophin protein is defective, rather than absent	• A milder clinical form of DMD	• Clinical diagnosis • Muscle biopsy • Exclude DMD	• Supportive care • Patients are wheelchair-bound by early adulthood • Although a milder course, prognosis remains poor

Myotonic dystrophy	• Autosomal dominant inheritance • Affects 1/8000 persons • Onset is usually in adolescence • Expansion of the trinucleotide repeat in the myotonic dystrophy gene results in an abnormal protein kinase	• Slow onset with progression of both striated and smooth muscle weakness and wasting • Myotonia: slow muscle relaxation after contraction (i.e., after handshake) • Distal muscle weakness • Cardiomyopathy • Cataracts • Club feet • Hypogonadism	• Clinical diagnosis • Genetic testing is available • Muscle biopsy • EMG helpful in adults	• Supportive care • Variable prognosis • May present as a floppy newborn infant (congenital myotonic dystrophy)
Fascioscapulohumeral muscular dystrophy	• Autosomal dominant inheritance • Onset is usually in adolescence	• Slow onset of facial weakness is the hallmark of this disease • Progression to variable proximal muscle weakness (shoulders, scapula)	• Clinical diagnosis • Genetic testing is available	• Supportive • Variable prognosis

CPK, creatine phosphokinase; EMG, electromyogram.

TABLE 9-8   NEUROMUSCULAR DISORDERS

DISORDER	ETIOLOGY/ DEMOGRAPHICS	CLINICAL	DIAGNOSIS	TREATMENT/NOTES
Spinal muscular atrophy (SMA) type I (Werdnig-Hoffman disease)	• Autosomal dominant inheritance • Degeneration of anterior horn cells	• Hypotonia (newborn floppy infant) • Head lag • Progressive muscle weakness • Hip dislocations • Tongue fasciculations • Normal intelligence • Gradual progression to restrictive lung disease, respiratory failure	• EMG • Muscle biopsy	• Supportive • There are 3 types of SMA (I-III): type I is the most severe with survival unlikely beyond age 2 y; types II and III are more benign forms with more gradual onset, severity, and prognosis • Most patients with SMA progress to respiratory failure and ventilator dependence
Myasthenia gravis	• IgG antibodies bind to and damage postsynaptic AChR • Disorder of neuromuscular conduction	• Weakness of eye and facial muscles, especially at end of day, when fatigue is more common • Ptosis/diplopia • Proximal muscle weakness • May present in school-age children who appear as if they cannot keep their eyes open	• Weakness will transiently improve with a dose of edrophonium (pathognomonic) • Circulating titers of IgG can be measured against AChR • EMG will show electrodecrements on repetitive nerve stimulation (the signal gets weaker as the nerve is stimulated)	• Supportive • Neostigmine and atropine can be used to increase muscle strength • Some patients have disease confined to eye and facial muscles • High incidence of thymomas
Transient neonatal myasthenia gravis	• IgG antibodies bind to and damage postsynaptic acetylcholine receptors • Disorder of neuromuscular conduction • Affects only newborn infants	• Signs develop shortly after birth • Hypotonia • Poor cry • Feeding difficulty	• Maternal history of myasthenia gravis • Edrophonium test	• Supportive • Neostigmine and atropine can be used to increase muscle strength • Self-limited course lasting 1-2 wk

	Etiology/Pathophysiology	Clinical Manifestations	Diagnosis	Treatment
Guillain-Barré syndrome (GBS)	• Idiopathic, however there is a high incidence with preceding *Campylobacter*, Epstein-Barr virus, mycoplasma, and coxsackievirus infections	• Ascending, symmetrical paralysis begins in the lower extremities • Paresthesias • Diminished or *absent reflexes* • May progress to respiratory weakness and possible failure	• CSF analysis reveals elevated total protein • Cytoalbuminologic disassociation in CSF: elevated protein level without pleocytosis • EMG testing reveals slowed nerve conduction manifested by an F-wave latency (returning signal from the nerve takes longer than the originating signal)	• Monitor baseline muscle strength and peak flow volumes • Intubation and mechanical ventilation may be necessary in severe cases to protect and maintain respiratory function • IVIG • Plasmapheresis for severe cases • Spontaneous resolution after 1-2 wk • Miller-Fisher variant of GBS involves cranial nerves: clinically presents with ophthalmoplegia, areflexia, ataxia
Infantile botulism	• Inhibits release of acetylcholine at somatic and autonomic synapses • Infantile form is associated with a history of honey or corn syrup ingestion (contains *C. botulinum* spores) • Children and adults generally develop symptoms after ingestion of preformed toxin	• Constipation • Bulbar palsies (suck, cry, feeding) • Ptosis, diplopia • Diminished or absent reflexes • Weakness, hypotonia • Poor feeding • Respiratory compromise	• Clinical diagnosis • EMG may be helpful • Isolation of *C. botulinum* or toxin in the stool	• Supportive • Human-derived botulism immune globulin • Avoid aminoglycosides as they may further potentiate the neuromuscular blockade

AChR, acetylcholine receptors; CSF, cerebrospinal fluid; EMG, electromyogram; IgG, immunoglobulin G; IVIG, intravenous immunoglobulin.

CENTRAL NERVOUS SYSTEM TUMORS

Central nervous system malignancies currently account for approximately 20% of all childhood cancers. Most brain tumors are primary lesions, occur in children 3 to 15 years of age, and are located in the posterior fossa. Brain tumors are classified by histology and anatomic location.

Presenting signs and symptoms are variable, depending upon the age at presentation and location of the tumor. Ataxia, loss of school performance, and behavioral changes are common with any type of brain tumor. Tumors in the posterior fossa usually manifest with signs and symptoms of increased intracranial pressure and obstructive hydrocephalus. CT and MRI aid the diagnosis of a suspected brain tumor. Treatment options include surgical resection, chemotherapy, and radiation therapy.

TABLE 9-9.   *INFRATENTORIAL TUMORS*

TABLE 9-10.   *SUPRATENTORIAL TUMORS*

`TABLE 9-9` *INFRATENTORIAL TUMORS*	
LESION	**CHARACTERISTICS**
Cerebellar astrocytoma (juvenile pilocytic astrocytoma)	• 15% of all pediatric brain tumors • Peak incidence in second decade of life • Usually invades the fourth ventricle and causes obstructive hydrocephalus • Presents with headache, vomiting, and ataxia • Excellent prognosis (>90% 5-y survival)
Brainstem glioma	• 10%-20% of all pediatric brain tumors • Peak incidence age 5-8 y • Destruction of cranial nerve nuclei • Diplopia, dysarthria, and dysphagia are common • Poor prognosis (20% 5-y survival)
Medulloblastoma/primitive neuroectodermal tumor (PNET)	• 15%-20% of all pediatric brain tumors • Tumor usually originates in the cerebellum • Both dissemination and tumor recurrence are common
Ependymoma	• Variable prognosis (50%-70% 5-y survival) • 5%-7% of all pediatric brain tumors • Peak incidence school age and adolescence • Lesions arise and invade the fourth ventricle with obstructive hydrocephalus • Variable prognosis (50% 5-y survival)

TABLE 9-10	SUPRATENTORIAL TUMORS
LESION	**CHARACTERISTICS**
Astrocytoma	• Small percentage of all pediatric brain tumors • Low-grade cerebral astrocytoma: low rate of metastatic disease, favorable prognosis • High-grade cerebral astrocytoma (anaplastic, glioblastoma multiforme): high rate of metastatic disease, poor prognosis
Germ cell tumors	• Small percentage of all pediatric brain tumors • Usually originate in the pineal or suprasellar region • Frequently spreads to the spinal cord • Associated with elevated levels of alpha-fetoprotein and human chorionic gonadotropin
Craniopharyngioma	• 5%-15% of all pediatric brain tumors • Benign tumors arising from remnants of Rathke pouch, located near the optic chiasm and anterior pituitary • Growth delay and diabetes insipidus are also common due to the location of the tumor (panhypopituitary function) • Surgical resection yields an excellent prognosis (>90% 5-y survival)

HEADACHE

Headaches are one of the most common complaints of children and account for a large number of pediatric office visits. There are three general categories of headaches: migraine, tension-type, and organic. A complete history is the single most valuable part of the assessment of a child who has headaches, and should include questions about aura, frequency, location, quality, duration, time of day, associated symptoms, precipitating or aggravating factors, other medical problems, and effect of analgesics on relieving the pain. Associated neurologic symptoms, such as visual and auditory disturbances, ataxia, focal weakness, seizures, personality changes, and deterioration in school performance, should raise suspicion of an organic etiology. Radiographic evaluation is generally not indicated unless an organic etiology is suspected (i.e., the patient does not respond to treatment as expected).

The precise cause of migraine is unknown. Serotonin transmission, vascular dysregulation, and intrinsic brain dysfunction have all been put forth as possible causes. Migraines are episodic in duration, frequency, and intensity. There is a genetic predisposition. Migraine headaches are commonly triggered by stress, anxiety, sleep disorders, menstruation, alcohol, chocolate, and cheese. There are four main types: migraine preceded by aura (classic migraine), migraine without aura (common migraine), complicated migraine (neurologic deficit persists during or after the headache), and migraine variants (benign positional vertigo, cyclic vomiting). Most migraines in children occur without aura. The characteristic symptoms include unilateral throbbing pain of moderate to severe intensity, which worsens with activity. Associated symptoms include nausea, vomiting, and photophobia. Patients may state that sleeping in a quiet, dark room relieves symptoms. Auras present prior to headache and consist of visual disturbances, parasthesias, vertigo, amnesia, confusion, and/or loss of consciousness.

The treatment of migraine headaches in children begins with avoidance of precipitating factors and foods. Children with common migraine headaches usually benefit from analgesics such as acetaminophen and nonsteroidal anti-inflammatories. In moderate to severe cases, more potent medications such as ergotamine preparations or serotonin agonists (i.e., sumatriptan) may be necessary. Narcotics are not usually indicated. Children who have severe, recurrent, debilitating headaches may benefit from prophylactic treatment with beta blockers, tricyclic antidepressants, or calcium-channel blockers.

Tension-type headaches are caused by muscular contraction. Patients usually describe a pressing, dull, band of tightness around the head. Headaches may be episodic or chronic in duration and frequency. Stress or psychosocial factors may play a precipitating role. Similar to migraine headache, the treatment of tension-type headache includes avoidance of precipitating factors and use of nonsteroidal anti-inflammatories. Biofeedback and relaxation therapies may also be useful.

Organic headaches result from structural, metabolic, or inflammatory disease processes. They are characterized by increasing severity, frequency, and duration over time. The classic example is the headache caused by a brain tumor, classically described as worse in the morning and relieved by vomiting. Medications have little effect on relieving the symptoms of organic headaches. Common benign organic etiologies include fever, upper respiratory tract infections, viral syndromes, influenza, sinusitis, and otitis media. A chronic pattern of a headache that is worse in the morning, increases in severity, and is minimally relieved by analgesic medications warrants further evaluation for an organic etiology.

CHAPTER 10

ALLERGY AND IMMUNOLOGY

IMMUNOLOGY

Role of the Immune System

The basic function of the immune system is to recognize and defend the host (self) from foreign substances or organisms (nonself). An *antigen* is a molecule that reacts with an antibody. Examples of antigens include bacterial cell wall proteins and penicillin. Normally, "self" molecules do not elicit an immune response. Malfunction of the immune system can result in a variety of disorders ranging from immunodeficiency to anaphylaxis.

Organization of the Immune System

The immune system can be divided into two basic categories, innate and adaptive.

The *innate* immune response is nonspecific, and often the first line of defense against an offending agent. Examples of the innate immune system include primary barriers to infection (hair, skin, cilia, gastric acid) as well as the primary cellular line of defense (neutrophils, macrophages, eosinophils, and mast cells.)

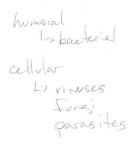

The *adaptive* immune response is specific in that it recognizes a particular antigen, produces a precise reaction, and then retains memory of the antigen for future interactions. Adaptive immunity is further divided into B-cell (*humoral*) and T-cell (*cellular*) components. Humoral immunity generally defends against bacterial infection, while cellular immunity defends against viruses, fungi, and parasites.

Immune-deficient children may require alteration of the standard vaccine schedule, as they often cannot receive live vaccines (i.e., varicella). The decision to defer vaccination depends on the child's specific disease, and is made on a case-by-case basis.

Immunoglobulins

Immunoglobulins (Ig) are secreted by B cells, usually in response to specific antigens. There are five types. IgG is the most prevalent immunoglobulin found in the serum, followed (in order) by IgA, IgM, IgD, and IgE.

| TABLE 10-1. | *IMMUNOGLOBULINS* |
| TABLE 10-2. | *SIGNS AND SYMPTOMS OF IMMUNE DEFICIENCY* |

183

TABLE 10-1   *IMMUNOGLOBULINS*

	BASIC STRUCTURE	CHARACTERISTICS	NOTES
IgG	• Monomer • 4 subclasses	• The most prevalent immunoglobulin • Enhances phagocytosis • Activates complement • Serum half-life = 30 d	• Accounts for 20% of total serum protein • Increased levels indicate late primary or current reactivated disease • Crosses the placenta
IgA	• Dimer • 2 subunits held together by a "j" chain	• Found in most secretions and body fluids (breast milk, saliva, mucus) • Most prevalent in epithelial cells	• Produced by the fetus • Does not cross the placenta
IgM	• Pentamer • 5 subunits held together by a "j" chain	• First response to a primary infection • Found in serum, mucosal surfaces, and breast milk • Serum half-life = 5 d	• Increased levels indicate current or recent primary infection, can also be seen in reactivation of some diseases • Does not cross the placenta
IgD	• Monomer	• Membrane-bound receptor on B cells	• Minimal clinical significance
IgE	• Monomer	• The least prevalent immunoglobulin • Involved with allergic and hypersensitivity reactions	• Produced by the fetus • Does not cross the placenta

(handwritten annotations: $t_{1/2} = 30d$; $t_{1/2} = 5d$)

TABLE 10-2   *SIGNS AND SYMPTOMS OF IMMUNE DEFICIENCY*

(handwritten note in left margin: produced by fetus / IgA / IgE / crosses placenta / IgG)

Fever (persistent)

Recurrent abscesses

Chronic diarrhea

Dermatitis

Chronic atelectasis

Recurrent/unusually severe presentations of common illnesses (i.e., pneumonia, sinusitis, meningitis), or isolation of unusual organisms

Infection with opportunistic pathogen

Failure to thrive

Malnutrition

Short stature

CGD
Chediak-Higashi
congenital leukocyte adhesion deficiency
Kostmann
Shwachman Diamond
myeloperoxidase deficiency
hyperimmune IgE syndrome (Job's)

IMMUNE DEFICIENCIES

Neutrophil Disorders

TABLE 10-3   *DISORDERS OF NEUTROPHIL FUNCTION*

CONDITION	ETIOLOGY	PRESENTATION	NOTES
Chronic granulomatous disease	• X-linked (majority) • Defect in phagocyte NADPH oxidase	• Infections with catalase + organisms (*S. aureus, E. coli, Serratia, Salmonella, Candida*) • Repeated skin infections • Fever • Lymphadenopathy	• NBT dye reaction • Oxidative burst testing • Prophylactic antibiotics (trimethoprim/ sulfamethoxazole)
Chediak-Higashi syndrome	• Autosomal recessive • Defect in neutrophil chemotaxis and degranulation	• Hepatosplenomegaly • Progressive neurodegenerative disease • Albinism • Neutropenia • Fever	• "Giant" granules are seen microscopically in neutrophils and eosinophils
Congenital leukocyte adhesion deficiency (LAD)	• Autosomal recessive • Defect in leukocyte migration and adhesion	• Leukocytosis • History of delayed umbilical cord separation • Recurrent serious bacterial infections • Gingivitis	• There is "normal" immune function • The "skin window test" evaluates the neutrophil ability to migrate and adhere to an area of inflammation • Look for adhesion markers on lymphocytes by flow cytometry
Kostmann syndrome	• Autosomal recessive • Impaired neutrophil maturation	• Monocytosis • Eosinophilia • Decreased absolute neutrophil count • Fever • Serious bacterial infections	• Treat with antibiotics, GCSF, and bone marrow transplantation

(Continued)

TABLE 10-3	DISORDERS OF NEUTROPHIL FUNCTION (CONTINUED)		
CONDITION	**ETIOLOGY**	**PRESENTATION**	**NOTES**
Shwachman-Diamond syndrome	• Autosomal recessive • Impaired neutrophil production	• Neutropenia • Pancreatic insufficiency • Recurrent infections • Malnutrition • Short stature	• Treat with antibiotics, GCSF, and bone marrow transplantation • Sweat testing is *normal*, in contrast to cystic fibrosis, which is high in the differential
Myeloperoxidase (MPO) deficiency	• Autosomal recessive • Complete absence of MPO from neutrophils • The most common disorder of neutrophils	• Mild bacterial infections • Mild fungal infections	• Absence of neutrophil MPO • Abnormal phagocyte function • NBT test may be abnormal, but oxidative burst will be normal
Hyperimmune E syndrome (Job syndrome)	• Autosomal dominant • Defect in neutrophil chemotaxis	• Increased IgE • Eczema • Noninflamed abscesses • Recurrent infections • Osteopenia	• Phagocyte function is normal

GCSF, granulocyte colony-stimulating factor; NADPH, nicotinamide-adenine dinucleotide phosphate; NBT, nitroblue tetrazolium dye test.

B-Cell Disorders

B cells develop in the bone marrow and differentiate into plasma cells that ultimately secrete immunoglobulins. B-cell disorders include problems in quantity (decreased numbers) and in function (normal amounts, but poor immunoglobulin production/function). B-cell deficiencies often manifest as opportunistic and serious bacterial infections. B-cell function can be tested by checking titers to organisms that the patient has been immunized against (i.e., tetanus or diphtheria).

TABLE 10-4.   B-CELL DISORDERS

T-Cell Disorders

T cells develop and mature in the thymus. T-cell deficiencies manifest with severe or recurrent viral, fungal, mycobacterial, and protozoal diseases.

TABLE 10-5.   T-CELL DISORDERS AND COMBINED LYMPHOCYTE IMMUNO-DEFICIENCY

TABLE 10-4	*B-CELL DISORDERS*		
CONDITION	**ETIOLOGY**	**PRESENTATION**	**NOTES**
X-linked agammaglobinemia (Bruton disease)	• X-linked • Abnormal B-cell maturation	• Absent B cells in serum • Low IgA, IgM, IgG, IgE • Recurrent pyogenic infections: empyema, osteomyelitis, meningitis • Paucity of lymphoid tissue (i.e., tonsils)	• Treat with antibiotics and monthly IVIG
Common variable hypogammaglobulinemia	• Deficient immunoglobulin production • Normal B-cell *quantity*	• Decreased IgA, IgG, IgM (variable levels) • Recurrent pyogenic infections: pneumonia, sinusitis • Diarrhea • Presents in adolescence/early adulthood • Hypertrophic lymphoid tissue	• *Giardia* infections common • Increased risk of autoimmune disease • Treat with antibiotics and monthly IVIG • Supportive care
Transient hypogammaglobinemia of infancy	• Delayed immunoglobulin production	• Normal quantity of B and T cells • Normal immune response to vaccines • Presents at age ≥6 mo • Recurrent pneumonia, otitis media • Mild disease	• IVIG in severe cases • Often resolves by age 3 y, but can persist up to age 7-8 y
Selective IgA deficiency	• The most common immunodeficiency • Decreased production of IgA	• Infections of the respiratory, gastrointestinal, and urogenital tracts	• Increased risk of autoimmune disease and malignancies • Possible fatal anaphylactic reactions when administered blood products containing IgA

IVIG, intravenous immunoglobulin.

TABLE 10-5   *T-CELL DISORDERS AND COMBINED LYMPHOCYTE IMMUNODEFICIENCY*

CONDITION	ETIOLOGY	PRESENTATION	NOTES
DiGeorge syndrome	• Abnormal development of the 3rd and 4th pharyngeal pouch, with resultant thymic aplasia • T-cell *deficiency* • Genetic defect on chromosome 22	• "CATCH 22" - **C**ongenital heart disease (aortic arch disease) - **A**bnormal ears - **T**hymus aplasia - **C**left palate - **H**ypocalcemia • *Candida* and *Pneumocystis* infections • Profoundly decreased T cells	• T cell (enumeration and subsets) • Antibiotic prophylaxis (trimethoprim/ sulfamethoxazole)
Wiskott-Aldrich syndrome	• X-linked • Impaired humoral/cellular immunity • Defective T-cell *function*	• Eczema • Thrombocytopenia/small platelets • Recurrent infections • Eosinophilia • Increased IgE • Other Ig levels normal • Bleeding	• Increased risk of malignancy • Splenectomy is helpful • Treat with antibiotics and IVIG • Bone marrow transplantation is curative
Ataxia-telangiectasia	• Autosomal recessive • Impaired humoral/cellular immunity • Defective T-cell *function* • Defective chromosomal repair	• Decreased IgA • Cerebellar ataxia • Oculocutaneous telangiectasias • Recurrent infection	• Increased risk of malignancy • Antibiotic prophylaxis • Bone marrow transplantation is curative
Severe combined immunodeficiency (SCID)	• Autosomal recessive • X-linked • Deficient T- and B-cell production from a variety of causes	• Thymic hypoplasia • Decreased lymphocytes • Decreased lymphoid tissue • Presents in newborn period with chronic diarrhea, FTT, opportunistic infections	• Flow cytometry and T-cell studies are the best tests to order • Poor prognosis • Treatment with antibiotics, IVIG, and bone marrow transplant

TABLE 10-5	T-CELL DISORDERS AND COMBINED LYMPHOCYTE IMMUNODEFICIENCY (CONTINUED)		
CONDITION	**ETIOLOGY**	**PRESENTATION**	**NOTES**
Major histocompatability complex (MHC) I/II deficiency ("bare lymphocyte syndrome")	• Autosomal recessive • Abnormal development/function of CD4/CD8 T cells	• Decreased CD4 and/or CD8 cells • Lymphopenia • Opportunistic infection • Chronic diarrhea • FTT	• Flow cytometry and T-cell studies are the best tests to order • Antibiotic prophylaxis

FTT, failure to thrive; IVIG, intravenous immunoglobulin.

HIV Basics

Transmission of HIV can occur in the following manners:

* Sexual contact.
* Exposure to contaminated blood/infected body fluid (i.e., genital secretions, breast milk), either through mucous membrane or via percutaneous inoculation. The risk of contracting HIV from a blood transfusion is estimated to be more than 1 in 600,000.
* Vertical transmission from mother to infant.

NEONATAL EXPOSURE

Infants who are born to HIV-positive mothers should undergo testing for HIV via DNA polymerase chain reaction (PCR) at birth, at age 1 to 2 months, and again at age 3 to 6 months. If the results of all three tests are negative, the infant is considered to be HIV negative. Regardless of the initial test results, all infants of HIV-positive mothers should be treated with zidovudine (AZT) for the first 6 weeks of life. In addition, HIV-positive mothers should receive antiretroviral therapy during pregnancy, and intravenous AZT during labor/delivery.

DIAGNOSIS OF NON-PERINATAL HIV

* For children 18 months of age or younger:
    * HIV DNA PCR remains the test of choice. Other detection methods (i.e., antibody detection) have higher rates of false negatives in this age group.
* For children older than 18 months:
    * Initial screening test: HIV enzyme immunoassay, which detects antibody to HIV. May take up to 6 months to develop antibody after infection.
    * Positive screening tests are confirmed by Western blots, to rule out false positive results.

- Tests performed less frequently to diagnose HIV include: detection of p24 antigen, HIV culture, and HIV PCR.

CLASSIFICATION

The Centers for Disease Control (CDC) criteria are based upon clinical and laboratory parameters. The patient's viral load is not taken into account by these criteria.

TABLE 10-6.   *CDC CLASSIFICATION OF HIV*

The CD4 count and total percentage of lymphocytes constitute the immunologic criteria. The patient's age is also taken into account. The criterion for absolute numbers is slightly higher in infants less than 1 year, and slightly lower in children 6 years and older, but the criterion for percentage of total lymphocytes is the same for all age groups. Examples:

- An HIV-positive child who is 4 years old, with a CD4 count of 750 (20% of total lymphocytes), lymphadenopathy, and recurrent otitis, would be categorized as CDC stage A2.
- A child who is CDC stage C3 is generally considered to have AIDS.

TABLE 10-6   *CDC CLASSIFICATION OF HIV*

CLINICAL CATEGORY	EXAMPLE		
N	Asymptomatic, or no more than one mild symptom		
A (mildly symptomatic)	Lymphadenopathy, recurrent otitis		
B (moderately symptomatic)	Chronic diarrhea, single invasive bacterial infection		
C (severely symptomatic)	Opportunistic disease, recurrent invasive bacterial infections, wasting		
IMMUNOLOGIC CATEGORY	AGE <1 Y	AGE 1-5 Y	AGE 6-12 Y
	Absolute CD4+ count (% of total lymphocytes)	Absolute CD4+ count (% of total lymphocytes)	Absolute CD4+ count (% of total lymphocytes)
1	≥1500 (25)	≥1000 (25)	≥500 (25)
2	750-1499 (15-24)	500-999 (15-24)	200-499 (15-24)
3	<750 (<15)	<500 (<15)	<200 (<15)

Modified from: Centers for Disease Control. Revised classification system for human immunodeficiency virus infection in children less than 13 years of age. MMWR 1994(43):1-10.

ANTIRETROVIRAL THERAPY (ART)

Deciding when/if to start a child on therapy is made on a case-by-case basis. There are three main classes of HIV drugs used in children:

1. Nucleoside reverse transcriptase inhibitors (NRTIs)
2. Non- nucleoside reverse transcriptase inhibitors (NNRTIs)
3. Protease inhibitors (PIs)

Highly active antiretroviral therapy (HAART) consists of three or more antiretroviral drugs. Standard combinations include two NRTIs and either an NNRTI or a PI.

Viral load is followed via RNA PCR. Therapy is considered successful if, after 4 to 6 weeks, the viral load is reduced by at least 1 log/90% (e.g., from 10,000 to 1,000 copies/M).

TABLE 10-7	*SIGNS/SYMPTOMS OF HIV*

HIV can present with any of the previously listed signs of immunodeficiency (Table 10-2). Additionally, HIV itself may cause any of the following symptoms.

Nephropathy
Hepatitis
Oral candidiasis
Depression of any hematologic cell line
Hypergammaglobulinemia (may manifest as normal total serum protein, with low albumin)
Encephalopathy
Encephalitis
Developmental delay

HYPERSENSITIVITY REACTIONS

TABLE 10-8. *HYPERSENSITIVITY REACTIONS*

Allergic Disorders

The most common allergic disorders include eczema, asthma, and allergic rhinitis. They occur in 20% to 30% of the population, and are IgE mediated. There is a large genetic component to allergic disorders. If one parent has an atopic disorder, the risk of the child having an atopic disease is 30%. If both parents have a history of atopic disorders, the child has a 50% to 70% risk of atopic disease. Eosinophilia may be an associated finding of any atopic disease.

TABLE 10-8	HYPERSENSITIVITY REACTIONS		
TYPE	**ETIOLOGY**	**PRESENTATION**	**TREATMENT/NOTES**
Type I (anaphylaxis, IgE mediated)	• IgE mediated • Histamine, heparin, leukotrienes, mast cells • Can be caused by bee stings, peanuts, and medications	• Hay fever • Hives • Status asthmaticus • Shock • Laryngeal edema	• Airway, breathing, circulation (ABCs)!! • SQ epinephrine • Histamine antagonists • Corticosteroids
Type II (cytotoxic, immunoglobulin mediated)	• IgG, IgM mediated • Involves activation of complement • Cellular lysis • Transfusion reactions	• Hemolytic anemia • Shock • Immune thrombocytopenic purpura	• Airway, breathing, circulation (ABCs)!! • Corticosteroids
Type III (immune-complex mediated)	• IgG, IgM mediated • Formation of antigen/antibody complexes	• Acute glomerulonephritis • Serum sickness	• Corticosteroids
Type IV (delayed, T-cell mediated)	• T-lymphocyte mediated • Does not involve antibodies	• Poison ivy • Poison oak • Contact dermatitis • Graft-versus-host disease	• Tuberculosis skin testing is an example of delayed-type hypersensitivity • Corticosteroids

Allergy Testing

A variety of methods are used to evaluate a patient for allergies. Identification and avoidance of allergens is the most important component of the management of allergic disorders.

SKIN TESTING

Identifies allergen-specific IgE. Diluted allergen is introduced into the skin (either intradermally or percutaneously) and interacts with mast cell–bound IgE. Cross-linking of IgE antibodies causes histamine release, resulting in a wheal and flare reaction within 15 to 20 minutes of injection. This test is usually performed in children over 6 months of age; younger children have an increased rate of false negatives, and have limited body surface area for testing.

Antihistamines (including H_2 blockers) and tricyclic antidepressants can produce false negative results, and should be withheld for 48 to 72 hours prior to testing. Topical steroids used at the injection site can also suppress skin test results. Inhaled corticosteroids and short-term systemic corticosteroids do not have any effect on skin testing. Skin testing should not be performed directly on actively eczematous skin.

IN VITRO TESTING

Measures serum levels of allergy-specific IgE. Commonly used methods include radioallergosorbent test (RAST) and enzyme-linked immunosorbent assay (ELISA). These tests are generally not as sensitive as skin testing in defining clinically pertinent allergens, and are indicated for patients who are not candidates for skin testing. Examples include patients who suffer from severe skin disease, cannot discontinue medications that interfere with skin testing, or have experienced severe anaphylaxis (skin testing can, in rare cases, cause anaphylaxis).

PATCH TESTING

Used to identify patients with contact dermatitis (i.e., from latex or nickel). A suspected agent is applied to the skin with an occlusive dressing and the area is evaluated 72 to 96 hours after application. The test is positive when the agent interacts with sensitized Langerhans cells in the skin, with subsequent T-cell activation, resulting in erythema and induration of the involved area.

Common Allergic Disorders

ALLERGIC RHINITIS (AR)

This disease occurs when allergens encounter nasal mucosa, bind to IgE antibody, and cause degranulation of superficial mucosal mast cells and basophils. This results in increased vascular permeability, tissue edema, congestion, and eventually nasal obstruction. Frequent symptoms include rhinorrhea, sneezing, and nasal pruritus. *Perennial* AR involves constant exposure to the offending agent; common causes include roaches, dust mites, and animal dander. *Seasonal* AR usually occurs in late spring and early summer from grass, trees, and weed pollen. Flowers are not typical causes of AR. Nasal swabs often demonstrate eosinophils. Treatment consists of identification and avoidance of offending agents, and the administration of antihistamines and/or intranasal steroids.

ATOPIC DERMATITIS

This disease is best described as a chronic, relapsing inflammatory skin disorder affecting 3% to 5% of children under 5 years of age. It is most frequent in patients with a personal or family history of atopic disease. In infants, commonly involved areas include the face and extensor surfaces; in older children and adults, flexural surfaces are most often involved. Clinically, patients will have a pruritic rash that is erythematous, crusted, or scaly in nature. Chronic irritation results in lichenification (thickening) of skin, and pigmentation changes (either hyper- or hypopigmentation). Treatment consists of identification and avoidance of offending agents, emollients, steroids, and treatment of superinfections. Excoriation is frequent, and superinfection may occur. Eighty to ninety percent of cases resolve by puberty.

FOOD ALLERGY

This group of disorders results from an abnormal immunologic response. The most common food allergies are to milk, wheat, soy, eggs, peanuts, tree nuts, and fish. This disorder should be distinguished from food *intolerance*, which is nonimmunologic in nature (i.e., lactase deficiency resulting in milk intolerance). Symptoms are variable and involve several systems:

- **Dermatologic**: Eggs, milk, wheat, peanuts, and fish are the most common causes of food-related skin disease. Frequent manifestations include urticaria, angioedema, and atopic dermatitis.
- **Gastrointestinal**: Cow milk, soy-based products, eggs, and wheat are the most common causes of gastrointestinal immune-mediated disorders. Symptoms include nausea, vomiting, abdominal pain, diarrhea, steatorrhea, enterocolitis, malabsorption, and allergic eosinophilic gastroenteropathy.
- **Respiratory**: Upper and lower respiratory tract symptoms, including anaphylaxis, have been reported with a variety of foods. Peanuts, tree nuts, and fish are the most frequently implicated. Both systemic and gastrointestinal manifestations may be present.

The only definitive treatment is identification and avoidance of offending agents. Children who have a history of an anaphylactic reaction should be given an autoinjectable epinephrine kit.

LATEX ALLERGY

Up to 3% of the general population may have an allergy to latex. Patients with spina bifida (frequent urinary catheterizations), health care workers, and those with a history of multiple surgeries (especially urinary tract surgery) are especially at risk. Contact dermatitis, immediate hypersensitivity (anaphylaxis), and irritant dermatitis (from occluded skin under the impermeable latex) are all possible manifestations. Identification of the allergy and avoidance of latex are the best therapy.

HYMENOPTERA ALLERGY

Stings from honeybees, bumblebees, yellow jackets, hornets, wasps, and fire ants can cause local and/or systemic reactions. Up to 5% of the population is at risk of anaphylaxis from insect stings. Children experience systemic reactions more often than adults, but fatal reactions are more common in adults. Systemic reactions include generalized urticaria, angiodema, laryngeal edema, bronchospasm, and cardiovascular collapse. Cutaneous symptoms account for 80% of systemic manifestations. The most frequent cause of death is upper respiratory tract obstruction. Treatment varies by age. Patients older than 16 years who have *any* systemic reaction should undergo immunotherapy. Children younger than 16 years who have a non-cutaneous systemic reaction should undergo immunotherapy. Children younger than 16 years who have only cutaneous symptoms are *not* candidates for immunotherapy. Regardless of age, all patients should be given an autoinjectable epinephrine kit. Immunotherapy does not completely eliminate the risk of future reactions.

CHAPTER 11

INFECTIOUS DISEASE

COMMON INFECTIOUS DISEASES

TABLE 11-1   *EAR, NOSE, AND THROAT INFECTIONS*

DISEASE	ETIOLOGY	CLINICAL PRESENTATION	DIAGNOSIS
Acute otitis media (AOM)	• *S. pneumoniae* • *H. influenzae* (nontypeable) • *M. catarrhalis* • Less common: *Mycoplasma*, viral, *S. aureus*	• Inflammatory fluid in middle ear *and* clinical signs such as fever, ear pain, vomiting, hearing loss	• Clinical • Tympanometry • Tympanocentesis to guide treatment if diagnosis in doubt
Otitis media with effusion (OME)	May be postinfectious, or due to viral URI, allergies	• Clear fluid in middle ear, without other localizing or systemic signs of infection	• Clinical
Otitis externa ("swimmer's ear")	• *P. aeruginosa* • *S. aureus*	• Purulent discharge • Pain with manipulation of pinna	• Clinical • Foul-smelling discharge • Narrowing of the ear canal
Sinusitis	• Inflammatory fluid within sinus cavity, thickening/inflammation of sinus mucosa • Same organisms as AOM	• Acute (0-10 d): purulent nasal discharge, + fever >39°C, facial pain/swelling • Subacute (10-28 d)/chronic (>28 d): persistent purulent nasal discharge, cough	• Clinical • CT scan if diagnosis in doubt • Plain films not likely to be helpful

TREATMENT	COMPLICATIONS	COMMENTS

• 1st: amoxicillin
• 2nd: amoxicillin/clavulanate
• 2nd- or 3rd-generation cephalosporin
• Trimethoprim/ sulfamethoxazole or macrolide for penicillin allergy
	• Facial nerve palsy
	• Mastoiditis
	• Brain abscess
	• Meningitis
	• Chronic otitis media:
	  - Tympanosclerosis
	  - Cholesteatoma
	  - Hearing loss
		• Predisposing conditions:
		  - Day care
		  - Exposure to cigarette smoke
		  - Family history
		  - Supine bottle feeding
		  - Craniofacial abnormalities
		• Change antibiotics if no improvement after 48-72 h
		• IV antibiotics if CNS involvement (including Bell palsy)
		• Prophylaxis in recurrent/chronic AOM

• Audiologic evaluation • Can observe for up to 3 mo • If lasts >3 mo, and patient's hearing is normal, can treat with antibiotics and continue to observe • If patient has hearing loss, and/or fails antibiotics, refer for tympanostomy tubes	• Hearing loss	• OME often mistaken for AOM, resulting in overtreatment and overuse of antibiotics
• Topical antibiotics • Topical steroids • Preventative measures important	• Cholesteatoma	• Prevention: drying solutions (vinegar/rubbing alcohol) • Earplugs *not* recommended (may abrade ear canal) • Make sure discharge is not from perforated AOM
Same antibiotics as AOM	• Periorbital cellulitis • Orbital cellulitis • Brain abscess • Meningitis • Cranial osteomyelitis	• Utility of decongestants and antihistamines is controversial

TABLE 11-2   *CONJUNCTIVITIS*

DISEASE	ETIOLOGY	CLINICAL PRESENTATION	DIAGNOSIS
Conjunctivitis	• Bacterial: *S. aureus, S. pneumoniae, H. influenzae* (type b and nontypeable) • Neonatal: gonorrhea, *Chlamydia* • Viral: adenovirus, HSV, VZV • Chemical • Allergic	• Itching, burning, irritated conjunctiva • Exudate • Chemosis • Unilateral presentation more suggestive of bacterial disease, but not pathognomonic	• Bacterial: culture of discharge • *Chlamydia*: scraping of conjunctiva for culture of intracellular organisms
Periorbital (preseptal) cellulitis	• Inflammation of the soft tissue anterior to the orbital septum • *S. pneumoniae, H. influenzae, M. catarrhalis, S. aureus,* anaerobes	• Erythema and swelling of the periorbital soft tissue • No limitation of eye movement, proptosis, or visual changes	• Clinical • If uncertain of extent of disease, CT scan helpful to rule out orbital cellulitis (see below)
Orbital (postseptal) cellulitis	• Inflammatory infectious process involving the anatomical orbit • Same organisms as preseptal cellulitis	• High fever • Proptosis • Blurry vision • Limitation of eye movements	• Clinical • CT scan useful to assess extent of disease

HSV, herpes simplex virus; VZV, herpes zoster virus.

TREATMENT	COMPLICATIONS	COMMENT
• Bacterial: antibiotic drops • Gonorrhea: IM ceftriaxone • *Chlamydia*: oral erythromycin • HSV/VZV: IV acyclovir, topical anti-viral, ophthalmology consultation • Viral: supportive care • Chemical: supportive care	• Rare • HSV keratitis can result in corneal scarring and blindness	• Do not substitute antibiotic eardrops for use in the eye, as they contain steroids that may be harmful to the eye • Must treat chlamydial conjunctivitis with systemic therapy, as topical therapy will not treat nasal carriage that could possibly lead to pneumonia
• Beta-lactamase–resistant penicillin (i.e., IV ampicillin/sulbactam, or oral amoxicillin/clavulanate) • Clindamycin acceptable for penicillin-allergic patients	• Progression to orbital cellulitis • Brain abscess • Meningitis • Cranial osteomyelitis	• Often associated with a history of undiagnosed sinusitis
• Beta-lactamase–resistant penicillin (i.e., IV ampicillin/sulbactam) • Clindamycin • Surgical drainage if indicated	• Orbital abscess • Optic nerve compression • Cavernous sinus thrombosis • Brain abscess • Meningitis • Cranial osteomyelitis	

TABLE 11-3   *PHARYNGITIS*

DISEASE	ETIOLOGY	CLINICAL PRESENTATION	DIAGNOSIS
Streptococcal pharyngitis*	*S. pyogenes* (group A streptococcus)	• Sudden onset of fever, tender cervical nodes, enlarged tonsils, exudate	• Rapid streptococcal antigen detection test • Throat culture
Mononucleosis*	• Epstein-Barr virus • Cytomegalovirus	• Usually older patients • Pharyngitis accompanied by fever, fatigue, hepatosplenomegaly	• Heterophile antibody (may be negative early in disease) • Epstein-Barr virus serology
Gonorrhea	*N. gonorrhoeae*	• Usually asymptomatic	• Throat culture
Viral	• Adenovirus • Coxsackie A/B • Influenza • Herpes simplex	• Vesicles, ulcerative lesions	• Clinical
Mycoplasma	*Mycoplasma pneumoniae*	• Usually manifests as upper respiratory tract infection with sore throat, otitis media, acute bronchitis	• Serology • Throat culture may take up to 3 wk
Diphtheria	*Corynebacterium diphtheriae*	• Respiratory distress, stridor, gray membrane covering posterior pharynx, fever (usually seen in immigrant or adopted child with incomplete vaccine status)	• Biopsy of membrane, or culture of mucosa beneath membrane
Peritonsillar abscess	• *S. pyogenes* (most common) • *S. aureus*	• Unilateral tonsillar enlargement • Uvula deviation • Hoarseness • Cervical lymphadenopathy • Torticollis	• Clinical • Culture
Retropharyngeal abscess	*S. aureus* (most common)	• Fever • Hyperextended neck	• Widening of retropharyngeal space (more than half the width of the cervical vertebrae)

PCN, penicillin.

*Patients with infectious mononucleosis may have a concurrent group A streptococcus (GAS) infection. Both of these illnesses present very similarly (fever, lymphadenopathy, tonsillar enlargement, exudates, palatal petechiae); therefore, you

TREATMENT	COMPLICATIONS	COMMENTS
• Penicillin VK • Clindamycin if PCN-allergic	• Rheumatic fever if untreated • Peritonsillar abscess	• Presence/absence of exudate *not* sufficient for diagnosis
• Supportive care • Steroids if severely enlarged tonsils	• Airway compromise if severely enlarged tonsils	• If patient develops rash after receiving amoxicillin for GAS pharyngitis, consider EBV • If EBV serology is negative, consider CMV serology
• IM ceftriaxone ×1	• Pelvic inflammatory disease if coexisting genital disease	• Consider treatment for *Chlamydia* • Screen for other sexually transmitted diseases
• Supportive care	• Dehydration if unable to drink	
• Mild disease: supportive care • Severe disease/pneumonia: azithromycin		
• Antitoxin • Erythromycin • Vaccination	• Case fatality 3%-23% in epidemics	• Vaccinate contacts who are not up to date • Treat all close contacts, regardless of vaccine status • Only toxin-producing strains can cause disease
• Beta-lactamase–resistant PCN • Aspiration of tonsil • Steroids if airway impingement	• Airway compromise • Dehydration if unable to tolerate oral fluids	• If recurrent abscess on *same side*, tonsillectomy indicated • Patient usually school age or older
• Surgical drainage • Antistaphylococcal antibiotic: nafcillin; clindamycin in PCN-allergic patient	• Airway compromise	• Patient usually preschool age or younger

must differentiate the two via laboratory testing. A positive GAS culture does *not* rule out mononucleosis, especially if the patient has hepatosplenomegaly

TABLE 11-4   *PNEUMONIA*

AGE GROUP	ETIOLOGY	CLINICAL PRESENTATION	DIAGNOSIS
Neonatal	• Group B strep • *E. coli* • *S. aureus* • *Listeria*	• Fever, tachypnea, nasal flaring, cough, hypoxemia, cyanosis	• CXR • Blood culture • Consider lumbar puncture
	Chlamydia trachomatis • Peak: age 2-19 wk	• "Staccato cough," tachypnea, conjunctivitis • Usually afebrile	• CXR with diffuse interstitial disease • Conjunctival scraping • Tissue culture
Pediatric	*Bordetella pertussis* (whooping cough) • Peak: age 1-3 mo, nonimmunized	• Catarrhal phase: upper respiratory symptoms • Paroxysmal stage: cough (with inspiratory "whoop") • Convalescent stage: resolution of symptoms	• CXR with interstitial pneumonia • Definitive diagnosis: culture of nasopharyngeal swab • Antigen detection from nasopharyngeal swab • CBC may show lymphocytosis
	Mycoplasma pneumoniae (age ≥5 y)	• Malaise, fever, cough • Rash not uncommon • Usually school age or older	• CXR with interstitial pneumonia • Fourfold increase in *Mycoplasma* antibody • IgM may persist for months after infection; detection on single sample does not confirm diagnosis • Cold agglutinin titers are not specific
	• *S. pneumoniae* • *S. aureus* • *H. influenzae* (nontypeable) • *N. meningitidis*	• Fever, tachypnea, cough, respiratory distress, cyanosis • May present only as fever in younger children ("occult pneumonia")	• CXR with lobar pneumonia • CBC: lymphocytosis, bandemia, neutrophilia • Blood culture • Sputum culture if etiology uncertain
	Chlamydia psittaci	• Fever, nonproductive cough, headache, wheezing	• CXR: interstitial pneumonia (may be out of proportion to clinical syndrome) • Fourfold increase in antibody titer
Viral	• Respiratory syncytial virus	• Fever, rhinorrhea, respiratory distress, poor feeding, apnea	• CXR: interstitial or lobar pneumonia • Antigen detection in nasopharyngeal secretions

TREATMENT	COMPLICATIONS	COMMENTS
• Ampicillin + gentamicin/ 3rd-generation cephalosporin for 10-21 d	• Sepsis • Bacteremia	
• Oral erythromycin (topical treatment of conjunctivitis not necessary)	• Otitis media • Conjunctivitis in neonates usually *not* scarring	• Mother may *not* have history of *Chlamydia*; be sure to test (and treat) mother if necessary
• Erythromycin • Consider inpatient observation in infants, who are at risk for severe disease	• Post-tussive vomiting common • Apnea in infants • Seizures • Encephalopathy	• See Table 11-20 for pre-/postexposure prophylaxis
• Macrolide (i.e., azithromycin, clarithromycin)	• May be severe in children with sickle cell disease, immunodeficiency, heart disease, and trisomy 21	• "Walking pneumonia": CXR appears disproportionately severe to clinical syndrome • More common than *S. pneumoniae* in school-aged/older children
• 2nd-/3rd-generation cephalosporin • Vancomycin for suspected resistant *S. pneumoniae*	• Pleural effusions common with *S. pneumoniae* • Pneumatoceles common with *S. aureus*	• *S. pneumoniae* disease on the decline since initiation of routine heptavalent vaccination
• Age up to 8 y: erythromycin • Age ≥8 y: tetracycline	• Pericarditis • Encephalopathy • Hepatitis	• *C. psittaci* transmitted by bird feces (parakeets, parrots, pigeons, turkeys) • Person-to-person spread by respiratory secretions
• Supportive care • Steroids and beta agonists are controversial	• Possible link to increased risk of asthma later in life	• Spread by contact with infected secretions • More severe in premature infants, and children with chronic cardiopulmonary disease or immunodeficiency • Palivizumab (mouse monoclonal antibody) should be given prophylactically to at-risk children

(Continued)

TABLE 11-4   *PNEUMONIA (CONTINUED)*

AGE GROUP	ETIOLOGY	CLINICAL PRESENTATION	DIAGNOSIS
Viral	• Influenza	• Fever, tachypnea, cough, myalgias, gastrointestinal symptoms	• Antigen detection in nasopharyngeal secretions
	• Parainfluenza • Herpes simplex virus • Adenovirus • CMV	• Fever, tachypnea, cough, respiratory distress, cyanosis • Broad range in severity of illness	• CXR with interstitial or lobar disease • Sputum culture • Serology available for selected diseases (i.e., CMV)

CBC, complete blood count; CMV, cytomegalovirus; CXR, chest radiograph.

TABLE 11-5   *URINARY TRACT INFECTIONS*

Definitive therapy should be guided by sensitivity results. Generally, neonates and septic or vomiting children should receive parenteral therapy initially, and can be changed to oral therapy when stable.

First urinary tract infection warrants diagnostic investigation in all children aged <2 y.

AGE GROUP	ETIOLOGY	CLINICAL PRESENTATION
Neonatal (0-2 mo)	• Group B Strep • *E. coli* • *Klebsiella*	• Fever, hypothermia, jaundice, lethargy, poor feeding
(2 mo-2 y)	• *E. coli* • *Klebsiella sp.*	• Fever, abdominal pain, dysuria, vomiting, secondary enuresis
(>2 y)	• *Enterococcus* • *E. coli* • Enteric gram-negatives (i.e., *Klebsiella, Serratia, Pseudomonas*)	• Dysuria, fever, urgency, polyuria, secondary enuresis

TREATMENT	COMPLICATIONS	COMMENTS
• Supportive care • Antivirals (see Table 11-20)		• Spread by contact and respiratory routes • See Table 11-20 for pre-/postexposure prophylaxis
• Supportive care • Specific therapy available for selected viruses (i.e., herpes)		

A voiding cystourethrogram is more sensitive than ultrasound for diagnosis of reflux disease. Dimercaptosuccinic acid scan is useful to detect renal scars or acute pyelonephritis. WBC/HPF >50 on urinalysis, high fever, vomiting, or high WBC should raise suspicion for pyleonephritis.

DIAGNOSIS	TREATMENT	COMPLICATIONS	COMMENTS
• Catheterized urinalysis with WBCs, blood, leukocyte esterase, nitrite • Urine culture/sensitivity	• Ampicillin + aminoglycoside/ 3rd-generation cephalosporin pending sensitivities	• Pyelonephritis • Sepsis • Renal scarring	• Galactosemia raises suspicion for *E. coli* • Blood culture should be performed, as most neonatal UTIs are hematogenous in origin • Consider lumbar puncture
• Urine culture	• Empiric therapy: 2nd/3rd-generation cephalosporin	• As above	
• Urine culture	• Empiric therapy: 2nd-/ 3rd-generation cephalosporin	• As above	• Consider *Staphylococcus saprophyticus* in sexually active adolescents

TABLE 11-6   *MENINGITIS*

DISEASE	ETIOLOGY	CLINICAL PRESENTATION	DIAGNOSIS

Neonatal	Early onset (<7 d):
	• Early-onset GBS
	• Early-onset *Listeria*
	• *E. coli*
	
	Late onset (≥7 d):
	• Late-onset GBS
	• Late onset *Listeria*
	• *E. coli*
	• *S. pneumoniae*
	• *S. aureus*
	• Other gram positives: *Enterococci, S. epidermidis*
	• Other gram negatives: *Citrobacter, Enterobacter, H. influenzae* type b
		• Fever, hypothermia, apnea, cyanosis, jaundice, lethargy, vomiting, poor feeding
		• Meningismus uncommon in neonates
		• Risk increased with:
		  - PROM >18 hours
		  - Other perinatal infections
		  - Prematurity
		  - Galactosemia (gram-negative infections)
			• CSF culture
			• CSF WBC >25/μL
			• CSF protein >30 mg/dL
			• CSF glucose <30 mg/dL
			• Gram stain
			• Latex agglutination is neither sensitive nor specific enough to reliably diagnose or exclude disease; useful for screen in pretreated patient

Older children/ adolescents	• *N. meningitidis* • *S. pneumoniae* • *H. influenzae* type b • *Enterococcus*	• Headache, photophobia, meningismus, vomiting, fever, rash	• CSF culture • CSF WBC >5/μL • CSF protein elevated • CSF glucose <60% serum glucose • Gram stain • Latex agglutination is neither sensitive nor specific enough to reliably diagnose or exclude disease; useful for screen in pretreated patient

TREATMENT	COMPLICATIONS	COMMENTS
• Empiric treatment: ampicillin and gentamicin *or* ampicillin and cefotaxime • Consider vancomycin if infant in nursery with indwelling catheter • Treat for 21 d	• Gram-negative infections (especially *Citrobacter* and *Enterobacter*) carry an increased risk of brain abscess • Seizures • Subdural effusions • Brain abscess • Cerebral edema • SIADH/central DI • Long-term sequelae: hearing loss (most common), motor/visual deficits, hydrocephalus	• Always consider concurrent meningitis with any infection in neonates (i.e., cellulitis, omphalitis, urinary tract infection) • Repeat lumbar puncture for gram-negative infections to document clearance
• Empiric therapy: 3rd-generation cephalosporin and vancomycin • Length of treatment is dependent upon causative organism	• As above • *H. influenzae most likely* to cause hearing loss • S. *pneumoniae* will cause *most severe* hearing loss	• *S. pneumoniae* and *H. influenzae* much less common now because of routine childhood vaccination against these organisms

(Continued)

TABLE 11-6   *MENINGITIS (CONTINUED)*

DISEASE	ETIOLOGY	CLINICAL PRESENTATION	DIAGNOSIS
Tuberculosis (TB)	*Mycobacterium tuberculosis*	• Fever, headache, meningismus, vomiting, cranial nerve palsies, seizures	• Choroidal tubercles on CT scan • Tuberculin skin test • CSF culture • CSF acid fast stain • CSF WBC 50-300/µL (mostly lymphocytes) • CSF protein markedly elevated • CSF glucose normal to low
Herpetic	• HSV types 1 and 2	• Neonatal: fever, irritability, seizures • Older children: fever, altered mental status, personality changes, seizures, focal neurologic deficits	• EEG: temporal lobe PLEDs (periodic, lateralizing, epileptiform discharges) is highly suspicious for HSV disease • CSF WBC normal to elevated • CSF protein elevated • CSF glucose normal • Negative Gram stain • PCR of CSF for HSV
Aseptic	• Nonpolio enteroviruses (causes ~85% of *all* meningitis) • Arboviruses • See comment column, right	• Same as bacterial meningitis	• Negative CSF culture • CSF WBC elevated • CSF protein normal • CSF glucose normal • PCR for enterovirus is now available

BCG, bacillus Calmette-Guérin; CSF, cerebrospinal fluid; DI, diabetes insipidus; GBS, group B streptococcus; HSV, herpes simplex virus; PCR, polymerase chain reaction; PROM, premature rupture of membranes; SIADH, syndrome of inappropriate antidiuretic hormone.

TREATMENT	COMPLICATIONS	COMMENTS
• 2 mo isoniazid, rifampin, pyrazinamide, and streptomycin, followed by 7-10 mo of isoniazid and rifampin (9-12 mo total treatment) *and* • Corticosteroids	• Seizures • Concurrent anticonvulsants and antiseizure meds increase risk of hepatotoxicity	• BCG vaccine is used to decrease TB meningitis (*not* pulmonary TB)
• IV acyclovir for 21 d	• High mortality rate if not treated promptly • Survivors of neonatal disease usually have some neurologic sequelae	• In neonatal disease, only ~30% of mothers will have a positive history of herpes • CSF culture for HSV usually unrevealing • PCR as sensitive as brain biopsy for diagnosis
• Consider empiric treatment until bacterial culture negative • Supportive care	• Minimal	• Other causes for culture-negative meningitis include: tuberculosis; spirochete or fungal disease; partially treated meningitis; herpes meningitis; HIV; focal intracranial infections (i.e., brain or subdural abscess)

TABLE 11-7   *BACTEREMIA*

Just as bacteremia may cause seeding and a secondary localized infection, the converse is true: bacteremia may be a consequence of a localized infection, especially osteomyelitis, septic arthritis, meningitis, pneumonia, urinary tract infections, and enteritis.

AGE GROUP	ETIOLOGY	CLINICAL PRESENTATION	DIAGNOSIS

Neonatal (0-3 mo)	• *E. coli*
	• Group B strep
	• *L. monocytogenes*
	• Gram-negatives:
	  - *Klebsiella*
	  - *Enterobacter*
	  - *Proteus*
	  - *Citrobacter*
	  - *Salmonella*
	  - *Pseudomonas*
		• Fever, hypothermia, apnea, cyanosis, jaundice, lethargy, vomiting, poor feeding	• Blood culture
			• CBC with leukocytosis, neutrophilia, bandemia

Pediatric (3 mo-3 y, occult bacteremia)	• *S. pneumoniae* • *H. influenzae* • *E. coli* • *Salmonella*	• Fever with mild clinical symptoms • Irritability, lethargy, abdominal pain, anorexia	• Blood culture • CBC with leukocytosis, neutrophilia, bandemia
Pediatric/ adolescent (>3 y)	• *N. meningitidis*	• "Meningococcemia" • Sudden onset of high fevers, headache, meningismus, petechial rash • Progression to purpura, hypotension, and shock is common • Outbreaks reported in college dorms and military camps	• Blood culture • Lumbar puncture • Organisms may also be cultured from: skin lesions, pleural fluid, synovial fluid • Nasopharyngeal cultures *not* recommended • Gram stain: "gram-negative diplococci" • Latex agglutination of spinal fluid may be helpful in pretreated patients

TREATMENT	COMPLICATIONS	COMMENTS
Empiric treatment: • Ampicillin and an aminoglycoside *or* • Ampicillin and 3rd- generation cephalosporin	• Hematogenous seeding of organism to cause localized infection (meningitis, osteomyelitis, pneumonia)	• Secondary to increased awareness, and maternal screening, neonatal group B strep infections are on the decline
• Ceftriaxone *or* • 3rd-generation cephalosporin	• As above	• Patient with underlying immunodeficiency, hemoglobinopathies more susceptible to *Salmonella*
• Penicillin G • Ceftriaxone or a 3rd- generation cephalosporin • Do not defer treatment of suspected case while waiting for confirmation	• Children with isolated meningitis associated with *decreased* mortality rate • Waterhouse-Friderichsen syndrome: adrenal hemorrhage, disseminated intravascular coagulation, purpura, shock, and death	• Spread by respiratory droplets • One of the most common causes of bacteremia in children/adolescents • See Table 11-20 for pre-/postexposure prophylaxis

TABLE 11-8   *INFECTIOUS DIARRHEA*

DISEASE	ETIOLOGY	CLINICAL PRESENTATION	DIAGNOSIS
Salmonella, non-typhi	• *S. paratyphi* • *S. enteriditis* • *S. typhimurium*	• Diarrhea (may be bloody), cramps, abdominal pain, fever • More severe disease in infants aged <3 mo, and patients with immunodeficiency, hemoglobinopathies, colitis, and chronic gastrointestinal disease	• Stool culture
Typhoid fever	• *Salmonella typhi*	• Fever, abdominal pain, hepatomegaly, splenomegaly, rose spots on trunk, altered mental status, meningismus • Diarrhea (may be bloody) is more common in younger children; may also present with constipation, or neither • Relative bradycardia (lower heart rate than expected for degree of fever) may be present	• Stool and/or blood culture • Bone marrow/urine culture • Leukopenia/leukocytosis, proteinuria, transaminitis, disseminated intravascular coagulation • Serology (Widal reaction) not helpful: high false-positive and false-negative rates
Shigellosis	• *Shigella sonnei* • *Shigella flexneri*	• Sudden onset of fever, watery/bloody diarrhea, cramps, tenesmus • Seizures	• Stool culture • Bacteremia rare • WBC or RBCs in stool suggestive of gut invasion, but not specific to *Shigella*
Campylobacter	• *Campylobacter jejuni*	• Fever, headache, cramps, nausea, vomiting • Diarrhea may be bloody, watery, with pus or bile noted	• Stool culture • Dark field microscopy of stool (low specificity; can be confused with *Vibrio*)
Escherichia coli	• Enterohemorrhagic (O157:H7)	• Bloody diarrhea • Severe abdominal pain	• Stool culture • Serologic testing available to O157:H7 serotype
	• Enterotoxigenic	• Fever in <1/3 • Watery diarrhea • Abdominal cramps	
	• Enteroinvasive	• Bloody diarrhea	
	• Enteropathogenic	• Bloody diarrhea	

TREATMENT	COMPLICATIONS	COMMENTS
• Supportive • Consider treatment for patients considered at risk for severe disease • Bacteremia should always be treated • Treatment choices include ampicillin, amoxicillin, or ceftriaxone	• Bacteremia • Sepsis • Meningitis	• Commonly transmitted by fecal contamination of poultry, red meat, eggs, dairy, produce • Turtles, iguanas, other reptiles are also reservoirs • High rates of resistance, follow sensitivities • Screen family members if symptomatic, or if family member at high risk for disease
• Ampicillin, amoxicillin, or ceftriaxone • Contact precautions until 3 stool cultures after treatment are negative	• GI hemorrhage • GI perforation • Pneumonia • Meningitis • Abscess formation	• Humans are only reservoir • High rates of resistance, follow sensitivities • Screen family members if symptomatic • Carriage state may occur
• TMP/SMX • Ampicillin • If able, may treat orally	• Dehydration/shock	• Humans are only reservoir • Low inoculum size required for disease
• Erythromycin or azithromycin will shorten length of illness	• Guillain-Barré syndrome • Septicemia in neonates	• Reservoir includes wild/domestic birds, young cats, dogs, hamsters • Contaminated water and milk products • Campylobactor and Yersinia infections may mimic appendicitis
• Supportive care • Consider TMP/SMX in severe disease	• Dehydration • O157:H7: hemorrhagic colitis • HUS	• Antibiotics may contribute to HUS • *E. coli* is most common cause of traveler's diarrhea

(Continued)

TABLE 11-8 *INFECTIOUS DIARRHEA (CONTINUED)*

DISEASE	ETIOLOGY	CLINICAL PRESENTATION	DIAGNOSIS
Yersinia	• *Yersinia enterocolitica*	• Enterocolitis: bloody diarrhea, fever • Acute presentation may mimic appendicitis with right lower quadrant pain, abdominal tenderness, and fever	• Stool culture • Culture of throat swabs, peritoneal fluid; blood cultures may also positive
Giardia	• *Giardia lamblia*	• Abdominal pain, foul-smelling stools, bloating, flatulence, anorexia • Many asymptomatic infections, especially in young children	• Stool examination for trophozoites/cysts • Antigen detection in stool • Examination of duodenal aspirate
Food poisoning	• *S. aureus* enterotoxin ingestion	• Abrupt onset of vomiting, cramps, diarrhea, fever 0.5-12 h after food ingestion • Generally lasts 24-48 h	• May recover staphylococci from stool or vomit • Can isolate toxin from suspected food

HUS, hemolytic-uremic syndrome; TMP/SMX, trimethoprim/sulfamethoxazole.

TABLE 11-9 *SEPTIC ARTHRITIS*

If not treated promptly, damage to growth plates may occur, especially in hip, where joint is contained in a capsule.

AGE GROUP	ETIOLOGY	CLINICAL PRESENTATION	DIAGNOSIS
Neonatal	• Group B strep • *S. aureus* • *N. gonorrhoeae* • *Enterobacter*	• Fever, irritability, vomiting, poor feeding	• Joint aspiration and culture • Blood culture • X-ray • CRP/ESR
Pediatric	• *S. pyogenes* • *S. aureus* • *H. influenzae*	• Fever, joint pain, joint swelling	• Joint aspiration and culture • Blood culture • X-ray • CRP/ESR
Adolescent	• *N. gonorrhoeae*	• Fever, sore throat, joint pain • Genital infection may be asymptomatic	• Joint aspiration and culture • Blood culture • X-ray • CRP/ESR • If joint culture negative, throat and genital cultures should be performed

CRP, C-reactive protein; ESR, erythrocyte sedimentation rate; PID, pelvic inflammatory disease.

TREATMENT	COMPLICATIONS	COMMENTS
• If septic, or immunocompromised, consider treatment with: 1st-generation cephalosporin or penicillin	• Hepatic, splenic abscess • Bacteremia • Post infectious: erythema nodosum, arthritis	• Reservoirs: pigs, milk products • Patients with iron overload especially susceptible
• Metronidazole • Alternative: albendazole	• Weight loss • Malabsorption • Anemia	• Reservoirs include humans, dogs, cats, beavers • High frequency with IgA deficiency • Treatment of asymptomatic carriers not recommended
• Supportive	• Dehydration	• Inadequate heating or storage of foods, especially meats, dairy, mayonnaise

TREATMENT	COMPLICATIONS	COMMENTS
• Ampicillin and aminoglycoside *or* • Ampicillin and 3rd-generation cephalosporin	• Bacteremia • Sepsis	• Often result of adjacent osteomyelitis
• Oxacillin • Consider gram-negative coverage in very young children	• Osteomyelitis (rare)	• *H. influenzae* now uncommon
• Ceftriaxone	• PID	• Patient should be treated for *Chlamydia* • May exist as either septic arthritis or sterile (reactive) arthritis • Most common in perimenstrual females

TABLE 11-10   *SEXUALLY TRANSMITTED DISEASES*

Any of these diseases may be completely asymptomatic.
Always treat patient's sexual partners.
Patients who are positive for either chlamydia or gonorrhea should be treated for both diseases, as these usually coexist.

DISEASE	ORGANISM	CLINICAL PRESENTATION	DIAGNOSIS
Gonorrhea	• *Neisseria gonorrhoeae*	• Urethritis, salpingitis, endocervicitis, pharyngitis	• Cervical culture (females) • Urethral culture (males) • Urine DNA detection
Chlamydia	• *Chlamydia trachomatis*	• Cervicitis, urethritis, endometritis, salpingitis	• Culture of epithelial cells from cervix/urethra • Urine ligase chain reaction
Genital herpes	• Herpes simplex virus (types 1 and 2)	• Vesicular or ulcerative lesions of genitalia (internal and/or external)	• Clinical • Antigen detection • Cell culture of lesions • Serology *not* helpful
Trichomonas	• *Trichomonas vaginalis*	• Frothy gray discharge, dysuria	• Wet mount demonstrates flagellated organisms • Culture also available
Syphilis	• *Treponema pallidum*	• Primary: painless ulcer at site of inoculation, or, in moister areas (i.e., anal folds); hypertrophic papular lesions (condyloma lata) • Secondary: maculopapular rash (palms and soles) • Tertiary: gummas and carditis • Neurosyphilis may occur at any stage	• Nontreponemal tests (VRDL/RPR) always require confirmation, many false positives; will usually revert to negative after treatment • Treponemal tests (FTA-ABS) more specific for syphilis; remains positive after treatment
Bacterial vaginosis	• *Gardnerella vaginalis* • *Mycoplasma hominis* • Decreased lactobacilli	• Thin malodorous vaginal discharge	• "Whiff test": fishy amine smell when mixed with potassium hydroxide • Vaginal pH >4.5 • Clue cells on wet mount are seen

Patients who have been diagnosed with one STD should undergo testing for chlamydia, gonorrhea, syphilis, hepatitis B, and HIV.

TREATMENT	COMPLICATIONS	COMMENTS
• Ceftriaxone IM × 1 *or* • Cefixime po × 1 *or* • Ciprofloxacin po × 1	• PID • Perihepatitis (Fitz-Hugh-Curtis syndrome)	• Frequent coinfection with *Chlamydia*
• Azithromycin po × 1 or • Doxycycline po × 7 d	• PID • Lymphogranuloma venereum: ulcerative genitalia lesions and painful lymphadenopathy	• Most common *bacterial* STD
• Acyclovir, valacyclovir, and famciclovir all decrease duration of shedding and symptoms	• Disseminated herpes can result in encephalitis and death	
• Metronidazole po × 1	• Rare	• Symptoms more severe in peri-menstrual period
• Primary disease: penicillin G IM × 1 • Secondary/tertiary disease: penicillin G IM q wk × 3 • Neurosyphilis: penicillin G IV q 4-6 h × 2 wk	• Progression of disease if untreated • May be transmitted to off-spring (congenital syphilis)	• Monitor VDRL 3, 6, and 12 mo after treatment to check for 4-fold decrease in titers
• Metronidazole po/intravaginal *or* • Clindamycin po/intravaginal	• PID	

(Continued)

TABLE 11-10   *SEXUALLY TRANSMITTED DISEASES (STDS) (CONTINUED)*

DISEASE	ORGANISM	CLINICAL PRESENTATION	DIAGNOSIS
Genital warts	• Human papilloma virus	• Broad range from (usually) asymptomatic to condyloma acuminata (cauliflower-like protrusion on external genitalia)	• Clinical appearance • White appearing when acetic acid applied • Biopsy
Chancroid	• *Haemophilus ducreyi*	• Painful, tender, non-indurated ulcerative lesion with exudate (may be single or multiple) • Bubo: painful unilateral inguinal lymphadenopathy	• Clinical • Gram stain and culture of lesion scraping

PID, pelvic inflammatory disease.

TABLE 11-11   *HERPES VIRUSES*

DISEASE	ETIOLOGY	CLINICAL PRESENTATION	DIAGNOSIS
Herpes simplex	• HSV 1 and 2 • Spread by direct contact with infected secretions or lesions, and vertically from mother to infant	• Genital lesions • Gingivostomatitis • Conjunctivitis/keratitis • Meningoencephalitis • Aseptic meningitis • Whitlow (distal finger) • Usually appears as painful vesicular lesions with an ulcerative base • Remains dormant in sensory nerve ganglia for life, with sporadic reactivation, especially in times of immunosuppression	• Viral culture of lesion is gold standard • Scraping of lesion base can be used to detect specific HSV antigens by DFA testing • PCR detects virus in cerebrospinal fluid (CSF culture is usually nonrevealing) • Serology unhelpful, due to ubiquity of disease • Tzanck prep not specific nor sensitive

TREATMENT	COMPLICATIONS	COMMENTS
• Usually spontaneously regress • Cryotherapy	• May lead to cervical cancer	• Most common STD
• High rate of coinfections with herpes virus, HIV, and syphilis • Azithromycin PO × 1 *or* • Ceftriaxone IM × 1	• Bubo may become fluctuant and drain	

TREATMENT	COMPLICATIONS	COMMENTS
• Genital outbreaks: oral antiviral therapy (acyclovir, famciclovir, valacyclovir) reduces viral shedding and duration of symptoms • If initial outbreak is severe enough to warrant hospitalization, then IV acyclovir is indicated • If ≥6 genital outbreaks/year, consider suppressive oral therapy • Gingivostomatitis: immunocompromised: IV/topical acyclovir; immunocompetent: oral acyclovir controversial, topical therapy of little benefit • Meningitis/encephalitis: IV acyclovir • Conjunctivitis/keratitis: topical agents: (i.e., trifluridine); consider IV acyclovir	• Disseminated herpes with visceral involvement can occur in immuno-compromised patients • High mortality in untreated CNS disease • Superinfection of eczematous lesions can occur (eczema herpeticum); will usually be described as superinfected eczema not responsive to conventional antibiotics	• Oral lesions involve the vermilion border (coxsackie and other oral vesicular lesions generally will spare the vermilion border) • See Chapter 1 for information on congenital herpes infection

(Continued)

TABLE 11-11   *HERPES VIRUSES (CONTINUED)*

DISEASE	ETIOLOGY	CLINICAL PRESENTATION	DIAGNOSIS
Chickenpox, zoster	VZV: • Spread by direct contact with infected chickenpox or zoster lesions, and by airborne respiratory secretions from chickenpox patient • Zoster patients may be infectious via respiratory secretions as well, but this is much more rare Chickenpox: • Incubation period: 14-16 d (range 10-21) • Patients are contagious starting 2 d before onset of rash, and until all lesions are crusted over	**Chickenpox:** • Classic "dew drop on a rose petal" presentation of pruritic vesicles in crops of various ages • Starts on trunk and spreads to extremities • May be accompanied by fever, fatigue, malaise **Zoster:** • Reactivation of latent virus in dorsal root ganglia • Vesicular eruption along dermatomes • Usually does not cross midline • Can involve face and eye, as well as body	• Clinical • Scraping of lesion base can be used to detect specific VZV antigens by DFA within 3-4 d of eruption • Paired acute and convalescent serum for VZV IgG
Roseola (exanthem subitum, sixth disease)	HHV-6 • Spread by contact with infected secretions (saliva) • Incubation period: 9-10 d	• Roseola: high fever up to 105°F in an otherwise asymptomatic patient, followed by the resolution of the fever and the prompt appearance of an erythematous maculopapular rash (accounts for 20% of HHV-6) • Many children with HHV-6 do not develop rash • Other symptoms include lymphadenopathy, upper respiratory symptoms, vomiting/diarrhea, and otitis media • 10%-15% develop febrile seizures	• Clinical • Laboratory testing cannot reliably differentiate between new and recurrent infections

TREATMENT	COMPLICATIONS	COMMENTS
• Healthy children: supportive care • IV acyclovir is recommended for otherwise healthy patients who are older than 12 y, have chronic skin/lung disease (i.e., eczema), are taking inhaled or oral steroids, or are on salicylate therapy • IV acyclovir recommended for all immunocompromised patients See section on postexposure prophylaxis for information on VZV-IVIG	• Bacterial superinfection/necrotizing fasciitis (group A streptococcus) is most common complication • Pneumonia • Encephalitis/meningitis • Arthritis, hepatitis, glomerulonephritis • Reye syndrome (encephalopathy and mitochondrial dysfunction) associated with viral illnesses and concurrent use of salicylates • Immunocompromised patients may present with hemorrhagic or progressive varicella, or disseminated zoster	• Varicella vaccine should be offered to all children aged ≥1 y who have not had documented varicella • See Chapter 1 for information on congenital varicella syndrome
• Supportive care	• Reactivation may occur in immuno-suppressed patients, with resultant bone marrow suppression, hepatitis, pneumonia, and central nervous system disease	• HHV-7 presents in a similar manner

(Continued)

TABLE 11-11 *HERPES VIRUSES (CONTINUED)*

DISEASE	ETIOLOGY	CLINICAL PRESENTATION	DIAGNOSIS
Infectious mononucleosis (IM)	• Epstein-Barr virus (herpes virus family) • Transmitted most commonly via saliva • Incubation period is 30-50 d	• Fever, upper respiratory symptoms • Exudative tonsillopharyngitis lasting >1 wk • Systemic symptoms: fatigue, tender lymphadenopathy, HSM • Suspect IM with any case of prolonged or severe case of pharyngitis	• Heterophile antibody positive (although many false negatives, especially early in disease, and in children aged <4 y) • VCA-IgM: appears at 3-6 wk (indicates acute infection, eventually clears) • VCA-IgG: 6-8 wk (positive for life, can indicate acute, recent, or past infection) • Anti-early antigen: 3-6 mo (indicates recent infection, eventually clears) • Anti-nuclear antigen: 6-8 mo (indicates past infection, eventually clears) • Blood count demonstrates lymphocytosis and atypical lymphocytes
Cytomegalovirus (CMV)	• Cytomegalovirus (herpes virus family) • Transmitted via secretions (saliva, urine), blood transfusions, sexually, and vertically (mother-infant transmission) • Incubation period unknown • Reactivation possible, and prolonged shedding (i.e., years) after infection common	• Asymptomatic infection most common in children • Heterophile-negative IM, especially in older adolescents • Immunocompromised/transplant patients: pneumonia, colitis, retinitis, hepatitis	• Serology: CMV IgM and IgG • Be aware that IgM can be positive with reactivated cases, and IgG is positive for life • Acute and convalescent titers more helpful than single assay • Culture (urine, blood, saliva); again, many patients will have prolonged excretion of CMV in body fluids in face of asymptomatic infection • Positive culture from organ tissue, however, is considered diagnostic • CMV antigen detection in WBCs used to detect infection in those patients with immunodeficiency

CMV, cytomegalovirus; CSF, cerebrospinal fluid; DFA, direct fluorescent antigen; EBV, Ebstein-Barr virus; HHV, human herpes virus; HSM, hepatosplenomegaly; HSV, herpes simplex virus; IVIG, intravenous immunoglobulin; PCR, polymerase chain reaction; VCA,

TREATMENT	COMPLICATIONS	COMMENTS

• Symptomatic treatment
• No contact sports for athletes until fully recovered, and no spleen is palpable (usually ~6 wk)
• Steroids should only be used if patient has tonsillar enlargement posing danger to airway, myocarditis, or massive splenomegaly with subsequent hemolysis
	• In susceptible patients, EBV is linked to:
	  - X-linked lymphoproliferative syndrome
	  - Burkitt lymphoma
	  - Nasopharyngeal carcinoma
	  - B-cell lymphoma
		• Treatment with amoxicillin or ampicillin (i.e., for misdiagnosed or superimposed streptococcal pharyngitis) yields a distinctive morbilliform rash

• Supportive care • Ganciclovir, foscarnet, and CMV intravenous immunoglobulin for selected conditions (i.e., transplant patients, retinitis, severe neonatal disease)	• Severe disease can result in permanent organ damage and/or death, usually in immunocompromised patients	• See Chapter 1 for information on congenital CMV

viral capsid antigen; VZV, varicella zoster virus.

TABLE 11-12   *SPIROCHETES*

DISEASE	ETIOLOGY	CLINICAL PRESENTATION
Lyme disease	• *Borrelia burgdorferi* • Vector: deer tick (*Ixodes scapularis* and *Ixodes dammini*)	• Early localized disease (3-31 d after bite): erythema migrans (an expanding erythematous target lesion), fever, headache, myalgias, arthralgias • Early disseminated disease (3-5 wk after bite): multiple target lesions, meningitis, conjunctivitis, carditis, arthralgias, headache, cranial nerve palsies • Late disease: arthritis (especially knees), CNS disease (polyradiculoneuropathy, encephalopathy)
Rocky Mountain spotted fever	• *Rickettsia rickettsia* • Vectors: wood tick (*Dermacentor andersoni*) and dog tick (*Dermacentor variabilis*) • Incubation period 2-14 d (mean: 7 d)	• Erythematous rash (vasculitic) starts on wrists/ankles, and spreads towards the trunk; frequently becomes petechial; palms and soles involved • Incubation period: 2-14 d (mean, 1 wk); rash usually appears by day 6 • Clinical: fever, *headache*, myalgias, and meningitis symptoms • Laboratory: anemia, thrombocytopenia, hyponatremia
Syphilis	• *Treponema pallidum* • Spread by sexual contact, or vertically from mother to infant • Incubation period 10-90 d (mean: 3 wk)	• Primary: painless ulcer at site of inoculation • Secondary: maculopapular rash (palms and soles) • Tertiary: gummas and carditis • Neurosyphilis may occur at any stage

EIA, enzyme immunoassay; IFA, immunofluorescence antibody; IHA, indirect hemagglutinin; RPR, rapid plasmin reagin; VDRL, Venereal

DIAGNOSIS	TREATMENT	COMMENTS

• EIA IgM and IgG (screening test, cross-reactions with other spirochete diseases, viral infections, and autoimmune diseases common); may be negative in early localized disease
• Western immunoblot (confirmatory): tests for immunoglobulins specific to Lyme
• IgM detectable 3-6 wk after infection, IgG takes weeks to months
• CNS disease: intrathecal *production* of Lyme antibody (not merely *presence* of antibody, which can be seen in patients without CNS disease)
	• Early localized disease:
	  <8 y old: amoxicillin × 2-3 wk
	  >8 y old: doxycycline × 2-3 wk
	• Early disseminated and late disease:
	  - Multiple erythema migrans: either amoxicillin or doxycycline for 3 wk
	  - Arthritis: same medication choices, for 28 d
	  - Recurrent/persistent arthritis, carditis, meningitis, encephalitis: IV ceftriaxone or IV penicillin for 2-3 wk
		• The tick must attach and feed for 24 h to transmit disease
		• If patient has negative serology, but clinical suspicion for early localized disease is high, can confirm diagnosis by documenting 4-fold increase in serum titers
		• Vaccine available for patients ≥15 y old at high risk of exposure

• Indirect IFA, EIA, and IHA most commonly used methods to detect rickettsial-group–specific antibodies • Antibody usually detectable by 7-10 d after disease • Four-fold increase in titer diagnostic • Usually not cultured, because of hazard to lab personnel	• Doxycycline (for children of all ages) • Treatment before day 5 of illness results in best outcome	• No rash in 20% • If untreated, can rapidly progress to shock, with meningitis, cardiac failure, renal failure, disseminated intravascular coagulation, and death
• Nontreponemal tests (VDRL/RPR): always require confirmation, many false positives; will usually revert to negative after treatment • Treponemal tests (FTA-ABS): more specific for syphilis; stay positive after treatment	• Primary disease: penicillin G IM × 1 • Secondary /tertiary disease: penicillin G IM q wk × 3 • Neurosyphilis: penicillin G IV q 4-6h × 2 wk	• Monitor VDRL 3, 6, and 12 mo after treatment to check for 4-fold decrease in titers • See Chapter 1 for information on congenital syphilis

Disease Research Laboratory.

TABLE 11-13   *STAPHYLOCOCCAL AND STREPTOCOCCAL SKIN DISEASES*

DISEASE	ETIOLOGY	CLINICAL PRESENTATION	DIAGNOSIS
Impetigo	• *S. pyogenes* • *S. aureus*	• Honey-colored crusts • Transmitted by direct contact • Bullous impetigo usually caused by *S. aureus*	• Nasopharyngeal swab • Culture of lesion
Scarlet fever	• *S. pyogenes* • *S. aureus*	• Fever, sore throat, abdominal pain precedes rash by 12-48 h • Blanching, erythematous sandpapery rash over entire body (may be painful in cases caused by staph) • Rash accentuated on flexural creases (Pastia lines) • Strawberry tongue, circumoral pallor, petechiae on uvula (in strep disease) • Rash desquamates several days after onset (staph disease has thicker flakes and more perioral peeling than strep disease) • Negative Nikolsky sign	• Clinical • Throat culture (or wound culture if appropriate) • ASO titer (may be normal in primary acute disease)
Scalded skin	• *S. aureus*	• Usually originates from respiratory illness, conjunctivitis, impetigo, circumcision sites • Prodrome: fever, irritability, vomiting • Erythroderma follows, with tenderness of skin • Bullous exfoliation occurs 1-3 d later, with positive Nikolsky sign	• Clinical • Culture of infective site (i.e., nasopharynx, wound) • Skin lesions *not* culture positive
Erysipelas	• *S. pyogenes*	• Infection of dermis and superficial lymphatics • Prodrome: fever, chills, +/- nausea, vomiting, headache • Painful, well-demarcated, erythematous plaque • Skin is edematous with orange peel appearance	• Clinical • Culture of advancing border of lesion, and nasopharynx • Septic patients: blood culture

TREATMENT	COMPLICATIONS	COMMENTS
• <10% BSA: topical mupirocin • ≥10% BSA, widespread lesions, bullous impetigo, or multiple affected contacts: oral antibiotics	• Acute glomerulonephritis is most common nonsuppurative complication of impetigo; not necessarily prevented by antibiotic treatment	• Children should not go to school/day care until treated for 24 h
• PCN • Clindamycin or macrolide if PCN allergic	• Rheumatic fever • Bacteremia/sepsis • Adenitis • Otitis • Sinusitis • Peritonsillar abscess	• Caused by erythrogenic exotoxin • Although throat is classic origin, may also originate in skin/wound infections (pharynx will be normal in these cases) • May also originate from carrier state
• Nafcillin or oxacillin	• Large areas of skin loss can result in dehydration and hypothermia • Superinfection	• Caused by hematogenous spread of exfoliative toxin • Shedding most pronounced near orifices
• PCN • Clindamycin or macrolide in PCN-allergic patients	• Bacteremia, with subsequent secondary lesions	

(Continued)

TABLE 11-13   *STAPHYLOCOCCAL AND STREPTOCOCCAL SKIN DISEASES (CONTINUED)*

DISEASE	ETIOLOGY	CLINICAL PRESENTATION	DIAGNOSIS
Toxic shock syndrome	• *S. aureus* • *S. pyogenes*	• Fever, hypotension, multiorgan system involvement • Staph: erythroderma, diarrhea, vomiting, myalgias, tampon use • Strep: painful localized site of infection, no rash or diarrhea as for staph • Both forms may be associated with invasive infection (i.e., pneumonia, endocarditis, osteomyelitis)	• Staph: fever, rash, hypotension, involvement of ≥3 organ systems, negative throat/CSF cultures, other diseases (i.e., measles) ruled out • Strep: hypotension, involvement of ≥2 organ systems, and isolation of *S. pyogenes*

ASO, antistreptolysin-O; BSA, body surface area; CSF, cerebrospinal fluid; PCN, penicillin.

TABLE 11-14   *PARASITES*

DISEASE	ETIOLOGY	CLINICAL PRESENTATION	DIAGNOSIS
Pinworms	• *Enterobius vermicularis* (roundworm) • Female lays eggs on perineal area at night • High rates of infection in day care, preschool and institutionalized children	• Perianal pruritis, especially at night • Loosely associated with bruxism and abdominal pain	• Visualization of worms in perianal region after child has fallen asleep • "Scotch tape test": collection of eggs on transparent tape, which are then microscopically examined
Ascariasis	•*Ascaris Lumbricoides* (roundworm) • Worm eggs are swallowed, hatch into larvae, and migrate to the lung, where they are coughed up, reswallowed, and mature into adults in the small intestine	• Usually asymptomatic • Anorexia, nausea, vomiting • Pneumonitis during worm migration through lung	• Microscopic examination of stool to detect eggs • Worms may be passed in stool, or occasionally through upper respiratory tract/mouth • May note eosinophilia on complete blood count

TREATMENT	COMPLICATIONS	COMMENTS
• Fluid management • Antistaphylococcal drug • Clindamycin to inhibit toxin production • Consider intravenous immunoglobulin • Surgery for necrotizing fasciitis	• Cases complicated by necrotizing fasciitis have higher mortality rates	• Toxin-mediated disease

TREATMENT	COMPLICATIONS	COMMENTS
• Mebendazole, single dose; may repeat treatment 2 wk later if still symptomatic • Alternatives: pyrantel pamoate, albendazole	• Worms may migrate to vaginal or urethral area erroneously, resulting in intraperitoneal infection, or infection of reproductive tract	• Consider treating family members as well
• Albendazole or • Mebendazole or • Pyrantel pamoate • Consider rechecking stool 3 wk after treatment if efficacy uncertain	• Intestinal obstruction, malabsorption with heavy worm burden; aberrant migration can cause bile duct obstruction, peritonitis • Administration of barbiturates, anesthetic agents can cause agitation of worms	• One of the most common infectious diseases in the world • Endemic in the tropics

(Continued)

TABLE 11-14   *PARASITES (CONTINUED)*

DISEASE	ETIOLOGY	CLINICAL PRESENTATION	DIAGNOSIS
Strongyloides	*Strongyloides stercoralis* (roundworm) • Worm larvae enter skin from infected soil, migrate through lymphatics to lungs, are coughed up, swallowed, and mature in the small intestine	• Pruritic papular rash at site of skin inoculation (usually feet) • Pneumonitis during worm migration through lung • Abdominal pain, vomiting, anorexia, nausea, diarrhea	• Microscopic examination of stool to detect larvae • Duodenal aspirate may also contain larvae • Serodiagnosis not widely available, cross-reactions are common • Eosinophilia on complete blood count common
Cysticercosis	• *Taenia solium* (pork tapeworm) • Eggs are ingested, larvae migrate throughout body, including brain, spinal canal, skin, eyes, and heart, and remain as an intermediate form	• Disease primarily manifests when cysts are present in CNS • Seizures, behavioral changes, cognitive decline • Pain, transverse myelitis, spinal compression from spinal disease • Decreased visual acuity from ocular disease	• CNS disease is diagnosed by characteristic findings on CT scan or MRI • Detection of antibody to *T. solium* in serum and CSF
Visceral larva migrans (VLM)	• *Toxocara canis* • Eggs shed by dogs and cats are ingested; larva penetrates the GI tract and migrates to lungs, liver, CNS, kidney, eye, and heart	• Low parasite burden may not result in symptoms • VLM may manifest as fever, wheezing, or seizures • Physical findings: hepatosplenomegaly, abnormal lung sounds, rash, lymphadenopathy • Ocular disease may present with decreased visual acuity, strabismus, periorbital swelling; usually *not* associated with visceral disease	• Enzyme-linked immunoassay (ELISA) to *T. canis* eggs • Increased isohemmaglutinin titers to A and B blood groups, accompanied by hypereosinophilia and hypergammaglobinemia • Liver biopsy may demonstrate larvae

TREATMENT	COMPLICATIONS	COMMENTS
• Albendazole *or* • Ivermectin *or* • Thiabendazole	• Larvae can penetrate colon wall and migrate through lymphatics to lungs to repeat life cycle; this process, called autoinoculation, can result in high worm burdens • Complications similar to *Ascaris* can also be seen	• Endemic in the tropics, southern and southwestern United States
• Symptomatic treatment for seizures • Corticosteroids • Antiparasitic therapy controversial, and may depend on whether there are viable cysts (vs. calcified lesions) in brain	• Cerebral infarction from vascular blockage • Autoinfection possible if patient infected with pork tapeworm	• Humans are the only definitive host • A leading cause of new-onset seizures in endemic areas • Ingestion of infected pork results in tapeworm infection; ingestion of eggs results in cysticerosis
• Mebendazole • Steroids are used in CNS disease and myocarditis	• Ocular disease difficult to cure	• Humans are end-stage hosts

(Continued)

TABLE 11-14	PARASITES (CONTINUED)		
DISEASE	ETIOLOGY	CLINICAL PRESENTATION	DIAGNOSIS
Scabies	• *Sarcoptes scabei* (dog mite) • Transmitted by direct contact with infected animal, person, or fomite • Eight legs	• Pruritic papular rash especially pronounced at skin folds (may be generalized in infants)	• Clinical • Scraping of terminal burrow may demonstrate mite, mite eggs, or mite feces
Head lice	• *Pediculus humanus capitis* (insect) • Transmitted by direct contact with infected person or fomite (i.e., hairbrush, hat) • Six legs	• Pruritic scalp most common symptom • May be completely asymptomatic	• Visualization of lice and/or nits on scalp, near hairline

TUBERCULOSIS (TB)

Definitions

- **TB Exposure**: Patient has had contact with suspected/known case of TB, negative tuberculin skin test (TST), no evidence of active disease.
- **Latent Tuberculosis Infection (LTBI)**: Patient with positive TST, no evidence of active disease.
- **TB Infection**: Patient has clinical or radiographic evidence of TB disease (pulmonary or otherwise). Not defined by presence or absence of positive TST.

Tuberculosis Skin Testing (TST)

Recommendations on the frequency of TST in children vary. Children who are HIV positive, or live with people who are HIV positive or have been incarcerated within

TREATMENT	COMPLICATIONS	COMMENTS
• 5% permethrin applied for 8-12 h, and then washed off • Apply from scalp to toes in infants; neck to toes in patients over 1 y old • Antihistamines to control pruritis • Lindane should be avoided, as it has potential for neurotoxicity	• Superinfection of lesions may occur • Norwegian scabies: large number of mites, widespread lesions; usually occurs in debilitated patients • Pruritus and skin lesions can persist for weeks after treatment, secondary to granulomatous reaction to mite feces and dead mites	• Treat clothing either by dry cleaning or placing in hot dryer • Treat family members
• 1% permethrin shampoo (kills eggs and adults) • Pyrethrin-based shampoos (low egg killing, so need to apply 1 wk later to kill newly hatched adults)	• Treatment should work quickly; if live lice visualized 24 h after treatment, review technique, and retreat • Permethrin resistance is becoming more prevalent	• Treat infected family members • Hair length, socioeconomic status, frequency of shampooing are *not* epidemiological factors • Removal of killed eggs (nits) is purely cosmetic, and not medically necessary

the past 5 years; children with a history of travel or who live with people who have a history of travel; children who immigrate to and from endemic countries; and children of migrant farm workers are considered to be in the highest risk group and require the most frequent screening.

Tuberculosis Skin Test (TST) Interpretation

Prior history of bacille Calmette-Guérin (BCG) vaccination should NOT influence the interpretation of TST results. TST should be reviewed 48 to 72 hours after placement. Routine anergy panels are not recommended. All patients with positive TST require a chest radiograph (CXR). A negative TST does NOT exclude TB disease.

Some general rules of thumb for deciding if a TST is positive are shown in Table 11-15.

TABLE 11-15. *TST RECOMMENDATIONS*

TABLE 11-15	TST RECOMMENDATIONS

False negatives maybe seen in immunosuppressed patients, concurrent viral illnesses (i.e., measles, varicella), disseminated TB.

TST RESULT	POSITIVE IF:
≥15 mm	Always positive, in all ages
≥10 mm	*Exposed to* high-risk populations (see above), children younger than 4 y, diseases associated with immune suppression (i.e., diabetes, chronic renal failure)
≥5 mm	Immunodeficiency, HIV positive, close contact with known or suspected case of tuberculosis, clinical or radiographic evidence of tuberculosis

Typical Clinical Scenarios

Following are typical scenarios concerning pulmonary TB in an otherwise normal patient. These recommendations do NOT apply to immunocompromised hosts, who often require longer periods of therapy.

- *TB exposure*: Place TST and start isoniazid (INH). Children less than 4 years of age should have a chest radiograph performed. If TST is negative, continue INH and place repeat TST after 3 months. (TST can take up to 3 months to convert to positive after exposure.) If second TST is negative, discontinue INH. If second TST is positive, continue treatment for positive TST (see below).
- *Positive TST, negative CXR (LTBI)*: Oral INH daily for 9 months, OR oral rifampin daily for 6 months.
- *Positive TST, positive chest radiograph (infection)*: Gastric aspirates or sputum should be collected for culture and sensitivity testing. Attempts should be made to find index case. Treatment options include:
  - Daily rifampin, INH, pyrazinamide for 2 months, followed by daily INH and rifampin for 4 more months
  - Daily rifampin, INH, pyrazinamide for 2 months, followed by twice weekly INH and rifampin for 4 more months.
  - Directly observed therapy is recommended to ensure compliance.

Congenital/Neonatal Tuberculosis

Only mothers with disseminated (i.e., extrapulmonary) disease pose a hazard to an infant in utero; mothers with pulmonary TB pose little risk to the fetus.

Infants with suspected congenital TB should be given a TST, a lumbar puncture, and a chest radiograph. Regardless of TST results (likely to be negative), quadruple therapy should be started: INH, rifampin, pyrazinamide, and streptomycin. Corticosteroids should be administered in cases of confirmed TB meningitis. Once the diagnosis is excluded, the infant should continue to receive INH and a repeat

TST should be placed at 3 to 4 months of age. If TST remains negative, the infant should complete 9 months of treatment. If TST converts to positive, workup for TB should be initiated. Separation from the mother is NOT necessary once infant is receiving INH and the mother is receiving therapy.

If an infant's mother/close contact has LTBI, the mother and household contacts should receive appropriate therapy, and the infant needs no further evaluation.

If an infant's mother/close contact has +TST/+CXR (TB infection), the infant should be separated until mother/contact is evaluated and receiving appropriate therapy. The infant should be managed as detailed above under the heading TB Exposure.

Infection Control

Most children with tuberculosis do not pose a public health risk, and do not require quarantine. Children who have TB-positive sputum, cavitary disease, laryngeal involvement, or widespread pulmonary disease should be quarantined (or hospitalized), until smears are improved, adequate therapy is ensured, and cough is resolved. Once these criteria are met, these children may attend school or daycare, and participate in regular activities.

EXANTHEMS

TABLE 11-16 *EXANTHEMS*

	CONJUNCTIVITIS	STRAWBERRY TONGUE	DESQUAMATION	LYMPHADENOPATHY	PALMS AND SOLES
Measles	+				+
Rubella	+			+	
Scarlet fever		+	+	+	+
Kawasaki	+	+	+	+	+
Varicella					
Smallpox					+
Epstein-Barr virus	+			+	
Coxsackie					+
Rocky Mountain spotted fever					+
Erythema multiforme	+		+		+

Active Immunization

Stimulates the immune system to mount an immune response to a desired pathogen, or by-product (i.e., toxin). Vaccines may be comprised of any one or combination of the components shown in Table 11-17.

TABLE 11-17	*VACCINE TYPES*
VACCINE TYPE	**EXAMPLES**
Inactivated bacteria	Whole cell pertussis, cholera
Bacterial component	*H. influenzae, S. pneumoniae* (capsular protein)
Live bacteria	Oral typhoid, bacille Calmette-Guérin
Inactivated virus	Rabies, intramuscular polio
Viral component	Hepatitis B, influenza
Live virus	Measles, mumps, rubella
Toxoid	Tetanus

Vaccines that contain protein as an antigen (i.e., *N. meningococcus* vaccine, which contains capsular protein) evoke a poor response in children less than 2 years of age. Protein antigens can be conjugated to a polysaccharide to elicit a better response in these children (i.e., *H. influenzae* vaccine, which is comprised of a capsular protein conjugated to a polysaccharide).

Most vaccines require multiple doses for maximal effect. Some vaccines confer lifelong immunity (i.e., varicella vaccine), and some vaccines require lifelong boosters (i.e., tetanus). The influenza vaccine is administered yearly, and its components are changed to reflect the antigenic drift in the community.

Passive Immunization

Passive immunization consists of parenteral administration of a specific immunoglobulin (Ig) product, usually consisting of human-derived antibodies. These are not administered as part of the usual scheduled immunizations. They may be administered as pre-exposure prophylaxis (i.e., hepatitis A Ig, RSV Ig), or post-exposure treatment (IVIG, varicella zoster Ig). Passive immunization with IVIG is also given to immunodeficient patients who are unable to mount an immune response to vaccines (i.e., advanced HIV, B-lymphocyte deficiencies).

Immunization Schedules

Vaccination history should be obtained at every office visit. Premature infants should be immunized according to their chronological age, even while hospitalized, unless contraindications exist. Missed or delayed immunizations in a child with proper documentation of prior vaccines do not require an additional administration or alteration of the vaccine schedule. If a dose is missed, the current schedule should continue with no additional dose.

*   *Missing documentation*: If a vaccination history is absent, or documentation is unavailable, the child should be considered to be nonimmunized, and vaccinated as such.
*   *Foreign adopted children*: Adopted children from other countries should comply with the U.S. immunization schedule. If written records are unavailable or unclear, serum titers should be drawn, and the child should be vaccinated against those diseases to which s/he is deemed susceptible.

Live Vaccines and Immune Globulin (Ig)

IV/IM Ig can interfere with the response to live-virus vaccines. If Ig is administered, the patient should not receive live vaccines for at least 3 months. The precise interval depends on the formulation and dosage of Ig administered. Additionally, if Ig is given within 14 days following administration of a live vaccine, serum titers should be checked after the appropriate interval, and the vaccine may be readministered as indicated. The exception to this rule is RSV Ig, which does not require alteration of the routine immunization schedule.

Measles and Tuberculin Skin Testing

Measles vaccine (either alone or in combination with mumps and rubella) may be given concurrently with TST. However, if measles vaccine is administered prior to TST, a 4-to-6 week waiting period is advised, as measles immunization may suppress the response to TST.

Measles and Varicella

Measles and varicella vaccines may be administered concurrently at separate sites. If they are administered on separate days, a 6-week waiting period is advised.

TABLE 11-18.   *MEASLES, MUMPS, AND RUBELLA*

TABLE 11-18   *MEASLES, MUMPS, AND RUBELLA*

DISEASE	ETIOLOGY	CLINICAL PRESENTATION	DIAGNOSIS
Measles (rubeola)	• Measles virus (para-myxovirus) • Spread by respiratory droplets • Incubation period 8-12 d • Contagious 3-5 d before onset of rash until 4 d after	• "The three Cs": cough, coryza, conjunctivitis • Koplik spots: gray white buccal mucosa lesions • High fever • Maculopapular rash starts ~2 d after above symptoms; starts on face and spreads distally	• Clinical suspicion • Detection of serum measles IgM *or* • Four-fold increase in serum measles IgG *or* • Isolation of virus from secretions
Mumps	• Mumps virus (paramyxovirus) • Spread by respiratory droplets • Incubation period 16-18 d • Contagious 1-2 d before gland swelling until up to 9 d after	• Swelling of ≥1 salivary gland (usually parotid) • Fever	• Isolation of virus from secretions • Four-fold increase in serum mumps IgG • Detection of serum mumps IgM • 50% will have spinal fluid pleocytosis
Rubella (German measles)	• Rubella virus (rubivirus) • Spread by respiratory droplets • Incubation period 14-23 d • Most contagious from up to 7 d before rash until 7 d after	• Fever • Suboccipital, cervical, and post-auricular lymphadenopathy • Generalized maculopapular rash that begins on the face (near hairline) and spreads distally • The rash has a classic 3-d course: initial rash fades while newer portions are forming	• Isolation of virus from secretions • Four-fold increase in serum rubella IgG, or seroconversion from IgG negative to IgG positive • Detection of serum rubella IgM

TREATMENT	COMPLICATIONS	COMMENTS
• Symptomatic treatment • Vitamin A for *hospitalized* children between 6 mo and 2 y of age, or children over 6 mo with/at risk for vitamin A deficiency, or immunodeficiency	• Most severe: pneumonia and neurologic disease (meningitis/encephalitis) • Subacute sclerosing panencephalitis: a rare (1/million), fatal neurodegenerative postinfectious disorder; presents mean of 7 y after diagnosis	• See Postexposure and Immunization sections for further information
• Supportive care	• Orchitis is a common complication in *post*pubertal males; it is usually unilateral, and therefore does not cause sterility • More severe disease in adults • CNS disease, arthritis, pancreatitis	• One dose of MMR will induce immunity to mumps in >95% of recipients • Nonimmunized exposed individuals should receive mumps vaccine
• Symptomatic treatment • Immunoglobulin may be considered in susceptible exposed women; however, it does not ensure that fetus will not be affected • MMR vaccine for exposed, nonpregnant close contacts within 72 h	• Noncongenital rubella is usually a benign illness • Polyarthralgias and polyarthritis common in adolescents	• See Neonatology section for discussion of congenital rubella • No cases of congenital rubella have ever been reported after inadvertent vaccination of a pregnant woman

Vaccination Contraindications

TABLE 11-19. *VACCINATION CONTRAINDICATIONS*

INFECTIOUS DISEASE PROPHYLAXIS AND TREATMENT

TABLE 11-20. *PRE-/POSTEXPOSURE PROPHYLAXIS/TREATMENT*

TABLE 11-19   *VACCINATION CONTRAINDICATIONS*

Complement-deficient patients should receive all routine vaccines, including live vaccines. Asplenic patients should receive all routine vaccines, including live vaccines. Additionally, asplenic patients should receive 23-valent pneumococcal vaccine and meningococcal vaccine after the second birthday.

VACCINE	CONTRAINDICATIONS
All vaccines	• History of an anaphylactic reaction to the vaccine • Moderate or severe systemic illness at the time of vaccination (upper respiratory illness, mild gastroenteritis, or current antibiotic therapy are *not* contraindications)
Diphtheria, tetanus, acellular pertussis (DTaP)	• Encephalopathy within 7 d of administration • Progressive neurologic disorder • *Precautions*: seizure within 3 d of vaccination, inconsolable screaming/crying for ≥3 h, unexplained temperature of ≥40.5°C within 48 h, collapse/shock-like state within 48 h
Oral polio vaccine (OPV)	• HIV positive • Immunosuppressed • Close contact with a person who is immunosuppressed • Pregnancy • The above patients CAN receive inactivated poliovirus vaccine (IPV), although response is not assured in immunodeficient patients
Measles, mumps, rubella (MMR)	• Recent IVIG treatment (see above) • Thrombocytopenia • Advanced HIV • Immunosuppressed • Pregnancy • Tuberculin skin test administered within past 4-6 wk • Egg allergy no longer considered a contraindication to MMR
Influenza	• Allergy to eggs or chicken protein
Varicella	• Recent IVIG treatment (see above) • Advanced HIV (consider for Stage A1 patients) • Immunosuppressed • Close contact with a person who is immunosuppressed • Pregnancy • Receiving salicylates

IVIG, intravenous immunoglobulin.

TABLE 11-20 PRE-/POSTEXPOSURE PROPHYLAXIS/TREATMENT

DISEASE	TREATMENT FOR PATIENT (EITHER INFECTED OR PRE-EXPOSURE)	TREATMENT FOR CONTACT (POSTEXPOSURE)	TIME CONSTRAINTS	COMMENTS
Diphtheria	• Erythromycin, antitoxin, vaccine (DTaP, DT, or dT, as appropriate) if not up to date	• Erythromycin, and vaccine if not up to date	• As soon as index case identified	• If compliance with erythromycin not assured, can give penicillin IM × 1 • Erythromycin is to eradicate nasal carriage
Influenza	• Influenza A: amantadine or oseltmavir • Influenza B: oseltmavir (age 1 y and older) or zanamivir (12 y and older)	• Amantadine (influenza A only) • Oseltmavir (influenza A and B)	• Start treatment for patient within 48 h for maximum efficacy	• Influenza vaccine *most effective* pre-exposure prophylaxis • Consider drug prophylaxis only in patients who are high risk: immunocompromised, health care worker, institutionalized, and lung/cardiac disease
Hepatitis A	• Pre-exposure: - Age <2 y: Hep A Ig ->2 y: Hep A vaccine	• Exposed within 2 wk: - Age <2 y: Hep A Ig ->2 y: Hep A Ig and Hep A vaccine • >2 wk after exposure: - Age <2 y: Hep A vaccine ->2 y: no treatment	• Hep A vaccine requires ~2-4 wk to onset of protection; if exposure is imminent (i.e., last-minute travel), give Hep A Ig as well	• For outbreaks in daycare centers with children in diapers, vaccinate ALL attendees and employees, as well as all new attendees and employees for the next 6 wk • If alll children in daycare are toilet trained, only close contacts and children in same room need to receive prophylaxis

(Continued)

TABLE 11-20   PRE-/POSTEXPOSURE PROPHYLAXIS/TREATMENT (CONTINUED)

DISEASE	TREATMENT FOR PATIENT (EITHER INFECTED OR PRE-EXPOSURE)	TREATMENT FOR CONTACT (POSTEXPOSURE)	TIME CONSTRAINTS	COMMENTS

Hepatitis B	• Hep B is a routine childhood immunization
	• Reduce risk by practicing safer sex, and reducing exposure to infective fluids
		• Hep B surface antigen + mother: infant receives HBIg and Hep B vaccine
		• Other exposure (blood products, rape victims):
		  – Nonimmunized/nonimmune: HBIg and Hep B vaccine
		  – Immunized: draw titers; if nonimmune, give HBIg and Hep B vaccine; if immune, no further treatment needed
			• HBIg likely provides ~ 14 d protection, an important point when counseling sexual partners of Hep B+ patients	• Hep B is not contraindication to breast-feeding, and do not need to wait until infant is immunized to begin breast-feeding

HIV	• Reduce risk by practicing safer sex, and reducing exposure to infective fluids	• If HIV status unknown (i.e., rape victim), and/or HIV and high-risk exposure: AZT/3TC +/-additional medication, depending on exposure type, for 4 wk	• AZT/3TC is most effective if initiated within 72 hours • Retest at 1, 3, and 6 mo	• Prophylaxis only indicated if high-risk exposure (i.e., *not* for a drop of blood on intact skin)
Measles	• Measles vaccine is a routine childhood vaccination • If young infant is traveling to measles-endemic area, may give monovalent vaccine as young as 6 mo	• Monovalent measles vaccine may be given to exposed infants as young as 6 mo • IM immunoglobulin	• Ig must be given within 6 d of exposure	• Infants immunized before their first birthday should be reimmunized with MMR according to normal schedule (at least 1 mo apart from initial measles vaccine) • Ig is indicated for nonimmune pregnant women, children less than 1 y old, and the immunocompromised (regardless of vaccine status)

Neisseria meningitidis	• Meningococcal vaccine available for high-risk individuals (asplenic, terminal complement deficiency, properdin deficiency, military recruits); may also be given to travelers and college students	• Rifampin po q 12h × 4 doses *or* • Ceftriaxone IM × 1 *or* • Ciprofloxacin po × 1 (18 y and older) • Eradicates nasal carriage	• Treat as soon as possible	• Don't forget to treat patient for nasal carriage as well • Prophylaxis indicated for CLOSE contacts: household members, child care, nursery schools, or exposure to nasopharyngeal secretions
Rabies	• Rabies vaccine available for high-risk individuals (veterinarians/animal health care workers, people who are leaving to live in endemic countries)	• Thoroughly clean wound • If animal is able to be observed for 10 d: rabies Ig only if animal develops symptoms of rabies • High-risk animal (see list, right), *and* no observation available: rabies IG in 5 doses	• Incubation period for rabies in humans is ~5-6 wk, but is ~4-5 d in most dogs/cats/ferrets • No human has ever fallen ill after the infecting animal was observed to remain healthy for 10 d	• Rodents (including rabbits) generally do *not* carry rabies • Dogs, cats, ferrets, bats, raccoons, foxes, coyotes DO carry rabies (both through bites and scratches contaminated with animal's saliva) • Consider tetanus vaccine
Tetanus	• Tetanus vaccine is a routine childhood vaccination	• Thoroughly clean wound • If tetanus status is unknown, or <3 tetanus vaccines: - Dirty wound: tetanus vaccine and tetanus Ig - Clean wound: tetanus vaccine		• Dirty wounds include those contaminated with dirt, soil, feces, or saliva; burns, frostbite, crush injuries, puncture wounds, and wounds >6 h old • Children <7 y: give DTaP as booster (or DT if pertussis contraindicated)

(Continued)

TABLE 11-20   PRE-/POSTEXPOSURE PROPHYLAXIS/TREATMENT (CONTINUED)

DISEASE	TREATMENT FOR PATIENT (EITHER INFECTED OR PRE-EXPOSURE)	TREATMENT FOR CONTACT (POSTEXPOSURE)	TIME CONSTRAINTS	COMMENTS
Tetanus		• If pt has had ≥3 tetanus vaccines: - Dirty wound: if last tetanus was within 5 y, no further treatment needed; if last dose >5 y ago, give booster - Clean wound: if last tetanus was within 10 y, no further treatment needed; if last dose >10 y ago, give booster		• Children >7 y: give dT as booster
Tuberculosis	• BCG vaccine given overseas, decreases incidence of meningitis, *not* incidence of pulmonary disease	• Exposed to active case: place PPD, start isoniazid • Children aged <4 y should have CXR performed • If repeat PPD in 3 mo is negative, discontinue therapy	• PPD may take up to 3 mo to convert to positive	• Treat for 3 mo even if initial PPD negative • If index case is known to be INH resistant, treat with rifampin
Varicella	• Varicella vaccine is a routine childhood vaccination • Infected patients are contagious 5 d before rash develops	• VZV vaccine • High-risk patients: VZIg • Quarantine high-risk patients who are exposed from postexposure days 8-21 (extended to day 28 if received VZIg, which prolongs incubation period)	• Vaccine must be given within 72 h • VZIg must be given within 96 h	• High-risk patients include: - Immunocompromised patients - Susceptible pregnant women - Any infant <28 wk gestation or <100 g - Infants >28 wk gestation with nonimmune mother - Infants whose mother developed VZV 5 d before delivery or 2 d after delivery

BCG, bacille Calmette-Guérin; CXR, chest radiograph; DTaP, diphtheria tetanus acellular pertussis; DT, diphtheria and tetanus (>7y); dT, diphtheria and tetanus (>7y); HB, hepatitis B, Hep, hepatitis; Ig, immunoglobulin; PPD, purified protein derivative; VZV, varicella zoster virus.

CHAPTER 12

HEMATOLOGY

TABLE 12-1.   *CLASSIFICATION OF ANEMIA*

Microcytic Anemia

IRON DEFICIENCY ANEMIA

ETIOLOGY: Iron deficiency is the most common cause of anemia worldwide. It is most frequently diagnosed between 6 and 24 months of age, due to depletion of iron stores combined with rapid growth and poor iron intake. There is a second peak during adolescence, due to acceleration of growth and loss of blood during menses.

TABLE 12-2.   *CAUSES OF IRON DEFICIENCY ANEMIA*

CLINICAL PRESENTATION: The dietary history is often significant for limited consumption of iron-rich foods (examples: meats, vegetables, fortified cereals). In newborns and infants, there may be a history of formula intolerance or consumption of large amounts of cow's milk, suggesting cow protein milk allergy and subsequent blood loss. Signs and symptoms in a child vary from the asymptomatic, to pallor, irritability and developmental delay. The anemia is usually discovered on routine screening blood

TABLE 12-1   *CLASSIFICATION OF ANEMIA*

MICROCYTIC	NORMOCYTIC	MACROCYTIC
• Iron deficiency	• Anemia of chronic disease	• B_{12} deficiency
• Thalassemia	• Early lead poisoning	• Folate deficiency
• Lead poisoning	• Early iron deficiency	• Reticulocytosis
• Copper deficiency	• Sickle cell anemia	
• Hereditary spherocytosis	• Renal failure	
• Sideroblastic		

TABLE 12-2	*CAUSES OF IRON DEFICIENCY ANEMIA*
Inadequate dietary intake	
Excessive cow's milk intake	
Gastrointestinal blood loss	
Protein intolerance	
Hemolytic anemia	
Pulmonary hemosiderosis	
Small bowel disease	
Chronic phlebotomy	

work. A history of chronic blood loss or guaiac-positive stools may also be present. In developing countries, hookworm infection is a major cause of iron deficiency.

TABLE 12-3.   *DIAGNOSIS OF IRON DEFICIENCY ANEMIA*

TREATMENT: Treatment is preceded by an investigation of the cause of the iron-deficient state. A routine CBC with both a serum iron level and saturation is generally sufficient (Table 12-3). Patients with suspected cow's milk protein allergy and associated blood loss should be changed to a diet consisting of a soy-based or elemental formula. Formula-fed infants should receive adequate iron fortification. Children who remain deficient should receive additional oral iron supplementation (4-6 mg elemental iron/kg/day).

LEAD POISONING

INCIDENCE: Estimates indicate that several million children in the United States have elevated lead levels (>15 μg/dL), and a smaller, but significant, number of children have levels over 25 μg/dL. The overall incidence in the United States is decreasing.

ETIOLOGY: Lead interferes with hemoglobin synthesis resulting in increased heme precursors and decreased hemoglobin production. Sources of intake include contaminated soil, paint (older houses), pipes made with lead soldering (older houses), lead-glazed pottery, or folk remedies.

TABLE 12-4.   *SIGNS AND SYMPTOMS OF LEAD POISONING*

DIAGNOSIS: The serum lead concentration obtained via venipuncture is preferred; fingerstick determinations can be falsely elevated by dust if the hand is not properly cleaned. Microcytic anemia with basophilic stippling may be present on the peripheral smear. Elevated free erythrocyte protoporphyrin (FEP) and zinc protoporphyrin (ZPP) may be present. An abdominal radiograph may reveal opaque lead particles in the gastrointestinal tract from an acute ingestion.

TREATMENT: The Centers for Disease Control and Prevention(CDC) recommends chelation therapy for serum lead concentration greater than 45 μg/dL. Oral chelation

TABLE 12-3   *DIAGNOSIS OF IRON DEFICIENCY ANEMIA*

Hemoglobin	↓
Mean corpuscular volume	↓
Serum iron	↓
Iron saturation	↓
Total iron-binding capacity	↑
Red cell distribution width	↑
Reticulocyte count	↓

TABLE 12-4   *SIGNS AND SYMPTOMS OF LEAD POISONING*

Abdominal pain

Anorexia

Chronic vomiting

Constipation

Microcytic anemia

Behavioral changes

Developmental delay

Speech delay

Sensorineural hearing loss

Encephalopathy

Seizures

Cerebral edema

Lethargy

therapy with succimer (DMSA), dimercaprol (BAL), or edetate calcium-disodium (EDTA) is employed depending upon severity of toxicity. Evaluation of the home environment with the assistance of the local health authorities is also important.

Macrocytic Anemia

TABLE 12-5.   *FOLATE DEFICIENCY VS. VITAMIN B$_{12}$ DEFICIENCY*

TABLE 12-5   *FOLATE DEFICIENCY VS. VITAMIN B$_{12}$ DEFICIENCY*

	FOLATE DEFICIENCY	**VITAMIN B$_{12}$ DEFICIENCY**
Characteristics	• Arrest of erythrocyte maturation	• Arrest of methionine formation
History	• Goat's milk diet • Broad-spectrum antibiotic use • Methotrexate use • Anticonvulsant use	• Small bowel disease • Bowel resection • Short gut syndrome • Celiac disease • Irritable bowel syndrome • Infection with the fish tapeworm *Diphyllobothrium latum*
Clinical presentation	• Glossitis • Megaloblastic anemia	• Pernicious anemia • Megaloblastic anemia • Demyelination of the dorsal column • Ataxia • Defects in proprioception • Defects in vibratory sensation
Diagnosis	• Red cell folate level • Hypersegmented neutrophils are seen on a peripheral blood smear	• Serum B$_{12}$ level • Schilling test: differentiates nutritional deficiency from intrinsic factor (IF) deficiency • Hypersegmented neutrophils are seen on a peripheral blood smear
Treatment	• Folate supplementation	• Parenteral B$_{12}$ supplementation

HEMOGLOBINOPATHIES

DEFINITION: A structural defect in hemoglobin production resulting in defective red blood cell formation and function.

TABLE 12-6.   *CLASSIFICATION OF HEMOGLOBIN*

THALASSEMIA

INCIDENCE: Varies with ethnicity. Beta thalassemia is most common in Italian, Greek, and African patients; alpha thalassemia is most common in African and Chinese patients. In North America, 20% of Asian immigrants have evidence of alpha thalassemia disease, and up to 6% of Mediterranean immigrants have evidence of beta thalassemia.

TABLE 12-6	CLASSIFICATION OF HEMOGLOBIN

TYPE	CHARACTERISTICS
A	• Predominant type of adult hemoglobin • Made up of 4 polypeptide chains, 2 α and 2 β chains
A$_2$	• Minor component of adult hemoglobin (~3%) • Made up of 2 α and 2 δ chains
C	• Most common in African Americans • Made up of 2 α and 2 abnormal β chains • May be homozygous (CC), combined with normal hemoglobin (HbC), or combined with sickle hemoglobin (Hb SC disease)
E	• Most common in persons from Southeast Asia • Made up of 2 α chains and 2 abnormal β chains
F	• Fetal hemoglobin • Made up of 2 α chains as those in HbA, plus 2 γ chains • The γ chain only differs from HbA by a few amino acids • Oxygen affinity of HbF is ↑ due to ↑ 2-3 diphosphoglycerate • Facilitates enhanced transplacental transport of oxygen to the fetus
H	• Most common in Asians • Made up of 4 β chains
S	• Sickle hemoglobin

Hb, hemoglobin.

ETIOLOGY: There is reduced or absent production of one or more hemoglobin chains. Adult hemoglobin normally consists of 4 chains (see Table 12-6). Thalassemia is a deficiency of one or more of these hemoglobin chains.

CLINICAL PRESENTATION: The patient presents with microcytic anemia, pallor, jaundice, and hepatosplenomegaly. A family history of anemia is frequent. Children with thalassemia develop characteristic "chipmunk" facies and frontal bossing due to bone marrow expansion. Recognize that prenatal fetal hemoglobin (HbF) is protective against the anemia and infants are usually free of symptoms until the transition of HbF to HbA at approximately 6 months of age. Some children may have delayed onset of this transition and present years later.

DIAGNOSIS: Hemoglobin electrophoresis is the gold standard. A peripheral blood smear reveals hypochromic, microcytic red blood cells. Tear drop and target cells may also be present.

TABLE 12-7.   *DIAGNOSIS OF THALASSEMIA*

TABLE 12-8.   *CLASSIFICATION OF THALASSEMIA*

TABLE 12-7	*DIAGNOSIS OF THALASSEMIA*
Hemoglobin	↓
Mean corpuscular volume	↓
Serum iron	↑
Iron saturation	↑
Total iron-binding capacity	↓
Red cell distribution width	↔
Reticulocyte count	↓
Red blood cells	↑

TABLE 12-8	*CLASSIFICATION OF THALASSEMIA*
CLASSIFICATION	**CHARACTERISTICS**
β-thalassemia trait	• Heterozygotes • Loss of one of the 2 β globin genes • ↓ HbA • ↑ HbA$_2$ • ↑ HbF • No evidence of clinical disease

TABLE 12-8	*CLASSIFICATION OF THALASSEMIA (CONTINUED)*

CLASSIFICATION	CHARACTERISTICS
β-thalassemia major	• Homozygotes • Loss of both β globin genes • ↓↓ HbA • ↓↓ HbA$_2$ • ↑↑ HbF • Severe clinical disease • Iron overload • Hemolytic anemia • Growth delay • Bone marrow expansion • Transfusion dependence • Chelation therapy
α-thalassemia trait	• Reduced synthesis of 2 α globin genes • Mild microcytic anemia
Hemoglobin H disease	• Loss of 3 of the 4 α globin genes • Severe impairment of globin synthesis • Excess tetramers of the β globin are produced (HbH) • ↑ HbF • Moderate microcytic anemia • Hemolytic anemia
Hydrops fetalis	• The most severe form of α-thalassemia • Loss of 4 α globin genes • Formation of excess γ globin chains (Bart hemoglobin) • ↓↓ HbA • ↓↓ HbA$_2$ • ↓↓ HbF • Catastrophic anemia • Edema • High-output cardiac failure • Neonatal demise

Hb, hemoglobin.

TREATMENT: Severity of disease directs treatment. Mild disease and asymptomatic carriers require no treatment. Those with thalassemia major require regular, frequent transfusions to prevent the development of extramedullary hematopoiesis, coarse facial features, and hepatosplenomegaly. The cumulative effect of repetitive transfusion is iron overload and resultant hemosiderosis. Iron chelation therapy for iron overload is mandatory. Splenectomy should be considered in moderate to severe cases. Patients with thalassemia major are at an increased risk for the development of postsplenectomy syndrome. This syndrome is characterized by severe infections with encapsulated organisms (*S. pneumoniae*, *H. influenzae*, *N. meningitidis*). Genetic counseling should be provided to affected individuals and prospective partners.

SICKLE CELL DISEASE (SCD)

INCIDENCE: 1 in 375 African American births.

ETIOLOGY: Transmission is by autosomal recessive inheritance. Patients with the disease are homozygous (one defective gene from each parent), while carriers are heterozygous (inheriting one defective gene and one normal gene). The defect results from substitution of the amino acid valine for glutamine in the sixth position of the beta globin chain on chromosome 11. The resultant product, hemoglobin S (HbS), has a shorter life span than normal hemoglobin (HbA) and irreversibly polymerizes at low oxygen tension. The defective hemoglobin is predisposed to clogging the microvasculature, producing the classic constellation of symptoms.

CLINICAL PRESENTATION: As with thalassemia, HbF is protective in infants. Children generally remain asymptomatic until after 6 months of age. Coexisting beta-thalassemia results in a less severe anemia, less hemoglobin polymerization, and fewer episodes of crisis. Children with sickle cell disease have impaired splenic function and are susceptible to an increased risk for infection.

TABLE 12-9.   *SIGNS AND SYMPTOMS OF SICKLE CELL DISEASE*

DIAGNOSIS: Hemoglobin electrophoresis is the gold standard for diagnosis. A microscopic analysis of the peripheral smear reveals sickle cells. Sickle cells are generally not seen in individuals with heterozygous trait. Newborn screening tests are in place in most states; however, false-negatives may occur due to the very small amount of HbS present at birth.

TABLE 12-10.   *DIAGNOSIS OF SICKLE CELL DISEASE*

TABLE 12-11.   *COMPLICATIONS OF SICKLE CELL DISEASE*

TABLE 12-9	SIGNS AND SYMPTOMS OF SICKLE CELL DISEASE

Abdominal pain

Splenomegaly (early)

Asplenia (late)

Gall stones

Back pain

Hemolysis

Vascular occlusion

Respiratory distress

Dactylitis

Headache

Pneumonia

Pallor

Scleral icterus

Cholecystitis

Osteomyelitis

TABLE 12-10	DIAGNOSIS OF SICKLE CELL DISEASE

Hemoglobin	↓
Mean corpuscular volume	↔ ↑
Reticulocyte count	↑
Red blood cells	↓

TREATMENT AND PROPHYLAXIS: Routine office visits and preventive health care maintenance are important. Antibacterial prophylaxis with penicillin VK starting at the time of diagnosis is standard practice. Pneumococcal and yearly influenza vaccines are administered to prevent life-threatening infections (the leading cause of death in sickle cell patients). Folic acid supplementation is also recommended. Hydroxyurea, an antineoplastic medication that may promote hemoglobin F synthesis, has also been used with some success. Bone marrow transplantation is curative.

TABLE 12-12. *SELECTED DEFECTS OF HEMATOPOIESIS*

TABLE 12-11   *COMPLICATIONS OF SICKLE CELL DISEASE (SCD)*

COMPLICATION	NOTES
Acute chest syndrome	• The leading cause of death in SCD • Dyspnea, fever, chest pain, tachypnea, hypoxemia • Treat with hydration, antibiotics and oxygen supplementation as needed • Add antibiotic coverage for atypical pneumonias (*Mycoplasma*) • Blood transfusions are often necessary in severe cases
Aplastic crisis	• Parvovirus B19 is the most common cause • Blood transfusions are often necessary in severe cases
Splenic sequestration	• Rapid, worsening anemia • Thrombocytopenia may be present • High incidence of recurrent episodes • Splenectomy may be necessary to prevent recurrence • Treat with hydration
Vaso-occlusive crisis	• Common first presenting sign of the disease • Very painful • Treat with hydration, analgesics, and oxygen supplementation as needed • Blood transfusions are often necessary in severe cases
Osteomyelitis	• *S. aureus* is the most common cause of osteomyelitis in SCD • *Salmonella* is another important cause of osteomyelitis in SCD
Dactylitis	• Painful swelling of the hands and feet • Common first presenting sign of SCD • Treat with analgesics and hydration
Priapism	• Very painful • Treat with IV hydration, analgesics, and oxygen supplementation as needed • Blood transfusions are often necessary in severe refractory cases
Stroke	• Treat with IV hydration and oxygen supplementation as needed • Blood transfusion is often necessary in severe cases
Infection with encapsulated organisms	• *S. pneumoniae* • *H. influenzae* • *N. meningitidis*
Avascular necrosis of the hip	• Presents with limping and knee pain

TABLE 12-12   *SELECTED DEFECTS OF HEMATOPOIESIS*

DEFECT	NOTES
Cyclic neutropenia	• Autosomal dominant • Neutropenia occurs every 18-21 d • Neutropenia accompanied by fever, oral ulcers, and malaise • Other cell lines may also be depressed (platelets, monocytes, lymphocytes) • Patients often have poor dentition from *C. perfringens* • Treat with granulocyte colony-stimulating factor (G-CSF)
Transient erythroblastopenia of childhood	• Follows a viral infection • Acquired depression of red cells only • Mean onset age 18-24 mo • Platelets and white count remain normal • Reticulocyte count will be low in early stages of disease, and increases as disease resolves • Normocytic anemia; may be asymptomatic until reaches severely low levels • Recovery within 2 mo is usual
Diamond-Blackfan anemia	• Congenital hypoplastic microcytic anemia • Family history in 20% • Mean age at presentation 2 mo • $\downarrow$ reticulocyte count, $\uparrow$ HbF • 20% have other congenital anomalies (dysmorphic facies, upper limb/hand defects) • Bone marrow shows nearly absent red cell precursors
Fanconi anemia	• Autosomal recessive • Pancytopenia, radial/thumb anomalies, short stature, café-au-lait spots • Chromosomal fragility, increased risks of malignancy (leukemias) • Bone marrow transplantation can be curative

HEMOLYTIC ANEMIA

HEREDITARY SPHEROCYTOSIS

DEFINITION: A structural red blood cell membrane disorder that results in a hemolytic anemia and splenic sequestration.

INCIDENCE: Most common hemolytic anemia in Northern Europeans, with a reported prevalence of 1 in 5000 in this population.

ETIOLOGY: Transmission is by autosomal dominant fashion in 75% of cases. An intracorpuscular membrane defect in spectrin or ankrin results in osmotic damage to the red blood cell membrane, resulting in intravascular hemolysis. The damaged red blood cells are sequestered and removed by the spleen.

CLINICAL PRESENTATION: A family history of splenectomy is often present. The clinical course is highly variable. Children generally present with hemolytic anemia, splenomegaly, abdominal pain, and jaundice. Severe cases may present with hyperbilirubinemia of the newborn. Gallstones are a common complication of the disease.

DIAGNOSIS: The osmotic fragility test measures the ability of the red blood cell membrane to withstand lysis in varying degrees of hypotonic solution. A peripheral blood smear reveals small spherical cells that lack normal biconcavity. The mean corpuscular hemoglobin concentration (MCHC) is elevated.

TABLE 12-13. *DIAGNOSIS OF HEREDITARY SPHEROCYTOSIS*

TREATMENT: Blood transfusions are indicated for severe anemia. Splenectomy is the treatment of choice for moderate to severe disease and may significantly improve quality of life.

GLUCOSE-6-PHOSPHATE DEHYDROGENASE DEFICIENCY (G-6PD)

DEFINITION: The enzyme glucose-6-phosphate dehydrogenase aids in the reduction of free radicals generated in the presence of oxidative stress. Deficiency of this enzyme leads to the generation of free radicals and hemolysis.

TABLE 12-13	*DIAGNOSIS OF HEREDITARY SPHEROCYTOSIS*
Hemoglobin	↔ ↓
Mean corpuscular volume	↓
Reticulocyte count	↑
Mean corpuscular hemoglobin concentration	↑

TABLE 12-14	*COMMON CAUSES OF HEMOLYSIS IN G-6PD DEFICIENCY*

Acute illness

Stress

Fava beans

Sulfur-containing antibiotics

Aspirin

Vitamin K analogues

Antimalarials

Methylene blue

CLINICAL PRESENTATION: The patient will present with an occasional mild hemolytic anemia when exposed to certain medications or foods. Pallor, jaundice, hyperbilirubinemia, dark urine, abdominal pain, back pain, and shock may be present in varying degrees.

TABLE 12-14. *COMMON CAUSES OF HEMOLYSIS IN G-6PD DEFICIENCY*

DIAGNOSIS: Made by assaying levels of G-6PD on a fresh blood sample.

TREATMENT: Prevention of hemolytic crisis by avoiding causes of hemolysis is important. Supportive care with hydration and blood product transfusion during the acute episode is often sufficient. G-6PD deficiency should be considered in neonates presenting with hyperbilirubinemia. G-6PD–deficient infants should be monitored carefully and phototherapy should be initiated early in the course.

BLEEDING DISORDERS

TABLE 12-15. *COMMON BLEEDING DISORDERS*

IMMUNE THROMBOCYTOPENIC PURPURA (ITP)

DEFINITION: A condition of isolated autoimmune platelet destruction.

ETIOLOGY: Circulating platelet antibodies bind to platelets, causing them to be removed in the spleen. Most patients recall a preceding viral syndrome up to 1 week prior to the presentation, suggesting an immune process.

PRESENTATION: The condition affects males and females equally. The patient presents with acute bruising, epistaxis, and diffuse petechiae. The bruising is often present in areas where trauma is not common.

TABLE 12-15   *COMMON BLEEDING DISORDERS*

	HEMOPHILIA A	HEMOPHILIA B	FACTOR XI DEFICIENCY	VON WILLEBRAND DISEASE
Deficiency	• Quantitative deficiency of factor VIII	• Quantitative deficiency of factor IX	• Quantitative deficiency of factor XI	• Quantitative deficiency of von Willebrand factor
Inheritance	• X-linked recessive	• X-linked recessive	• Variable modes	• Autosomal dominant
Common presentation	• Neonatal bleeding • Easy bruising • Hemarthrosis • Prolonged PTT, normal PT	• Neonatal bleeding • Easy bruising • Hemarthrosis • Prolonged PTT, normal PT	• Prolonged/heavy bleeding after dental extraction • Prolonged PTT, normal PT	• Mucosal bleeding • Prolonged/heavy bleeding with menses • Prolonged bleeding after dental extraction • Prolonged PTT, normal PT
Treatment	• Factor replacement • Desmopressin	• Factor replacement	• Fresh frozen plasma	• Cryoprecipitate

PT, prothrombin time; PTT, partial thromboplastin time.

DIAGNOSIS: Isolated severe decrease in platelet count. Bone marrow aspirate or biopsy is rarely indicated.

TREATMENT: Avoid antiplatelet medications. Options include corticosteroids and/or intravenous immunoglobulin (IVIG), both of which act to decrease the process of antibody-mediated platelet destruction. Anti-D immune globulin has been used as well. Splenectomy should be considered in refractory cases. Platelet transfusions are indicated in life-threatening emergencies (e.g., intracranial hemorrhage). Precaution against trauma is necessary until the platelet count returns to near normal.

CHAPTER 13

ONCOLOGY

LEUKEMIA

ACUTE LYMPHOBLASTIC LEUKEMIA (ALL)

DEFINITION: A malignant disorder of lymphocyte development and regulation. It is the most common malignancy of childhood.

ETIOLOGY: Multifactorial with a genetic predisposition. There is a peak incidence between 2 and 6 years of age. There is an increased risk in males, Caucasians, and children with Down and Fanconi syndromes.

TABLE 13-1	SIGNS AND SYMPTOMS OF ACUTE LYMPHOBLASTIC LEUKEMIA

Pallor

Fatigue

Fever

Bruising

Petechiae

Mucosal bleeding

Epistaxis

Lymphadenopathy

Hepatosplenomegaly

Leukopenia

Thrombocytopenia

Anemia

DIAGNOSIS: Suggested on peripheral blood count and smear by the presence of suppression of at least one major cell line (leukopenia, anemia, thrombocytopenia) and the presence of circulating blasts. Diagnosis is made definitively by bone marrow aspiration and biopsy.

TABLE 13-2. *PROGNOSTIC FACTORS FOR ACUTE LYMPHOBLASTIC LEUKEMIA*

TREATMENT: Chemotherapy. There is a role for allogeneic bone marrow transplantation in relapsed ALL or those with Philadelphia chromosome [9:22] markers.

ACUTE MYELOGENOUS LEUKEMIA (AML)

DEFINITION: A malignant disorder affecting myeloid differentiation during hematopoiesis. AML is much less common than ALL (approximately 500 children are diagnosed per year in the United States).

ETIOLOGY: Multifactorial with a genetic predisposition. There is an increased risk in children with Down syndrome, Fanconi anemia, and radiation exposure, and in those who have received prior chemotherapy.

CLINICAL PRESENTATION: Symptoms are similar to the presentation of ALL. They often correlate with the suppression of hematopoietic cell lines (anemia, pallor, bruising, petechiae; fever, splenomegaly, and lymphadenopathy). There are some variants of promyelocytic AML that may present with disseminated intravascular coagulation (DIC.)

DIAGNOSIS: The diagnosis of AML is made by bone marrow aspiration and biopsy revealing a homogeneous population of myeloblasts. The presence of Auer rods (small, pink intracellular inclusions) is pathognomonic for AML. The diagnosis

TABLE 13-2 *PROGNOSTIC FACTORS FOR ACUTE LYMPHOBLASTIC LEUKEMIA*

CRITERIA	STANDARD RISK	HIGH RISK
Age at diagnosis	1-10 y	<1 y, >10 y
WBC at presentation	<50,000/mL	>50,000/mL
Cytogenetic markers	• Trisomy 4,10,17 • Translocation [12:21]	• Trisomy 5 • Translocation [8:14], [9:22], [4:11], [1:19]
Prognosis	80%-85% 5-y survival	Variable, but poorer than standard-risk patients

may also be suggested on peripheral blood smear by the suppression of at least one major cell line (leukopenia, anemia, thrombocytopenia) with the presence of circulating blasts.

TREATMENT: Chemotherapy to induce remission is standard. Increased disease-free survival has been seen with allogeneic bone marrow transplantation. The 5-year survival is considerably less than that of ALL, possibly reaching 50%. Poor prognostic indicators include a presenting white blood cell count higher than 100,000/mL, monosomy 7, and the development of AML as a secondary malignancy.

TUMOR LYSIS SYNDROME

DEFINITION: Hyperkalemia, hyperphosphatemia, and hyperuricemia occurring as a result of rapid tumor lysis. It is most common with leukemia, lymphoma, and malignancies with a high circulating blast count.

ETIOLOGY: The rapid destruction of malignant blasts releases cell contents. May be spontaneous or induced by chemotherapy.

TABLE 13-3	*METABOLIC SIGNS OF TUMOR LYSIS SYNDROME*
ABNORMALITY	**TREATMENT/NOTES**
Hyperuricemia	• Hydration • Allopurinol (xanthine oxidase inhibitor) - Prevents formation of new uric acid
Hyperphosphatemia	• Hydration • Phosphate-binding resins
Hyperkalemia	• Hydration • Calcium gluconate (stabilizes myocardial cells) • Potassium-binding resins • Loop diuretics • Inhalational beta agonists • Insulin, glucose

Hypocalcemia	• Hydration
	• Calcium supplementation only if:
	  - Symptomatic hyperkalemia
	  - Symptomatic hypocalcemia

TREATMENT: The most important first-line therapy is vigorous hydration. Tumor lysis syndrome can rapidly progress to acute renal failure warranting emergent dialysis.

SOLID TUMORS

TABLE 13-4   *NEUROBLASTOMA VS. WILMS TUMOR*

	NEUROBLASTOMA	WILMS TUMOR
Definition	• Malignant proliferation of neural crest cells	• Malignant proliferation of nephrons
Age at onset	• Median age 1.5 y	• Median age 4 y

Presentation	• Abdominal mass
	• Fever
	• Weight loss
	• Hypertension
	• Opsoclonus (dancing eyes)
	• Myoclonus (dancing feet)
	• Periorbital ecchymosis (from tumor spread)
	• Horner syndrome
		• Abdominal flank mass
		• Fever
		• Weight loss
		• Hematuria
		• Hemihypertrophy
		• Associated with:
		  - Aniridia
		  - Hypospadias
		  - Solitary kidney

Diagnosis	• Ultrasound • CT scan • Tumor biopsy • Mass arises from adrenals, sympathetic nerve chain • Increased urinary catecholamines (homovanillic and vanillylmandelic acid) • Mass crosses the midline • Often metastatic at diagnosis • MIBG scan positive	• Ultrasound • CT scan • Tumor biopsy • Mass arises from kidneys • Mass usually does not cross the midline • Variable metastatic disease • MIBG scan negative • Defect on chromosome 11

TABLE 13-4 *NEUROBLASTOMA VS. WILMS TUMOR (CONTINUED)*

	NEUROBLASTOMA	WILMS TUMOR
Treatment	• Chemotherapy • Excisional surgery • Radiation therapy	• Excisional surgery • Chemotherapy • Radiation therapy

Prognosis	• Poor prognosis associated with:
	  1. N-myc amplification
	  2. Increased serum ferritin
	• Earlier stages: 90% 3-y survival
	• Advanced stages: 30%-40% 3-y survival
		• Earlier stages: 90% 3-y survival

MIBG, metaiodobenzyl guanidine.

SKELETAL TUMORS

TABLE 13-5 *OSTEOSARCOMA VS. EWING SARCOMA*

	OSTEOSARCOMA	EWING SARCOMA
Definition	• A malignant tumor of osteoid origin • Most common malignancy of bone in children	• A small round cell bone tumor of neural crest cells • Second most common malignancy of bone in children
Age at onset	Second decade of life	70% <20 y of age
Presentation	• Fever • Weight loss • Bone pain	• Fever • Weight loss • Bone pain

(Continued)

TABLE 13-5   *OSTEOSARCOMA VS. EWING SARCOMA (CONTINUED)*

	OSTEOSARCOMA	EWING SARCOMA

Diagnosis	• X-ray "<u>sunburst</u>" appearance
	• Lytic erosive lesion (metaphysis)
	• MRI
	• Biopsy
	• Most common sites:
	  1. Distal femur
	  2. Proximal tibia
	  3. Proximal humerus
		• X-ray "<u>onion skin</u>" appearance
		• Lytic erosive lesion (diaphysis)
		• MRI
		• Biopsy
		• Most common sites:
		  1. Distal extremities
		  2. Proximal extremities
		  3. Pelvis

Treatment	• Chemotherapy • Surgical resection • Limb salvage	• Chemotherapy • Radiation therapy • Surgical resection
Prognosis	• Approximately 60%-70% 5-y survival (without metastatic disease)	• Approximately 50%-85% 2-y survival (without metastatic disease)

SIGNS AND SYMPTOMS

TABLE 13-6   *CAUSES OF AN ANTERIOR MEDIASTINAL MASS*

"THE FOUR T's"
Thymoma
Teratoma
Thyroid disease
Terrible lymphoma

| TABLE 13-7 | *CAUSES OF LYMPHADENOPATHY* |

Malignant
  Lymphoma
  Leukemia
  Other malignancy
Infectious
  Bacterial lymphadenitis
  Viral syndrome
  Infectious mononucleosis
  Cytomegalovirus
  Toxoplasmosis
  Tuberculosis
  Dental abscess
  Cat scratch disease
  Syphilis
  Herpes simplex virus
  Rubella
  Human immunodeficiency virus
  Coccidioidomycosis
  Histoplasmosis
  Blastomycosis
  Plague
Inflammatory
  Systemic lupus erythematosus
  Juvenile rheumatoid arthritis
  Kawasaki syndrome

TABLE 13-8	*CAUSES OF HEPATOSPLENOMEGALY*

Extramedullary hematopoiesis

Lymphoma

Leukemia

Lymphoproliferative disorder

Malignancy

Infectious mononucleosis

Cytomegalovirus

Human immunodeficiency virus

Toxoplasmosis

Sickle cell disease

Thalassemia

Gaucher disease

Hemochromatosis

Biliary atresia

Budd-Chiari syndrome

Galactosemia

Congestive heart failure

Cardiogenic shock

TABLE 13-9	*CAUSES OF PETECHIAE*

Viral infection (most common cause)

Malignancy

Aplastic anemia

Medications

Sepsis

Early meningococcemia

Rickettsial infections (Rocky Mountain spotted fever)

Immune thrombocytopenic purpura

Disseminated intravascular coagulation

Systemic lupus erythematosus

Juvenile rheumatoid arthritis

CHAPTER 14

ENDOCRINOLOGY

Neonatal Physiology

The thyroid gland is the first endocrine gland to develop (24th day of gestation). It originates from pharyngeal epithelium, and is attached to the tongue by the thyroglossal duct. The fetus acquires the ability to synthesize thyroid hormone at 10 to 12 weeks of gestation. Immediately following delivery there is a surge of thyroid-stimulating hormone (TSH), followed by an increase in thyroid hormone that lasts for 24 to 36 hours. Newborn screening for thyroid disorders is performed after 48 hours of life to allow for the resolution of this surge. TSH and thyroid hormone levels in premature infants are lower than term infants and newborn screening in this age group should be interpreted with care.

Postnatal Physiology

TSH is produced by the pituitary gland, and stimulates release of thyroid hormone (thyroxine) from the thyroid gland. There are two general types of thyroid hormone, T3 and T4. The thyroid gland is the primary source for T4. Monodeiodination of T4 in the peripheral tissues largely produces most of the T3 and reverse T3 (rT3). Although T3 is present in a lower concentration than T4, it is more metabolically active. Thyroid hormone is carried in the blood by thyroid-binding globulin (TBG). Disorders of the thyroid can be divided into hypothyroidism and hyperthyroidism.

Hypothyroidism

Hypothyroidism is defined as deficient synthesis or activity of thyroid hormone. The etiology may be congenital or acquired.

CONGENITAL HYPOTHYROIDISM

ETIOLOGY: Congenital hypothyroidism occurs in 1 out of every 4000 live births. The most frequent cause (85%) is dysgenesis of the thyroid gland. Other important causes include defective synthesis of thyroxine and thyroglobulin, and defective TSH production due to hypothalamic/pituitary defects. Transient congenital hypothyroidism may occur secondary to maternal factors including TSH receptor-blocking antibody, ingestion of antithyroid medication, radiation treatment, or severe iodine deficiency. Hypothyroid newborns are often overweight (more than 4 kg), and are frequently postmature (gestational age >42 weeks).

TABLE 14-1.   *SIGNS AND SYMPTOMS OF CONGENITAL HYPOTHYROIDISM*

DIAGNOSIS: Most newborn infants with hypothyroidism appear normal. Newborn screening consists of a two-tiered laboratory approach. First, T4 is measured on filter paper blood spot. If the T4 level is less than the 10th percentile, the second step is the measurement of TSH on filter paper. If TSH is elevated, a thyroid panel should be obtained for further evaluation. Thyroid ultrasonography and I^{123} scans can confirm the presence of an ectopic gland or thyroid dysgenesis. An abnormal I^{123} scan in the presence of a normal-sized thyroid gland is most consistent with maternal antithyroid antibodies or thyroid dyshormonogenesis.

TREATMENT: Hypothyroid infants should receive hormone replacement with L-thyroxine. Long-term cognitive function should be monitored carefully as thyroid hormone is largely responsible for brain development.

ACQUIRED HYPOTHYROIDISM

Acquired hypothyroidism most frequently occurs after the newborn period and is usually caused by Hashimoto thyroiditis. Other important causes include severe

TABLE 14-1	*SIGNS AND SYMPTOMS OF CONGENITAL HYPOTHYROIDISM*
Poor feeding	
Constipation	
Macroglossia	
Protuberant abdomen	
Umbilical hernia	
Puffy face	
Goiter	
Jaundice	
Hypothermia	
Sepsis	
Large open fontanelles	

iodine deficiency, radiation exposure, antithyroid medications, lithium, infiltrative diseases of the thyroid, and TSH deficiency. TSH deficiency is frequently due to damage to the pituitary from head trauma, tumors, granulomatous disease, infections, irradiation, and postpartum hemorrhage (Sheehan syndrome).

TABLE14-2. *SIGNS AND SYMPTOMS OF ACQUIRED HYPOTHYROIDISM*

HASHIMOTO THYROIDITIS

Hashimoto thyroiditis is the most common thyroid disorder of childhood. This autoimmune disorder is characterized by lymphocytic infiltration of the thyroid gland with associated antithyroid antibodies (specifically, antiperoxidase and antithyroglobulin antibodies). Hashimoto thyroiditis affects girls more frequently than boys with a peak incidence during adolescence. This condition is common in children with Turner and Down syndromes. Diagnosis is made by demonstration of antimicrosomal and antiperoxidase antibodies in the serum. In early stages of disease, T3, T4, TSH, and free T4 (FT4) levels may all be normal. In later stages, hormone levels are usually decreased with an elevated TSH. Treatment is with hormone replacement (L-thyroxine).

Hyperthyroidism

Hyperthyroidism is defined as excess concentrations of free thyroid hormones (usually T4) causing thyrotoxicosis. The condition is usually acquired, but may be present in the newborn period.

TABLE 14-2	*SIGNS AND SYMPTOMS OF ACQUIRED HYPOTHYROIDISM*
Cold intolerance	
Fatigue	
Dry skin	
Constipation	
Weight gain	
Growth failure	
Muscle weakness	
Menstrual irregularities	
Myxedema	
Alopecia	
Developmental problems	
Poor school performance	
Goiter	

ACQUIRED HYPERTHYROIDISM

Nearly 90% of acquired cases of hyperthyroidism are due to Graves disease (toxic nodular goiter). Other important causes include early phases of Hashimoto and de Quervain thyroiditis.

GRAVES DISEASE

DEFINITION: Graves disease is acquired hyperthyroidism due to the stimulation of the thyroid gland by anti-TSH thyroid receptor antibodies.

ETIOLOGY: Graves disease occurs more frequently in girls than boys, with the peak incidence during adolescence.

CLINICAL PRESENTATION: Lid lag and lid retraction are frequently the first symptoms of the disease.

TABLE 14-3.   *SIGNS AND SYMPTOMS OF GRAVES DISEASE*

DIAGNOSIS: The diagnosis of Graves disease is made by demonstration of thyroid receptor, antiperoxidase, and antithyroglobulin antibodies, as well as elevated serum T3 and T4 and decreased TSH levels. Radionuclide scanning reveals increased I^{123} thyroid uptake.

TREATMENT: Treatment options include propylthiouracil (PTU) and methimazole (MMI). PTU blocks the synthesis of T4 to T3 as well as the coupling of iodotyrosines and organic binding of iodide, thereby reducing synthesis of thyroid hormones. MMI blocks

---

TABLE 14-3   *SIGNS AND SYMPTOMS OF GRAVES DISEASE*

Lid retraction
Lid lag
Proptosis
Exophthalmos
Goiter
Weight loss
Heat intolerance
Fatigue
Tachycardia
Diarrhea
Tremors
Hyperreflexia
Proximal muscle weakness
Menstrual irregularities
Poor school performance

the coupling and organic binding of iodine only. PTU is preferred during pregnancy, as it does not cross the placenta. The most frequent side effect of antithyroid medications is granulocytopenia. MMI may cause aplasia cutis of the fetal scalp. Beta blockers are useful for symptomatic relief of tachycardia, palpitations, and anxiety attacks. Radioactive ablation with I^{131} and thyroidectomy are reserved for refractory cases.

DE QUERVAIN THYROIDITIS (TRANSIENT SUBACUTE THYROIDITIS)

de Quervain thyroiditis is a self-limited disorder characterized by painful enlargement of thyroid gland. The etiology is believed to be secondary to viral infection. Presenting symptoms include low-grade fever, earache, neck swelling, and tenderness. The disorder is characterized by an early phase of transient hyperthyroidism, followed by a period of transient hypothyroidism. In contrast to Graves disease, uptake on I^{123} radionuclide scan is decreased due to inflammatory gland destruction. de Quervain patients do not have antithyroid receptor antibodies.

NEONATAL HYPERTHYROIDISM

In neonates, hyperthyroidism is usually transient and found most frequently in children born to mothers with Graves or Hashimoto disease, due to the transplacental passage of TSH receptor antibody.

TABLE 14-4. *SIGNS AND SYMPTOMS OF NEONATAL HYPERTHYROIDISM*

On diagnostic evaluation, the thyroid profile reveals elevated T4 and suppressed TSH. Treatment with iodine, beta blockers, and prednisone may provide symptomatic relief until maternal antibody levels abate. Long-term cognitive function should be carefully monitored.

Thyroid Nodules

Thyroid nodules are usually evaluated by radionuclide scanning. "Hot" nodules (increased uptake) are usually benign; "cold" nodules (decreased uptake) are more worrisome for a malignant process. Papillary carcinoma is the most common type of thyroid cancer in childhood.

TABLE 14-4	SIGNS AND SYMPTOMS OF NEONATAL HYPERTHYROIDISM
	Tachycardia
	Hypertension
	Irritability
	Flushing
	Poor feeding and weight gain
	Craniosynostosis
	Symmetric intrauterine growth retardation
	Goiter

DISORDERS OF THE PARATHYROID GLAND

Parathyroid hormone (PTH) and vitamin D regulate body calcium. Both work together to stimulate osteoclasts to reabsorb calcium and phosphate from the bone. In the kidney, PTH increases calcium absorption and phosphate excretion. PTH also stimulates the production of 1,25-dihydroxyvitamin D (active form of vitamin D). Vitamin D increases the absorption of calcium and phosphate by the intestine.

Hypoparathyroidism

Deficient PTH activity results in hypocalcemia and hyperphosphatemia. Several genetic syndromes are associated with hypoparathyroidism (see below). The disorder may also occur as a transient process in newborns, or as an acquired illness. Most of the symptoms are due to hypocalcemia. Patients with hypoparathyroidism have decreased serum PTH, hypocalcemia, hyperphosphatemia, normal 25-hydroxyvitamin D level, and decreased 1,25-dihydroxyvitamin D levels. Urine testing reveals an increased calcium to creatinine ratio and hypophosphaturia. EKG demonstrates a prolonged Q-T interval. Treatment consists of supplementation with 1,25-dihydroxyvitamin D and calcium.

TABLE 14-5.   *SIGNS AND SYMPTOMS OF HYPOPARATHYROIDISM*
Genetic syndromes are associated with hypoparathyroidism:

* *DiGeorge syndrome* (see Chapter 16) and velocardiofacial syndromes are classically associated with hypoparathyroidism, due to aplasia of the parathyroid glands.
* *Albright hereditary osteodystrophy* (pseudohypoparathyroidism) is caused by a

TABLE 14-5	*SIGNS AND SYMPTOMS OF HYPOPARATHYROIDISM*
Muscle cramps	
Headache	
Hyperreflexia	
Tetany	
Abdominal pain	
Constipation	
Irritability	
Lethargy	
Apneic spells	
Seizures	
Cardiac dysrhythmias	
Delayed eruption of teeth	

defective PTH receptor. Affected patients have short stature, obesity, round face, and short 4th metacarpal. PTH levels are *elevated*, in contrast to other forms of hypoparathyroidism, in which the PTH is low.

- *Familial autoimmune polyglandular syndrome type I* is characterized by Addison disease, hypoparathyroidism, chronic mucocutaneous candidiasis, and vitiligo.

ACQUIRED CAUSES OF HYPOPARATHYROIDISM

Acquired hypoparathyroidism results from destruction of the parathyroid glands. Common causes include surgery and infiltration and destruction of parathyroid glands (i.e., from Wilson disease, hemochromatosis, or radiation). PTH production may also be suppressed in patients with hypomagnesemia.

TRANSIENT HYPOPARATHYROIDISM

Transient hypoparathyroidism is typically found in preterm infants, infants of diabetic mothers, and in maternal hypercalcemia during pregnancy.

Hyperparathyroidism

Hyperparathyroidism results from excessive release of PTH. This condition may also be seen in association with genetic syndromes, as an acquired illness, or in response to primary vitamin D dysregulation. Most symptoms are due to hypercalcemia. Patients with hyperparathyroidism have elevated serum PTH levels, elevated 1,25-dihydroxyvitamin D levels, hypercalcemia, and hypophosphatemia. Urine testing reveals a decreased calcium to creatinine ratio and hyperphosphaturia. EKG demonstrates a short Q-T interval. Treatment consists of the administration of calcium-binding agents and removal of any existing tumors.

TABLE 14-6	SIGNS AND SYMPTOMS OF HYPERPARATHYROIDISM
Weakness	
Weight loss	
Nausea	
Vomiting	
Abdominal pain	
Headache	
Lethargy	
Depression	
Bone pain	

GENETIC CAUSES OF HYPERPARATHYROIDISM

- *Multiple endocrine neoplasia* (MEN) *I and II* are associated with parathyroid adenomas.
- In *familial hypocalciuric hypercalcemia*, PTH production is suppressed by serum hypercalcemia.

ACQUIRED CAUSES OF HYPERPARATHYROIDISM

Parathyroid adenoma is the most common cause of primary hyperparathyroidism in childhood (85% of all cases). Other important causes include hypertrophy of the parathyroid glands and other parathyroid hormone–secreting tumors. Hyperparathyroidism may also occur in patients with chronic renal insufficiency and primary vitamin D deficiency.

DISORDERS OF THE ADRENAL GLAND

FIGURE 14-1. *ADRENAL GLAND.*

FIGURE 14-2. *ADRENAL STEROIDOGENESIS.*

ADDISON DISEASE

DEFINITION: Addison disease is defined as primary adrenocortical deficiency.

ETIOLOGY: Addison disease is caused by the destruction or dysfunction of the adrenal cortex. Both glucocorticoid and mineralocorticoid function are affected. Autoimmune

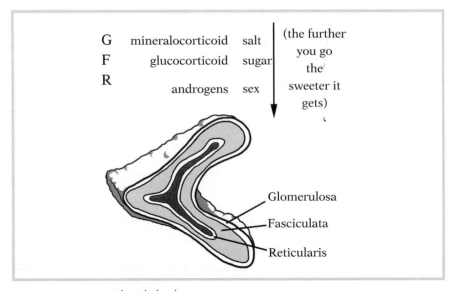

— **FIGURE 14-1** — Adrenal gland.

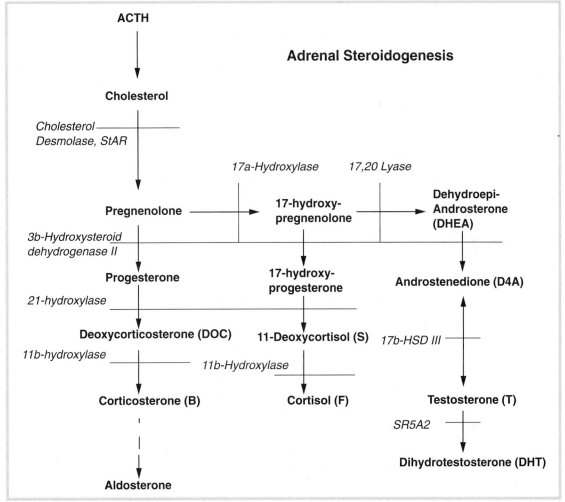

— **FIGURE 14-2** — Adrenal steroidogenesis.

destruction of the adrenal gland accounts for nearly 80% of cases. Other important causes include destruction of the gland by infection (i.e., HIV or tuberculosis), and hemorrhage.

CLINICAL PRESENTATION: Common presenting features include weakness, fatigue, poor appetite, and weight loss. Physical exam reveals hyperpigmentation (exposed skin, palmar creases, pressure areas, knuckles) due to high circulating levels of ACTH. Vitiligo and muscle wasting are frequently present. Adrenal crisis may occur, characterized by nausea, vomiting, diaphoresis, and orthostatic hypotension.

DIAGNOSIS: Laboratory evaluation reveals increased ACTH levels, hyperkalemia, hyponatremia, hypoglycemia, low cortisol, low aldosterone, and elevated renin. Eosinophilia is common.

TREATMENT: Treatment consists of glucocorticoid and mineralocorticoid replacement, with stress doses of glucocorticoids during periods of stress, infection, and adrenal crisis.

CUSHING SYNDROME

ETIOLOGY: This constellation of signs and symptoms occurs after exposure to elevated levels of glucocorticoids. More than 99% of cases are iatrogenic (exogenous), due to administration of steroids. Children with severe asthma and rheumatologic disease are commonly affected. Endogenous (non-iatrogenic) causes of Cushing syndrome are divided into ACTH-dependent and ACTH-independent forms. ACTH-dependent forms usually result from ACTH-producing pituitary tumors. The excess ACTH stimulates increased production of cortisol. ACTH-independent forms result from inappropriately increased production of cortisol by adrenal tumors such as adrenal adenoma and adrenal carcinoma. (Adrenal tumors are the most common cause of Cushing syndrome in infancy and the first few years of life.)

TABLE 14-7.   *SIGNS AND SYMPTOMS OF CUSHING SYNDROME*

DIAGNOSIS: The evaluation of the patient with suspected Cushing syndrome begins with serum cortisol levels. Serum cortisol levels are normally highest in the morning,

TABLE 14-7	*SIGNS AND SYMPTOMS OF CUSHING SYNDROME*
	Moon facies
	Buffalo hump
	Supraclavicular fat pads
	Truncal obesity
	Growth failure
	Purple stretch marks
	Easy bruising
	Osteopenia
	Osteoporosis
	Hypertension
	Hirsutism
	Irregular menses
	Impaired glucose metabolism and hyperglycemia
	Impaired immune function

and lowest in the evening. In patients with Cushing syndrome, both morning and evening serum cortisol levels are elevated. Additionally, 24-hour urinary free cortisol level is also elevated. The dexamethasone suppression test is used in patients with endogenous Cushing syndrome to determine if it is ACTH dependent or independent. In ACTH-dependent Cushing syndrome, cortisol is suppressed by a low-dose dexamethasone test. In ACTH-independent Cushing syndrome, cortisol is suppressed by a high-dose dexamethasone test. Plasma ACTH should also be measured. If a tumor is suspected, imaging studies (i.e., abdominal CT or head MRI) should be performed.

TREATMENT: Treatment is based upon the etiology.

PSEUDO-CUSHING SYNDROME

This condition is diagnosed when a patient's symptoms and laboratory tests reveal abnormalities seen in patients with Cushing syndrome, without elevated glucocorticoid levels. Common causes of pseudo-Cushing syndrome include obesity, anorexia nervosa, depression, and acute stress. Another important cause of pseudo-Cushing syndrome is exposure to alcohol in breast milk.

CONGENITAL ADRENAL HYPERPLASIA (CAH)

CAH occurs in several forms, all linked by impaired glucocorticoid and/or mineralocorticoid synthesis. The disease is inherited in an autosomal recessive fashion. Low cortisol levels cause chronically elevated ACTH and subsequent overstimulation of the dysfunctional adrenal cortical tissue. Of the five main enzymes in the adrenal gland that convert cholesterol into cortisol and aldosterone, deficiency of 21-hydroxylase (OHD) and 11b-hydroxylase are the most frequently encountered and are primary causes of female pseudohermaphroditism. The 21-OHD form is the most common type of CAH (accounting for 90% of cases), occurs late in cortisol synthesis, and causes the channeling of accumulating steroid precursors into androgen synthesis pathways. There are two forms of CAH due to 21-OHD, classical and nonclassical. In classical CAH, there is complete or near complete deficiency of the 21-hydroxylase enzyme and it can present as either salt-wasting or simple virilizing phenotype. Approximately 75% of classical CAH patients have the salt-wasting form resulting from impairment of aldosterone synthesis. In the classical form, 46,XX females present at birth with degrees of virilization of external genitalia ranging from clitoromegaly to a phallic urethra. In the nonclassical form, there is no genital ambiguity at birth.

TABLE 14-8. *CONGENITAL ADRENAL HYPERPLASIA*

PHEOCHROMOCYTOMA

DEFINITION: Pheochromocytoma is a catecholamine-secreting tumor that arises from the chromaffin cells (neural crest derivatives) of the adrenal medulla.

ETIOLOGY: This condition is usually unilateral and occurs in males more often than females, most often before 14 years of age. In children, pheochromocytomas produce mostly norepinephrine. There is a genetic predisposition to pheochromocytoma, and familial cases tend to be bilateral. Diseases commonly associated with pheochromocytoma include neurofibromatosis, von Hippel-Lindau, tuberous sclerosis,

TABLE 14-8   *CONGENITAL ADRENAL HYPERPLASIA (CAH)*

FORM	LABORATORY FINDINGS	SERUM HORMONE LEVELS
21-OHD classic *Salt-wasting form*	• Hyperkalemia • Hyponatremia • Elevated renin	• Increased 17-OHP • Increased androgens • Decreased cortisol • Decreased to absent aldosterone
Simple virilizing form	• Normal aldosterone • Normal renin • Normal electrolytes	• Increased 17-OHP • Increased androgens • Decreased cortisol
21-OHD nonclassic		
11b-OHD	• Hypokalemia • Hypernatremia • Decreased renin	• Increased DOC • Increased androgens • Decreased cortisol • Decreased aldosterone
3-b-HSD	• Hyperkalemia • Hyponatremia	• Increased 17-OHP • Decreased androgens • Increased DHEA • Decreased cortisol • Decreased aldosterone

CLINICAL PRESENTATION	GENITALIA AT BIRTH	NOTES
• 46,XX females may present at birth with virilization of external genitalia ranging from clitoromegaly to phallic urethra • Aldosterone deficiency causes electrolyte imbalance, causing vomiting, failure to thrive, and possibly cardiovascular collapse	• Females appear ambiguous • Males appear normal with hyperpigmentation of scrotum	• 75% of classic CAH patients have salt-wasting form
• 46,XX females may present at birth with virilization as in the salt-wasting form • Postnatal virilization in males	• Females appear ambiguous • Males appear normal with hyperpigmentation of scrotum	• May present in adrenal crisis during stress • Increases in 17-OHP and androgens are markedly higher in simple virilizing form than in nonclassic CAH
• Presents in childhood with growth acceleration and bone advancement • Virilization, amenorrhea, and infertility present later in life	• Normal genitalia at birth in both sexes	• Presents later in life with virilization, amenorrhea, and infertility • This is a milder form of CAH
• Hypertension • Hypokalemic alkalosis	• Females appear ambiguous • Postnatal virilizing in males	• Second most common type of CAH (accounts for 5% of cases)
Early in life: • Weight loss • Dehydration • Salt wasting • Shock • Adrenal crisis • Cardiovascular collapse	• Females: virilization at birth, i.e., clitoromegaly and rarely labial fusion • Males: ambiguous genitalia, micropenis, perineal hypospadias, and bifid scrotum	• Complete loss of enzyme activity is associated with severe salt wasting • Partial loss is usually not associated with salt wasting

(Continued)

TABLE 14-8   *CONGENITAL ADRENAL HYPERPLASIA (CAH) (CONTINUED)*

FORM	LABORATORY FINDINGS	SERUM HORMONE LEVELS
17-OHD	• Hypokalemia • Hypernatremia • Decreased rennin	• Decreased androgens • Decreased cortisol • Increased corticosterone (B) • Increased DOC • Decreased aldosterone
StAR deficiency *(lipoid hyperplasia)*	• Hyperkalemia • Hyponatremia • Elevated renin	• All steroids decreased including aldosterone

ACTH, adrenocorticotrophic hormone; DHEA, dehydroepiandrosterone; DOC, deoxycorticosterone; 21-OHD, 21-hydroxylase; 11b-OH, 11b-hydroxylase; 3-b-HSD, 3b-hydroxysteroid dehydrogenase; 17-OHD, 17-hydroxylase; 17-OH, pregnenolene (precursor of17-OHP); 17-OHP, 17-hydroxyprogesterone; StAR, steroidogenic acute regulatory protein.

Sturge-Weber, and multiple endocrine neoplasias (MEN IIA, MEN IIB). Symptoms often are episodic in nature.

TABLE 14-9.   *COMMON SIGNS AND SYMPTOMS OF PHEOCHROMOCYTOMA*

DIAGNOSIS: The evaluation includes the measurement of urinary catecholamines (epinephrine, norepinephrine), homovanillic acid (HVA), vanillylmandelic acid (VMA), and dopamine and metanephrine in a 24-hour specimen collected during an acute episode. Imaging studies to localize a tumor include abdominal MRI, CT, and I^{131} MIBG scans.

TREATMENT: Surgical removal of the tumor is standard therapy.

CLINICAL PRESENTATION	GENITALIA AT BIRTH	NOTES
• Hypertension • Males present with micropenis, gynecomastia • Females present with primary amenorrhea and lack of secondary sexual characteristics	• Females are normal appearing • Males have a female phenotype with blind-ending vagina, and abdominal or inguinal testis	• 17-hydroxylation is not required for aldosterone synthesis, so only cortisol and androgen synthesis are impaired • Aldosterone levels are decreased because increased DOC suppresses renin
		• Despite cortisol insufficiency, these patients do not experience adrenal crisis because elevated levels of corticosterone induce glucocorticoid activity
• Males present with female genitalia (sex-reversal) • Both sexes present with salt-wasting in infancy	• Females are normal appearing • 46,XY males have female phenotype, underdeveloped Wolffian ducts and severe salt wasting	• Complete deficiency of all adrenal steroid hormones • Most rare and severe defect of adrenal steroidogenesis (fatal in 2/3 of patients during infancy)

TABLE 14-9   *COMMON SIGNS AND SYMPTOMS OF PHEOCHROMOCYTOMA*

Hypertension (uniformly present)
Headaches
Nausea
Vomiting
Abdominal pain
Palpitations
Postural hypotension
Diaphoresis
Pallor

DISORDERS OF SEX DETERMINATION

Human intersex disorders result from discordance between genetic sex, gonadal sex, and sexual phenotype. There is a wide range of disorders, ranging from virilization in otherwise normal females to true hermaphrodism. Disorders of sex differentiation are among the most common birth defects, occurring in about 7 of 1,000 live births.

Fetal Sexual Development

Embryos of both sexes initially develop in an identical fashion. Sex differentiation typically proceeds in the direction of female development unless genes located on the Y chromosome (the sex-determining region of the Y chromosome [SRY]) are activated, prompting male development. The internal genitalia in both sexes arise from a dual duct system—the Wolffian and Müllerian ducts. Once this bipotential gonad is determined to become testes, the differentiation of the genital ducts (internal genitalia) begins through the action of anti-Müllerian hormone (AMH) and testosterone. In males, testosterone is secreted by the Leydig cells and promotes the development of Wolffian duct derivatives (vas deferens, seminal vesicles, and epididymis). In females the absence of testosterone secretion causes regression of Wolffian ducts and development of Müllerian ducts into the uterus, fallopian tubes, and the upper third of the vagina. Unlike internal genitalia, external genitalia in both sexes develop from common lineage (genital tubercle, genital folds and swellings, and urogenital sinus). The genital tubercle is the origin of the clitoris in the female and the glans penis in the male. The urogenital swellings become the labia majora or the scrotum. The genital folds develop into either the labia minora or the shaft of the penis.

Disorders of Gonadal Differentiation

FEMALE PSEUDOHERMAPHRODISM

Female pseudohermaphrodism can best be described as a genetic female (XX) with ambiguous or male virilization of the external genitalia. Ovaries, uterus, and fallopian tubes are present. There are several disorders that present with this phenotype.

- **Complete 46,XX Gonadal Dysgenesis**: The presence of streak gonads, normal internal and external female genitalia, and lack of stigmata of Turner syndrome characterize this phenotype. It is either sporadic or inherited as an autosomal recessive trait.
- **Turner Syndrome**: This disorder typically results from complete or mosaic X monosomy (45,XO or 45,XO/46,XX). Characteristic somatic stigmata include webbing of the neck, broad chest, horseshoe kidneys, cardiovascular abnormalities (aortic stenosis), and short stature. Turner patients have normal female genitalia, but do not develop secondary sex characteristics because their streak gonads do not produce estrogen.

MALE PSEUDOHERMAPHRODISM

A male pseudohermaphrodite is a genetic male (XY) with ambiguous or female virilization of the external genitalia. Testes are present. There are several disorders that present with this phenotype.

- **46,XY Complete Gonadal Dysgenesis**: Individuals have streak gonads. Absence of secondary sex characteristics and amenorrhea are apparent during puberty.
- **Mixed 46,XY Gonadal Dysgenesis**: Characterized by dysgenetic gonads, mixed internal organs (Müllerian and Wolffian structures), and ambiguous genitalia.

TRUE HERMAPHRODISM

A true hermaphrodite can have both ovarian and testicular tissue separately, or more frequently together in one gonad called ovotestis. The most common karyotype is 46,XX, followed by 46,XX/46,XY mosaicism and 46,XY. True hermaphrodites have ambiguous genitalia ranging from near-normal female to normal male genitalia. The internal ducts are usually appropriate for the gonad (ovary or testis). The presence of ovotestis is more frequently associated with fallopian tube development rather than a vas deferens or epididymis; rarely, both types of ducts are present.

KLINEFELTER SYNDROME (46,XXY)

This disorder is characterized by nondisjunction in the developing zygote resulting in 24,XX ova or 24,XY sperm. Patients with Klinefelter syndrome present with a large arm span, small testes, subnormal testosterone level, excessive growth of the lower extremities, and the presence of under-virilization during adolescence.

Internal and External Genital Differentiation Disorders

ANDROGEN INSENSITIVITY SYNDROME

Androgen insensitivity syndrome (AIS), an X-linked inherited disorder, is characterized by failure of normal masculinization of the external genitalia in chromosomally male individuals. Failure of virilization can be either complete (CAIS) or partial (PAIS), depending on the severity of the androgen receptor defect. In utero, the XY fetus makes testosterone prompted by a functional SRY gene. However, the defective AR does not respond to androgen stimulation, and the fetus develops as a phenotypic female. At birth, 46,XY patients have phenotypic female genitalia, testes present in the inguinal canal or abdomen, a blind vaginal pouch, and absent or rudimentary Müllerian or Wolffian ducts. During puberty, the patient develops breast tissue, but remains with scant or absent body hair. The diagnosis is frequently made at this time because of primary amenorrhea. Gonadectomy is standard because of the risk for malignant tumors of the testis (mostly seminoma) in 5% to 10% of cases.

STEROID 5-α-REDUCTASE DEFICIENCY

This enzyme converts testosterone to dihydrotestosterone (DHT), an androgen responsible for the masculinization of the external genitalia in males. Affected 46,XY phenotypic individuals present at birth with ambiguous genitalia and are usually assigned the female gender if undiagnosed. Marked virilization during puberty characterized by penile growth and absence of gynecomastia often lead the individual to change her gender identity and become male.

Puberty begins with activation of the hypothalamic-pituitary-gonadal axis, resulting in an increase in the frequency and amplitude of leuteinizing hormone–releasing hormone (LHRH) secretion. LHRH stimulates the release of leuteinizing hormone (LH) and follicular-stimulating hormone (FSH). LH and FSH then stimulate the growth of the ovaries and testes, as well as the production of sex steroids (estradiol in females and testosterone in males). The onset of puberty is a result of the increase in baseline serum LH and FSH values. The onset and duration of puberty varies in both sexes and is dependent on genetic and environmental factors (malnutrition, strenuous physical conditioning). Puberty is divided into five stages, called sexual maturity rating (SMR) stages (also known as Tanner stages). Children should be assessed at each well child visit.

TABLE 14-10	SEXUAL MATURITY RATING STAGES OF PUBERTAL DEVELOPMENT*	
	BOYS	**GIRLS**
SMR stage 1	• No sexual development	• No sexual development
SMR stage 2	• *Testicular enlargement* • Scrotum becomes reddened, thinner, and more textured • Sparse, fine, downy hair at base of phallus or scrotum (pubarche)	• *Breast budding* beneath the areola (thelarche) • Sparse, fine, downy pubic hair over mons and labia majora (pubarche)
SMR stage 3	• *Penile length enlargement* • Testicles continue to enlarge (>4 mL volume) • Pubic hair is coarse, more curly, and pigmented	• Breast development beyond the areola, no protrusion of papilla or nipple • Pubic hair is coarse, more curly, and pigmented • Physiologic vaginal discharge • *Peak height velocity occurs*
SMR stage 4	• *Peak height velocity occurs* • Penis (length *and* circumference) and testicles continue to enlarge • Pubic hair is denser and curled, although not adult distribution or density	• *Menarche occurs* • Nipple and areola form secondary mound distinct from breast contour • Pubic hair is denser and curled, although not adult distribution or density
SMR stage 5	• Pubic hair extends to inner thighs, with adult density • Penis and testicles are adult size	• Pubic hair extends to inner thighs, with adult density • Nipple and areola no longer distinct from breast contour

*Important characteristics in italics.

The average age at the onset of puberty (SMR stage 2) is 11 to 11.5 years for both boys and girls. Progression from SMR stage 2 to stage 5 can take from 2.5 to 5 years to complete, with wide variation among individuals. Menarche generally occurs approximately 2 years after thelarche. The mean age at menarche is 12.9 years in Caucasians and 12.2 years in African-Americans. Anovulatory cycles are common in the 12 to 18 months after menarche. Irregular menses due to anovulatory cycles is most common within the first year of menarche.

In females, the growth spurt begins within 1 year of breast budding, and peak height velocity (PHV) occurs in SMR stage 3. In males, the growth spurt begins later, and the PHV does not occur until SMR stage 4. The average PHV in males is 10 cm/y; in females, the PVH is 9 cm/y. Males are ultimately taller than females due to more years of prepubertal growth, and a higher PVH.

Precocious Puberty

Precocious puberty is characterized by the onset of secondary sex characteristics before the youngest accepted age. In females, sexual development before 7 years in Caucasians and before 6 years in African-Americans is considered precocious. In boys, sexual development before 9 years of age is considered precocious regardless of race. Incidence of precocious puberty is about 1 in 10,000 and is more frequent in females than males. There are two forms of precocious puberty: central precocious puberty and pseudoprecocious puberty.

- **Central Precocious Puberty (CPP):** Results from premature activation of hypothalamic-pituitary-gonadal axis, triggering secretion of the pituitary gonadotropin hormones and subsequent gonadal development. In females, 90% of cases are idiopathic. In males, 90% of cases are due to central nervous system abnormalities.

TABLE 14-11. *CAUSES OF CENTRAL PRECOCIOUS PUBERTY*

- **Pseudoprecocious Puberty (PPP):** Results from extra pituitary secretion of gonadotropins, or less frequently from autonomous secretion of sex steroids (ovaries or adrenals). Evaluation should include a determination of the size of the gonads at the time of presentation, which can differentiate the possible underlying etiology. Specific investigations (see Table 14-13) should be tailored to the presenting clinical signs and symptoms.

TABLE 14-12. *CAUSES OF PSEUDOPRECOCIOUS PUBERTY*

TABLE 14-13. *EVALUATION OF PRECOCIOUS PUBERTY*

TREATMENT OF PRECOCIOUS PUBERTY

The effective treatment of precocious puberty is important to decrease psychological trauma, and to avoid premature closure of the growth plates, which can result in short stature.

TABLE 14-14. *TREATMENT OF PRECOCIOUS PUBERTY*

TABLE 14-11	*CAUSES OF CENTRAL PRECOCIOUS PUBERTY*

- Tumors
  - Hypothalamic tumors
  - Craniopharyngioma
  - Hamartoma (produces GnRH)
  - Astrocytoma
- Neurofibromatosis
- Septo-optic dysplasia
- Arachnoid cyst
- Hydrocephalus
- Head trauma
- Cerebral palsy
- Encephalitis or meningitis
- Radiation

GnRH, gonadotropin-releasing hormone.

TABLE 14-12	*CAUSES OF PSEUDOPRECOCIOUS PUBERTY*

GONAD SIZE	POSSIBLE CAUSES
Prepubertal gonads	• Congenital adrenal hyperplasia (21-hydroxylase or 11-hydroxylase deficiency) • Ovarian cysts • Granulosa cell tumors • Leydig cell tumors
Enlarged gonads	• Germinomas (secrete hCG hormone, identical to LH) • McCune-Albright syndrome (associated findings include hyperpigmented macules and polyostotic fibrous dysplasia) • Familial testotoxicosis (as in McCune-Albright syndrome, there is abnormal activation of the LH receptor)

hCG, human chorionic gonadotropin; LH, luteinizing hormone.

TABLE 14-13   *EVALUATION OF PRECOCIOUS PUBERTY*

TEST	PURPOSE/INTERPRETATION
Bone age	• Bone age is advanced compared to chronological age in precocious puberty
Pelvic ultrasound	• Evaluation for ovarian tumor or cyst
Head MRI	• Evaluation for central nervous system abnormality
Adrenal CT	• Evaluation for adrenal lesion (i.e., in suspected CAH)
Adrenal androgens	• CAH may present with growth acceleration, penis enlargement, clitoromegaly, and pubic hair • Evaluation should include 17-OHP
Alpha-fetoprotein and beta-hCG	• These tumor markers may be elevated in hepatoblastoma, germinomas, yolk sac tumors, teratocarcinomas and chorioepitheliomas
Serum gonadotropins	• In CPP, LH and FSH are increased • In PPP, LH and FSH are decreased
GnRH stimulation test	• In CPP, administration of GnRH results in increased secretion of LH and FSH • In PPP, administration of GnRH does *not* alter secretion of LH and FSH

CAH, congenital adrenal hyperplasia; CPP, central precocious puberty; FSH, follicle-stimulating hormone; GnRH, gonadotropin-releasing hormone; hCG, human chorionic gonadotropin; LH, luteinizing hormone; 17-OHP, 17-hydroxyprogesterone; PPP, pseudoprecocious puberty.

TABLE 14-14   *TREATMENT OF PRECOCIOUS PUBERTY*

TREATMENT	MECHANISM OF ACTION
Gonadotropin-releasing agonists (leuprolide)	• Chronic administration suppresses the pulsatile release of LH/FSH from the pituitary, reversing secondary sex characteristics • Also decreases height velocity and rate of bone maturation
Aromatase inhibitors	• Decreases the conversion of testosterone to estradiol (estradiol accelerates bone maturation and early epiphyseal closure)
Surgery	• Used in PPP to remove causative tumors

FSH, follicle-stimulating hormone; LH, luteinizing hormone; PPP, pseudoprecocious puberty.

Pubertal Development Disturbances

• **Premature Thelarche**: A benign condition characterized by unilateral or bilateral breast development without other signs of sexual maturation. Laboratory investigations are within normal limits. Reassurance and observation are sufficient.

• **Premature Pubarche**: A benign condition characterized by early appearance of pubic hair, axillary hair, and less commonly body odor or acne. Plasma levels of adrenal androgens (DHEA, DHEA-S, D4A, testosterone, 17-OHP) are comparable to values found in children with pubic hair (SMR stage 2).

• **Gynecomastia**: A relatively common condition in both newborns and adolescent boys. It is self-limited in 90% of the cases. The most frequent cause is physiologic disturbances during the newborn period, or during puberty. The condition can also be pathologic due to an imbalance between testosterone and estrogen concentrations (see Table 14-15).

TABLE 14-15.   *PATHOLOGIC CAUSES OF GYNECOMASTIA*

Delayed Puberty

Delayed puberty is characterized by the failure to exhibit signs of pubertal development by age 14 in males and by age 13 in females. About 2.5% of healthy adolescents

TABLE 14-15	*PATHOLOGIC CAUSES OF GYNECOMASTIA*
CAUSE	**EXAMPLES**
Decreased testosterone production	• Klinefelter syndrome • Kallmann syndrome • Hypopituitarism • Hyperprolactinemia
Increased conversion of androgens to estrogens	• Obesity • Liver disease • Adrenal tumors • Estrogen-secreting tumors
Drugs/medications	• Marijuana • Isoniazid • Ketoconazole • Dilantin • Spironolactone • Estrogen-containing cosmetics

are diagnosed with delayed puberty. This condition occurs more frequently in males. The most common cause is constitutional pubertal delay. A family history of "late bloomers" is often present. A majority of cases have no underlying disorder. Cases that have an organic etiology can be divided into those with elevated gonadotropins, and those with low or normal gonadotropins.

Males should be evaluated for pubertal delay if they exhibit minimal testicular growth (length under 2.5 cm by 14 years of age), lack of pubic hair by age 15 years, or if genital development is incomplete 5 years after adrenarche. Females should be evaluated if there is no pubarche by age 14 years, menarche has not occurred by age 16, or if menarche has not occurred within 5 years of thelarche.

- *Elevated* gonadotropins (FSH and LH) are seen in gonadal failure, defective gonadal steroidogenesis, and steroid receptor defects. Gonadal failure can be seen in genetic syndromes (Turner syndrome, Klinefelter syndrome), gonadal dysgenesis, premature ovarian failure, or destruction of the gonads (i.e., radiation therapy). Defective gonadal steroidogenesis and steroid receptor defects include CAH due to 3-beta-hydroxysteroid dehydrogenase, CAH due to 17-alpha-hydroxylase deficiency, and complete androgen resistance
- *Low/normal* gonadotropins (FSH and LH) are seen in a wide variety of conditions, including malnutrition, chronic disease, strenuous exercise, CNS tumors, hypothyroidism, hyperprolactinemia, Prader-Willi syndrome, Kallmann syndrome, and Cushing syndrome.

The evaluation depends on the clinical presentation. Baseline gonadotropins (LH and FSH), testosterone and estradiol, chromosomal analysis, and MRI of the head can be useful in pinpointing an organic cause for delayed puberty.

DISORDERS OF GROWTH

Growth Hormone

Growth hormone (GH) is produced by the pituitary gland. GH synthesis and secretion are controlled by the counter regulatory action of two hypothalamic hormones: (1) growth hormone releasing hormone (GHRH), which stimulates GH synthesis and secretion; and (2) somatostatin, which inhibits GH synthesis and secretion. GH stimulates production of insulin-like growth factor-1 (IGF-1). A cascade of growth disorders can result from defects in GH production, regulation, and action (GH resistance due to GH receptor/postreceptor defects).

All children should have height and weight measured at each well child visit. A growth chart that includes measurements at birth and growth velocity over a period of time is the most valuable tool in assessing a child's growth. The heights and weights of parents, siblings, and grandparents are helpful to fully evaluate the child with a growth disorder. This information can be used to calculate target height.

TABLE 14-16.   *CALCULATION OF TARGET HEIGHT*

TABLE 14-16	*CALCULATION OF TARGET HEIGHT*

- Female: target height = (mother's height (cm) + father's height (cm) − 13 cm) divided by 2
- Male: target height = (mother's height (cm) + 13 cm + father's height (cm)) divided by 2

Short Stature

Short stature is defined as height more than 2 standard deviations below the mean (or less than the 3rd percentile) for gender. There are several disorders that can cause short stature:

- *Constitutional growth delay (CGD)* is the most common cause of short stature. Children with CGD usually have a family history of "late bloomers." Overall growth velocity is normal, but puberty and bone age are delayed. Ultimate height potential is eventually achieved. Reassurance is all that is necessary.
- *Familial short stature* is characterized by normal growth velocity, age-appropriate bone age, and a predicted adult height close to target height (based on parental heights).
- *Endocrinopathies*, including GH deficiency, hypothyroidism, Cushing syndrome, adrenal insufficiency, and panhypopituitarism, can result in short stature. Children often have a drop-off on the growth curve around the time of presentation.
- *Genetic syndromes*, including Turner syndrome, Noonan syndrome, Prader-Willi syndrome, and Down syndrome, are associated with short stature. Depending on the syndrome, the child may have short stature from birth.
- *Skeletal dysplasias* (i.e., achondroplasia, osteogenesis imperfecta) are often associated with short stature.
- *Chronic illnesses* that cause increased metabolic needs or malnutrition can cause secondary short stature. Common examples include cystic fibrosis, congenital heart disease, chronic renal failure, and inborn errors of metabolism.

Diagnostic evaluation is based on the clinical presentation. Often, a thorough history and review of the growth chart are sufficient to diagnosis CGD or familial short stature. Treatment of short stature depends on the underlying cause. Administration of growth hormone until epiphyses are closed is indicated in selected conditions, including GH deficiency, Turner syndrome, renal failure, and Prader-Willi.

Tall Stature

Tall stature is defined as height more than 2 standard deviations above the mean for gender. It occurs as frequently as short stature, but is not often brought to medical attention. Familial tall stature is the most common etiology. Other possible causes include excess GH secretion (gigantism), Marfan syndrome, and Klinefelter syndrome. Only gigantism is associated with elevated levels of GH. All other conditions have normal to low GH levels.

METABOLIC BONE DISORDERS

RICKETS

ETIOLOGY: Rickets results from a softening and weakening of newly formed bone secondary to poor mineralization. Rickets is primarily caused by vitamin D deficiency although less frequently calcium and phosphate deficiency can play a role in the pathogenesis. Vitamin D is normally absorbed from food and/or produced by the skin's exposure to sunlight. Vitamin D is then twice hydroxylated, first in the liver (to 25-hydroxyvitamin D) and then in the kidneys to the active form, 1,25-dihydroxy-vitamin D. Vitamin D hydroxylation is stimulated by PTH. (Remember, PTH also stimulates osteoclasts to reabsorb calcium and phosphate from bone, and increases calcium absorption and phosphate excretion in the kidney.) When vitamin D levels fall, PTH is secreted to maintain normocalcemia.

The active form of vitamin D:
- Promotes absorption of calcium and phosphorous from the intestine.
- Increases reabsorption of phosphate in the kidney.
- Regulates release of calcium and phosphate from bone.

TABLE 14-17.   *CAUSES OF RICKETS*

TABLE 14-18.   *SIGNS AND SYMPTOMS OF RICKETS*

FIGURE 14-3.   *RICKETS*

TABLE 14-17	*CAUSES OF RICKETS*
CAUSE	**CHARACTERISTICS**
Vitamin D deficiency and/or defective metabolism	• Nutritional vitamin D deficiency: poor intake, malabsorption (especially fat malabsorption) • Deficient sunlight exposure • Deficient vitamin D metabolism: 1-alpha-hydroxylase deficiency (vitamin D–dependent rickets type I), renal disease • Vitamin D receptor/post receptor defect (vitamin D–dependent rickets type II) • Drugs (phenobarbital, phenytoin) • Liver disease (impaired 25-hydroxylation of vitamin D)
Impaired renal reabsorption of phosphorus	• X-linked hypophosphatemic rickets (decreased proximal renal tubular phosphate resorption with low/normal vitamin D and PTH levels) • Fanconi syndrome • Renal tubular acidosis
Low calcium/phosphorus intake	• Dietary calcium deficiency (rare) • Dietary phosphorus deficiency (rare after infancy)

TABLE 14-18	*SIGNS AND SYMPTOMS OF RICKETS*

Bone pain or tenderness

Generalized muscular hypotonia

Short stature

Craniotabes along suture lines

Frontal bossing

Rachitic rosary

Harrison groove

Bowlegs and knock-knees

Epiphyseal enlargement of wrists/ankles

Greenstick bone fracture

Kyphoscoliosis

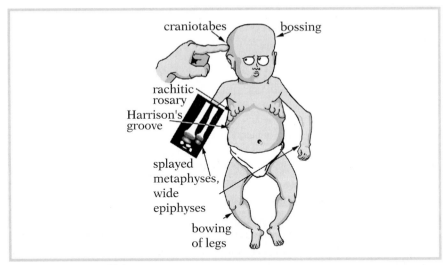

– FIGURE 14-3 – Rickets.

DIAGNOSIS: The diagnostic evaluation of rickets begins with serum calcium, phosphorus, PTH, vitamin D levels, and urine collection for calcium and phosphorus. Alkaline phosphatase is usually elevated. Urine measurements of calcium and phosphorus show hypocalciuria and hyperphosphaturia. Radiographs of the long bones show metaphyseal widening and cupping.

TABLE 14-19. *LABORATORY FINDINGS IN RICKETS*

TABLE 14-19 *LABORATORY FINDINGS IN RICKETS*

	CA	P	PTH	25-VIT D	1,25-VIT D	TREATMENT
Nutritional	↓	↓	↑	↓	↑↓	Vitamin D_3
Vit D–dependent type I	↓	↓	↑	=	↓	1,25 D_3
Vit D–dependent type II	↓	↓	↑	=	↑	1,25 D_3
Chronic renal disease	↓	↑↓	↑	↓	↓	1,25 D_3
Liver disease	↓	↓	↑	↓	↓	Vitamin D_3
X-linked hypophosphatemia	=	↓	=	=	=↓	Phosphorus, 1,25 D_3
Prematurity	↓	↓	↑	↓	↑	Ca, Phosphorus, Vit D_3
Anticonvulsants	↓	↓	↑	↓	↓	Vitamin D_3

TREATMENT: Treatment of rickets consists of oral vitamin D supplementation for 2 to 3 months. Patients with hypophosphatemic rickets require oral phosphate supplementation as well.

HYPOGLYCEMIA

Hypoglycemia is defined as a blood glucose lower than 60 mg/dL.

TABLE 14-20. *SIGNS AND SYMPTOMS OF HYPOGLYCEMIA*

NEONATAL HYPOGLYCEMIA

Neonatal hypoglycemia causes symptoms in 1 to 3 babies per 1,000 live births. The incidence is greater in neonates with high-risk criteria, including prematurity, hypothermia, hypoxia, intrauterine growth retardation, small/large for gestational age, and infants of diabetic mothers. Neonates are more susceptible to hypoglycemia, especially during the first 72 hours of life, due to inadequate muscle, lipid, and glycogen stores, and immature regulation of gluconeogenesis and ketogenesis. Major long-term sequelae of prolonged hypoglycemia include neurologic damage, mental retardation, recurrent seizures, and personality disorders.

Other important causes of hypoglycemia include endocrine disorders (i.e., hyperinsulinism, glucagon deficiency, panhypopituitarism, growth hormone deficiency, ACTH deficiency), metabolic disorders, amino acid and organic acid disorders, and storage diseases.

HYPERINSULINISM

Hyperinsulism is the most common cause of nonketotic hypoglycemia in young children. It may be acquired (i.e., infant of diabetic mother) or genetic. Genetic

TABLE 14-20	*SIGNS AND SYMPTOMS OF HYPOGLYCEMIA*

INFANTS	CHILDREN
• Hypotonia	• Headache
• Lethargy	• Mental confusion
• Apathy	• Behavioral changes
• Poor feeding	• Anxiety
• Jitteriness	• Tremulousness
• Seizures	• Visual disturbances (diplopia)
• Congestive heart failure	• Dysarthria
• Cyanosis	• Seizures
• Apnea	• Ataxia
• Hypothermia	• Stroke
	• Coma
	• Diaphoresis
	• Tachycardia
	• Pallor

hyperinsulinism usually results from a genetic defect of islet-cell regulation, and usually requires near-total pancreatectomy.

HYPERGLYCEMIA

DIABETES MELLITUS (DM)

DEFINITION: Diabetes mellitus is a group of metabolic disorders characterized by hyperglycemia due to defects in insulin secretion, insulin action, or both. In diabetes mellitus, abnormalities in carbohydrate, fat, and protein metabolism result from deficient action of insulin on target tissues. There are two types of DM: type 1 and type 2.

• **Type I (Juvenile-Onset Diabetes):** Characterized by pancreatic beta-cell destruction leading to insulin deficiency. The etiology of type 1 DM may be immune mediated (anti-insulin autoantibodies, anti-islet cell autoantibodies), or idiopathic. Both types have strong HLA associations with DR3 and/or DR4 molecules. The inheritance of both DR3 and DR4 carries the greatest risk for diabetes. There is strong evidence that not only genetic factors but also environmental factors contribute to the etiology of type 1 DM. If one twin from a pair develops type 1 DM, then 60% of both monozygotic and 8% of both dizygotic twins will develop type 1 DM at some point in their lifetimes. The risk of type 1 DM in the offspring of diabetic mothers is 2% to 3% and in the offspring of diabetic fathers is 5% to 6%. If both parents have DM, the risk is 30%. Patients with type 1 DM are prone to other autoimmune disorders (Hashimoto thyroiditis, Addison disease, and vitiligo).

• **Type II (Adult-Onset Diabetes):** Characterized by insulin resistance and usually associated with obesity. The islet cells of the pancreas in patients with type II diabetes continue to produce insulin, but the patient does not respond appropriately, resulting in persistent hyperglycemia. Risk factors for developing type II DM include increasing age, weight gain, physical inactivity, hypertension, hyperlipidemia, and a history of gestational diabetes during childbirth. Important additional conditions that may indirectly result in type II DM include endocrine disorders (Cushing syndrome, hyperthyroidism), pancreatic disorders (cystic fibrosis, pancreatitis, hemochromatosis, abdominal trauma), medications (beta agonists, glucocorticoids), infections (congenital rubella, cytomegalovirus, mumps) and genetic syndromes (Down, Turner, and Klinefelter). There is a stronger genetic predisposition to type II DM with greater than 80% concordance in monozygotic twins. Type II DM occurs more frequently in Hispanics, African Americans, and Native Americans.

TABLE 14-21. *SIGNS AND SYMPTOMS OF DIABETES MELLITUS*

DIAGNOSIS: The evaluation of DM usually begins with the measurement of random and fasting blood glucose levels. Hyperglycemia is defined as a fasting blood glucose higher than 126 mg/dL and a random blood glucose higher than 200 mg/dL. An abnormal oral glucose tolerance test (OGTT) is characterized by a 2-hour blood glucose higher than 200 mg/dL after a measured oral challenge of glucose. The serum measurements of insulin and islet cell autoantibodies as well as the presence of glutamic acid decarboxylase (GAD65) antibodies are useful in the evaluation of type I DM.

COMPLICATIONS: Complications of DM include retinopathy, nephropathy, renal failure, peripheral neuropathy, and atherosclerosis (most frequent cause of death in type II)

DIABETIC KETOACIDOSIS (DKA)

DKA is the most frequent presenting complaint in over 25% of newly diagnosed type I DM patients. DKA in previously diagnosed DM patients is most commonly caused by infection, poor compliance. and puberty. Clinical signs and symptoms of DKA include metabolic acidosis (elevated anion gap), hyperglycemia, ketonuria, glycosuria, hyponatremia, and hypophosphatemia. Hyperkalemia may be noted on serum samples secondary to concomitant acidosis, but the patient generally has a total body deficit of potassium. Hyponatremia is a compensatory response to the increased osmolar load imposed by profound hyperglycemia and is frequently falsely exaggerated secondary to hyperlipidemia. For each 100 mg/dL increase in serum glucose over 100 mg/dL, there is an appropriate decrease in serum sodium of 1.6 mEq/L. For each 1 gm/dL increase in triglycerides, there is a false sodium decrease of 2 mEq/L.

TABLE 14-21	*SIGNS AND SYMPTOMS OF DIABETES MELLITUS*

Malaise

Polyuria

Nocturia

Polydipsia

Polyphagia

Weight loss

Candidiasis

Failure to thrive

Abdominal pain

Vomiting

Fruity-smelling breath (ketones)*

*Ketoacidosis is not a common presentation in type II diabetes unless the patient is under stress.

Severity of dehydration should be assessed in all patients with DKA and should be considered to be at least 10%. Isotonic intravenous fluids (i.e., normal saline) should be administered as bolus therapy prior to administration of medications (insulin, bicarbonate). After appropriate fluid resuscitation, an insulin infusion (0.05-0.1 units/kg/hour) is generally necessary to resolve the ketoacidosis and correct the serum pH. Glucose is added to the intravenous fluids after the serum glucose decreases to less than 250 mg/dL. Additionally, potassium supplementation is necessary, as insulin will drive potassium intracellularly. Intravenous fluids are titrated using glucose to control the blood glucose levels. The insulin infusion is titrated to control the ketoacidosis by monitoring blood pH, serum bicarbonate, and ketones. Serum ketones clear before urine ketones. The patient should be closely monitored for signs and symptoms of acute cerebral edema (headache, blurry vision, vomiting, lethargy), which is a rare but devastating complication of DKA.

CHAPTER 15

INBORN ERRORS OF METABOLISM

ORGANIC ACID DISORDERS (ORGANIC ACIDEMIAS)

Organic acidemias (organic acidurias) are disorders characterized by the excretion of non–amino organic acids in urine. Most result from deficient enzyme activity at a specific step in amino acid catabolism (typically branched-chain amino acids or lysine). Organic acidemias usually present in the first weeks of life with vomiting, feeding difficulties, dehydration, lethargy, and neurologic symptoms (hyper- or hypotonia, seizures, and coma). Massive ketosis and metabolic acidosis are the hallmarks of organic acidemias. Laboratory investigation reveals a high anion gap acidosis, elevated ammonia, ketones, and hypoglycemia. Neutropenia may also be present. Urine organic analysis is the first step in diagnosis. Organic acids found in urine provide a high degree of suspicion for the specific pathway involved and are nearly always abnormal during acute illness. During crisis, the treatment consists of carnitine supplementation and intravenous glucose to help reverse the catabolic state. Bicarbonate may be administered for correction of the metabolic acidosis. Long-term treatment usually includes specific dietary restrictions.

TABLE 15-1. *ORGANIC ACID DISORDERS*

297

TABLE 15-1   *ORGANIC ACID DISORDERS*

DISORDER	ENZYME DEFECT	CLINICAL PRESENTATION	NOTES
Glutaric acidemia (type I)	• Glutaryl-CoA dehydrogenase	• Macrocephaly • Encephalopathic crises • Hypotonia • Dystonia • Choreoathetosis • Subdural fluid collections • Metabolic acidosis	• Elevated lysine and tryptophan • Decreased carnitine • Elevated glutaric acid in urine • Elevated lactate • Treat with a restricted diet, carnitine and riboflavin supplementation
Isovaleric acidemia	• Isovaleryl CoA dehydrogenase	• Characteristic body odor of "sweaty feet" • Vomiting • Seizures • Coma • Ketoacidosis • Hepatomegaly • Pancytopenia • Neutropenia • Thrombocytopenia	• Elevated leucine • Elevated isovaleric acid • Elevated ammonia • Elevated lactate • Increased anion gap • Treat with high-calorie, protein-restricted diet • Carnitine and glycine supplementation may be useful
Methylmalonic acidemia	• Methylmalonyl-CoA mutase	• Hepatomegaly • Hypotonia • Hypoglycemia • Seizures • Lethargy • Ketoacidosis • Pancytopenia • Neutropenia • Thrombocytopenia • Increased ketones	• Elevated glycine • Elevated ammonia • Elevated lactate • Treat with a protein-restricted diet, carnitine supplementation • May respond to vitamin B_{12}

TABLE 15-1	ORGANIC ACID DISORDERS (CONTINUED)		
DISORDER	**ENZYME DEFECT**	**CLINICAL PRESENTATION**	**NOTES**
Propionic acidemia	• Propionyl-CoA carboxylase	• Hepatomegaly • Hypoglycemia • Hypotonia • Seizures • Lethargy • Neutropenia • Ketoacidosis • Pancytopenia • Neutropenia • Thrombocytopenia	• Elevated glycine • Elevated propionic acid • Elevated ammonia • Elevated lactate • Treat with a protein-restricted diet and carnitine supplementation • May respond to biotin
Classic maple syrup urine disease	• Branched-chain alpha-ketoacid dehydrogenase	• Maple syrup urine odor • Hypertonicity • Opisthions • Seizures • Hypoglycemia • Ketoacidosis	• Elevated serum valine, isoleucine, leucine • Elevated alloisoleucine (diagnostic) • Decreased alanine • Treat acutely with dialysis • Long-term treatment with diet low in valine, isoleucine, and leucine

DISORDERS OF AMINO ACID METABOLISM

Disorders of amino acid metabolism such as phenylketonuria (PKU), homocystinuria, hereditary tyrosinemia, and alkaptonuria represent a significant percentage of all inborn errors of metabolism and have a characteristic clinical presentation. Laboratory evaluation will reveal normal anion gap, normal serum pH, and normal ammonia levels. Diagnosis can be confirmed by measuring plasma amino acids and testing the urine for metabolites characteristic of the specific disorder.

TABLE 15-2.   AMINO ACID DISORDERS

TABLE 15-2   *AMINO ACID DISORDERS*

DISORDER	ENZYME DEFECT	CLINICAL PRESENTATION	NOTES
Alkaptonuria	• Homogentisic oxygenase	• Black-colored urine • Darkening of sclerae, cornea, ear cartilage • Arthritis • Valvular disease	• Accumulation of homogentisic acid • Diagnose by measuring homogentisic acid in urine • No treatment available • Vitamin C is recommended for older children and adults
Hereditary tyrosinemia type I (hepatorenal tyrosinemia)	• Fumarylacetoacetate hydrolase	• Failure to thrive • Vomiting • Fever • Hepatomegaly • Bleeding (hematuria, melena) • Hypoglycemia • Hyperbilirubinemia • Transaminitis • Renal tubular acidosis (Fanconi type) • Acute episodes of neuropathy • Fishy urine odor	• Elevation of serum tyrosine • Elevated succinylacetone in urine (diagnostic) • Tyrosinemia also occurs in liver failure and scurvy • Treat with low-tyrosine, phenylalanine diet, liver transplantation • Patients have increased risk of hepatocellular carcinoma • Most frequent in Quebec
Classic homocystinuria	• Cystathionine synthase	• Tall, thin body habitus similar to Marfan syndrome • Arachnodactyly • Ectopia lentis (downward dislocated lens) • Mental retardation • Seizures • Thromboembolic disease • Skeletal abnormalities (kyphosis, scoliosis)	• Accumulation of methionine and homocysteine in blood, urine • May respond to B_6 and/or B_{12} therapy

DISORDER	ENZYME DEFECT	CLINICAL PRESENTATION	NOTES
Phenylketonuria (PKU)	• Phenylalanine hydroxylase	• "Mousy" or musty urine odor • Normal appearing at birth • Fair skin, blue eyes • Mental retardation • Microcephaly • Vomiting • Hyperactive deep tendon reflexes	• Brain damage results from buildup of phenylalanine • Newborn screening will detect most cases; the patient must be fed protein before screening is performed • Always rule out tetrahydrobiopterin deficiency when evaluating a patient for PKU (affects metabolism of phenylalanine) • 80% of infants born to mothers with elevated phenylalanine at risk for IUGR, microcephaly, dysmorphy facies, MR and congenital malformations (heart defects) • Treat with dietary restriction of phenylalanine-containing foods (for life)

TABLE 15-2   *AMINO ACID DISORDERS (CONTINUED)*

UREA CYCLE DEFECTS

Urea cycle defects are disorders of ureagenesis characterized by elevated serum ammonia. The overall prevalence is 1 in 30,000 births. The majority of urea cycle defects present during the first days of life with lethargy, seizures, coma, and respiratory alkalosis. The clinical presentation may be confused with sepsis. Disorders of ureagenesis should be differentiated from other disorders that present with hyperammonemia (fatty acid oxidation and organic acid disorders). Laboratory investigation frequently reveals a normal anion gap, respiratory alkalosis, and hyperammonemia. Metabolic alkalosis may also be present in cases of prolonged vomiting. Diagnosis can be confirmed by measurement of plasma amino acids and urinary organic acids. Emergency treatment consists of intravenous glucose, sodium benzoate, and sodium phenylacetate to aid nitrogen excretion through alternate pathways. Long-term treatment consists of dietary restriction of nitrogen, supplementation of deficient amino acids, as well as administration of sodium phenylacetate and sodium benzoate. The most common disorders are summarized in Table 15-3.

TABLE 15-3.   *UREA CYCLE DEFECTS*

TABLE 15-3   *UREA CYCLE DEFECTS*

DISORDER	ENZYME DEFECT	CLINICAL PRESENTATION	NOTES

Ornithine tran-scarbamylase (OTC) deficiency	• Ornithine transcarbamoylase	• Poor feeding
		• Vomiting
		• Tachypnea
		• Hypothermia
		• Hypotonia
		• Seizures
		• Hepatomegaly
		• Encephalopathy
			• OTC is X-linked recessive
			• CPS is autosomal recessive
			• Both OTC and CPS have the following in common:
			  - Normal anion gap
			  - Respiratory alkalosis
			  - Elevated glutamine and alanine
			  - Decreased citrulline and arginine
			• The only difference is CPS presents with decreased orotic acid and OTC has elevated orotic acid in the urine
			• Treatment:
			  - High-calorie diet
			  - Protein restriction
			  - Citrulline supplementation

Carbamyl phosphate synthetase deficiency (CPS)	• Carbamyl phosphate synthetase		

Argininosuccinic aciduria	• Argininosuccinate lyase (ASL)		• Elevated citrulline
			• Elevated argininosuccinic acid
			• Elevated glutamine and alanine
			• Friable hair (trichorrhexis nodosa)
			• Treatment:
			  -High-calorie diet
			  -Protein restriction
			  -Arginine supplementation

Arginase deficiency	• Arginase	• Developmental regression
		• Spastic quadriplegia
		• Seizures
		• Choreoathetotic movements
		• Hepatomegaly
			• Usually no symptoms in the newborn period
			• Does not result in severe hyperammonemia
			• Plasma amino acid analysis reveals only elevated arginine
			• Treatment
			  -High-calorie diet
			  -Protein restriction

DISORDERS OF CARBOHYDRATE METABOLISM

Disorders of carbohydrate metabolism affect glucose homeostasis and cellular energy production. Patients typically present with hypoglycemia, elevated lactate levels, and hepatomegaly. The most common disorders are summarized in Table 15-4.

TABLE 15-4   *DISORDERS OF CARBOHYDRATE METABOLISM*

DISORDER	ENZYME DEFECT	CLINICAL PRESENTATION	NOTES

Galactosemia	Galactose 1-phosphate uridylyl transferase
	
	(Galactokinase deficiency extremely rare and presents with cataracts)
		• Hepatomegaly
		• Hypoglycemia
		• Cataracts
		• Jaundice
		• Gram-negative sepsis
		• Reducing substances are positive in the urine in babies fed regular formula
			• Incidence 1: 60,000
			• Diagnosis:
			  - Measurement of enzyme levels in red blood cells (performed by newborn screening)
			  - Elevated serum galactose 1-phosphate levels
			  - Elevated urinary galactitol
			• Treatment: galactose, and lactose-free diet (lactose = glucose + galactose); soy formula preferred as it doesn't contain galactose

Hereditary fructose intolerance	• Deficiency of fructose 1-phosphate aldolase (aldolase B)	• Often presents after initiation of fruit juice to infant
		• Vomiting
		• Hypoglycemia
		• Jaundice
		• Hepatomegaly
		• Proximal RTA
			• Diagnosis:
			  - Serum aldolase B activity
			  - Genetic testing is available
			• Accumulation of fructose-1-phosphate
			• Treatment: avoid fructose, sorbitol, and sucrose
			• Sucrose is broken down to fructose and glucose

GLYCOGEN STORAGE DISEASES

Glycogen is synthesized as a storage form of glucose by the liver and kidney and has a significant role in energy supply for the body. Glycogen storage diseases (GSD) are a group of inherited metabolic disorders in which genetic enzyme deficiencies block glycogen degradation, leading to excess accumulation of glycogen within the body.

Symptoms vary by GSD type and may include muscle cramps and wasting, enlarged liver, and hypoglycemia. Disruption of glycogen metabolism also affects other biochemical pathways as the body seeks alternative fuel sources, which can lead to the accumulation of abnormal metabolic by-products that can damage the kidneys and other organs. GSD can be fatal, but the risk hinges on the type of GSD. The most common disorders are summarized in Table 15-5.

TABLE 15-5   *GLYCOGEN STORAGE DISEASES*

DISORDER	ENZYME DEFECT	CLINICAL PRESENTATION	NOTES
Von Gierke disease (type I glycogen storage disease)	• Glucose-6-phosphatase • Prevents the release of glucose during glycogenolysis and gluconeogenesis	• Hypoglycemia • Lactic acidosis • Hyperuricemia • Hyperlipidemia • Coagulopathy • Hepatomegaly • Doll-like face • Short stature • Enlarged kidneys • Fanconi syndrome • Hepatic adenomas	• Gout develops secondary to renal insufficiency • Administration of glucagon during hypoglycemia has no response • Increased creatinine kinase • Treatment consists of frequent glucose feeds during the day and continuous glucose feeds at night via nasogastric tube; feeds can be supplemented with cornstarch (uncooked cornstarch releases glucose over a longer period of time) • Fructose and sucrose restriction
Pompe disease (type II glycogen storage disease)	• Lysosomal acid 1,4-glucosidase • Prevents the degradation of glycogen to glucose	• Macroglossia • Hypotonia • Hepatomegaly • Hypertrophic cardiomyopathy • Congestive heart failure • Shortened PR interval	• Poor prognosis due to cardiorespiratory failure if the disorder presents in infancy • No specific treatment available • High-protein diet may be beneficial
Cori disease (type III glycogen storage disease)	• Debranching enzyme	• Hypotonia • Hepatomegaly • Hypoglycemia	• Symptoms may abate at puberty • Myopathy and cardiomyopathy may develop later in life

TABLE 15-5   *GLYCOGEN STORAGE DISEASES (CONTINUED)*

DISORDER	ENZYME DEFECT	CLINICAL PRESENTATION	NOTES
McArdle disease (type V glycogen storage disease)	• Muscle phosphorylase	• Muscle cramps • Exercise intolerance • Weakness • Myoglobinuria	• Predominantly affects skeletal muscle • Increased creatine kinase • Increased ammonia levels • Treatment with dietary supplementation of glucose during periods of exertion • Good prognosis

PEROXISOMAL DISORDERS

Peroxisomes are small cellular particles that are involved in beta-fatty oxidation of very long chain fatty acid (VLCFA), metabolism and synthesis of bile acids, and myelin phospholipids (plasmalogens). Most peroxisomal disorders have decreased plasmalogen and bile acids, along with elevated VLCFA. All peroxisomal disorders carry a poor prognosis with death at an early age.

TABLE 15-6   *PEROXISOMAL DISORDERS*

CONDITION	CLINICAL FEATURES	NOTES
X-linked adrenoleukodystrophy	• Hyperactivity • Deterioration of school performance • Seizures • Ataxia • Blindness • Weakness • Primary adrenal insufficiency	• Frequently presents as a slow progressive course of neurologic deterioration making diagnosis challenging • Affects cerebral white matter • Affects males only (X-linked)
Zellweger syndrome	• Craniofacial dysmorphism • Large anterior fontanel • Mental retardation • Seizures • Hypotonia • Retinal degeneration • Renal cysts • Hepatomegaly • Stippling of epiphyses • Cataracts	• Cerebrohepatorenal syndrome • CNS dysmyelination

SPHINGOLIPIDOSES

The sphingolipidoses are characterized by deficiency of the acid hydrolases that degrade specific lipids in lysosomes. Clinical presentation is variable and may consist of progressive mental and motor deterioration leading up to death. Adult-onset disease usually has a milder course. There are two categories of sphingolipidoses:

TABLE 15-7   *SPHINGOLIPIDOSES*

DISORDER	ENZYME DEFECT	CLINICAL PRESENTATION	NOTES
Fabry disease	• α-Galactosidase	• Burning pain in the hands and feet • Angiokeratomas (clusters of ectatic blood vessels) • Corneal opacities • Paresthesias • Autonomic dysfunction	• X-linked recessive • Symptoms do not present until late childhood to early adulthood • Variable severity of disease
Gaucher disease	• Glucocerebrosidase	• Splenomegaly • Thrombocytopenia • Bleeding • Bone pain	• Ashkenazi Jews are most frequently affected • The most common lysosomal storage disease • Gaucher cells are present in bone marrow • Bone marrow transplantation is curative • Enzyme replacement therapy (glucocerebrosidase) is available
Krabbe disease	• Galactosylceramide β-galactosidase	• Tonic spasms • Infantile irritability • Developmental delay • Regression of milestones • Blindness • Seizures	• Prognosis poor • Demyelination disorder
Metachromatic leukodystrophy	• Arylsulfatase A	• Regression of milestones • Seizures • Blindness	• "Brown" or "red" staining of cortical tissue on histopathology • Demyelination disorder

(1) storage disease–type sphingolipidoses, including Tay-Sachs, Gaucher, Fabry, and Niemann-Pick diseases, are characterized primarily by storage of uncleaved substrate in neurons and other cell types, and (2) leukodystrophy-type sphingolipidoses, including Krabbe disease and metachromatic leukodystrophy, are characterized by impairment of a biochemical process necessary for myelin development or maintenance. The most frequently encountered disorders are summarized in Table 15-7.

TABLE 15-7   *SPHINGOLIPIDOSES (CONTINUED)*

DISORDER	ENZYME DEFECT	CLINICAL PRESENTATION	NOTES

Niemann-Pick disease	• Sphingomyelinase	• *Macular cherry red spot*
		• Hepatosplenomegaly
		• Developmental delay
		• Seizures
			• There are 3 types of Niemann-Pick disease:
			  1. Type A: early infantile onset with severe neurologic manifestations
			  2. Type B: milder disease process with later onset and absent neurologic manifestations
			  3. Type C: not actually a sphingolipidosis, but a disorder of cholesterol transport; characterized by hepatomegaly and severe neurologic manifestations

Sandhoff disease	• β-Hexosaminidase • α-Hexosaminidase	• *Macular cherry red spot* • Macrocephaly • Developmental delay • Loss of previously acquired milestones • Seizures • Blindness	• Often confused with Tay-Sachs disease but is not frequent among Ashkenazi Jews
Tay-Sachs disease	• α-Hexosaminidase	• *Macular cherry red spot* • Exacerbated startle reflex • Developmental delay • Loss of previously acquired milestones • Hypotonia • Blindness	• Ashkenazi Jews most frequently affected

MUCOPOLYSACCHARIDOSIS (MPS)

These disorders primarily affect the catabolism of sulfated components of gly-cosaminoglycans (GAGs) in connective tissue. The main components of GAGs, dermatan sulfate, heparin sulfate, and keratin sulfate, accumulate within the connective tissue and ultimately affect cellular structure and function. The clinical presentation and severity of these disorders are highly variable. The evaluation is generally initiated with screening for urine glycosaminoglycans.

TABLE 15-8   *MUCOPOLYSACCHARIDOSIS*

DISORDER	ENZYME DEFECT	CLINICAL PRESENTATION	NOTES
MPS type I (Hurler syndrome)	• α-Iduronidase	• Coarse facial appearance • Macroglossia • Umbilical hernia • Respiratory insufficiency • Hepatosplenomegaly • Cardiomyopathy • Developmental delay • Loss of developmental milestones • Skeletal dysplasias • Cataracts • Progressive hearing loss	• There are 3 subtypes of MPS type I based on severity of symptoms • Hurler is most severe of the MPS type I subtypes • Variable prognosis usually dependent on the degree of cardiomyopathy • Developmental delay evident by end of 1st year • Death in early childhood is frequent
MPS type II (Hunter syndrome)	• Iduronate-2-sulfatase	• Coarse facial appearance • Umbilical hernia • Respiratory insufficiency • Hepatosplenomegaly • Developmental delay • Loss of developmental milestones • Progressive hearing loss	• X-linked recessive inheritance • Absent cataracts • Absent cardiomyopathy • Milder disease with survival beyond childhood • Onset typically at ages 2-4 y

TABLE 15-8	MUCOPOLYSACCHARIDOSIS (CONTINUED)		
DISORDER	**ENZYME DEFECT**	**CLINICAL PRESENTATION**	**NOTES**
MPS type III (Sanfilippo A syndrome)	• Heparan *N*-sulfatase	• Coarse facial features are mild or absent • Developmental delay • Respiratory insufficiency • Chronic diarrhea • Hyperactivity • Aggressive behavior	• There are 4 subtypes of MPS type III based on severity of symptoms • Sanfilippo A is most severe subtype • Survival is generally beyond childhood
MPS type IV (Morquio A syndrome)	• *N*-acetylgalactosamine-6-sulfatase	• Severe skeletal dysplasias • Short stature • Odontoid dysplasia • Genu valgum • Cloudy corneas • Normal intelligence	• There are 2 subtypes of MPS type IV based on severity of symptoms • Morquio A is most severe subtype • Onset at ages 1-3 y • Odontoid dysplasia can be neurologically devastating if not recognized and treated

DISORDERS OF HEME BIOSYNTHESIS (PORPHYRIAS)

Porphyrias are disorders of abnormal heme biosynthesis and metabolism. Heme biosynthesis occurs almost entirely in the liver and bone marrow and is composed of eight specific reactions, each catalyzed by a specific enzyme. Accumulation of porphyrin precursors results in clinical manifestations of the neurologic and integumentary systems. The two most frequent disorders are summarized in Table 15-9.

TABLE 15-9. *PORPHYRIAS*

TABLE 15-9   *PORPHYRIAS*

DISORDER	ENZYME DEFECT	CLINICAL PRESENTATION	NOTES
Acute intermittent porphyria	• Hydroxymethylbilane (HMB)-synthase	• Neurovisceral crises are the hallmark of this disorder characterized by crampy, diffuse abdominal pain and peripheral neuropathies • Psychiatric disorders • Autonomic dysfunction • Seizures	• Autosomal dominant inheritance • Frequently manifests during or after puberty • Certain medications (barbiturates, carbamazepine, oral contraceptives, griseofulvin), low-calorie diets, and alcohol consumption can precipitate an acute crisis • Screen the urine for delta-aminolevulinic acid (Δ-ALA) and porphobilinogen (PBG) during a neurovisceral crisis to aid in the diagnosis • Treatment during an acute crisis consists of intravenous glucose and hematin once daily for 4 d • Prenatal diagnosis is available
Porphyria cutanea tarda	• Hepatic uroporphyrinogen (URO)-decarboxylase	• Cutaneous photosensitivity • Bullae and vesicles manifest on the skin after minor trauma • Hyperpigmentation	• Most common form of porphyria • Iron overload (thalassemia, chronic liver disease) contributes to the severity of the disease • Elevated plasma porphyrins • Treatment involves avoidance of precipitating medications, alcohol, and fasting • Phlebotomy to reduce hepatic iron stores improves symptoms

FATTY ACID OXIDATION DISORDERS

Fatty acid oxidation takes place in the mitochondria and plays an essential role in energy production. During gluconeogenesis, fatty acids are used for hepatic ketone synthesis and for oxidation in muscle. Fatty acids are the preferred fuel for the heart and skeletal muscle during exercise. Nearly all of the defects present in early infancy as life-threatening episodes of hypoketotic hypoglycemic coma following decreased intake during an acute illness. In disorders involving long-chain and VLCFA metabolism, chronic skeletal myopathy and cardiomyopathy are present. Treatment includes dietary restriction of fatty acids, carnitine supplementation, and administration of glucose-containing intravenous fluids during acute episodes.

TABLE 15-10   *FATTY ACID OXIDATION DISORDERS*

DISORDER	ENZYME DEFECT	CLINICAL PRESENTATION	NOTES
MCAD	• Medium-chain acyl-CoA dehydrogenase	• Hypoketotic hypoglycemia • Seizures • Encephalopathy	• Presents after stress or long fasting • Increased risk of SIDS • Elevated ammonia
			• Elevated lactate • Abnormal liver enzymes • Low carnitine • Dicarboxylic aciduria • No skeletal or cardiomyopathy • Treat with glucose-containing IV fluids and carnitine • Fat restriction in diet

(Continued)

TABLE 15-10   *FATTY ACID OXIDATION DISORDERS (CONTINUED)*

DISORDER	ENZYME DEFECT	CLINICAL PRESENTATION	NOTES
LCAD	• Long-chain acyl-CoA dehydrogenase	• Hypoketotic hypoglycemia • Seizures • Encephalopathy • Skeletal myopathy • Dilated hypertrophic cardiomyopathy • Hepatomegaly	• Presents after stress or long fasting • Elevated ammonia • Elevated lactate • Elevated creatinine kinase • Low carnitine • Dicarboxylic aciduria • Treat with glucose-containing IV fluids and carnitine • Fat restriction in diet
VLCAD	• Very long-chain acyl-CoA dehydrogenase		

SIDS, sudden infant death syndrome.

CHAPTER 16

GENETICS

AUTOSOMAL DISORDERS

Autosomal genetic disorders affect the non-sex chromosomes, and occur in 1 out of every 500 individuals in the general population. Males and females are affected equally. Autosomal disorders are transmitted from an affected parent to an affected child or, less frequently, can be the result of a new mutation. Family members often show different symptoms, features, or severity of the same autosomal disorder (variable penetrance or expression). Occasionally, an individual with an autosomal disorder shows no symptoms of the condition (nonpenetrance). These disorders may occur in a dominant or recessive fashion.

Autosomal Dominant Disorders

An autosomal dominant disorder is expressed in a person who has only one altered copy of the gene. The chance of an affected parent transmitting the disorder is 50%. The affected genes are transmitted through several generations if the disease allows survival to childbearing years. Additionally, these disorders frequently occur due to a spontaneous mutation.

TABLE 16-1	AUTOSOMAL DOMINANT DISORDERS	
CONDITION	**CLINICAL FEATURES**	**NOTES**
Achondroplasia	• Large head • Frontal bossing • Flat nasal bridge • Rhizomelic shortening • Normal intelligence	• Associated with advanced paternal age • High incidence of spontaneous mutations

(Continued)

TABLE 16-1	AUTOSOMAL DOMINANT DISORDERS (CONTINUED)	
CONDITION	**CLINICAL FEATURES**	**NOTES**
Albright hereditary osteodystrophy	• Pseudohypoparathyroidism • Short stature • Obesity • Short 4th metacarpal	
Apert syndrome	• Craniosynostosis • Syndactyly • Proptosis • Acrocephaly (cone-shaped head)	• Hearing and vision loss • Defect located on chromosome 10
Beckwith-Wiedemann syndrome	• Macrosomia • Macroglossia • Omphalocele	• Duplication of paternal chromosome 11p • Hypoglycemia is common
Crouzon syndrome	• Craniosynostosis • *No* syndactyly • Acrocephaly (cone-shaped head)	• Hearing and vision loss • Defect located on chromosome 10
Ehlers-Danlos syndrome	• Hyperextensible joints • Stretchy skin • Bruises easily	• Defect in collagen
Holt-Oram syndrome	• Atrial septal defect • Absent or hypoplastic thumb • 3-jointed thumbs	
LEOPARD syndrome	• **L**entigines • **E**KG abnormality • **O**cular hypertelorism • **P**ulmonic stenosis • **A**bnormal genitalia • **R**etarded growth and development • **D**eafness	
Marfan syndrome	• Tall, thin males • Increased arm span • Decreased upper to lower segment ratio • Dislocated upward lens • Arachnodactyly	• Risk for aortic dissection • Defect in fibrillin

TABLE 16-1   *AUTOSOMAL DOMINANT DISORDERS (CONTINUED)*

CONDITION	CLINICAL FEATURES	NOTES
Noonan syndrome	• Short stature • Pectus excavatum • Webbed neck • Low-set ears • Pulmonic stenosis	• Defect located on chromosome 9 • Normal karyotype • Often confused with Turner syndrome • May be seen in females and males
Neurofibromatosis type I	• Café-au-lait spots • Neurofibromas • Lisch nodules • Axillary freckles • Optic glioma • Scoliosis • Pseudoarthrosis of tibia	• Defect located on chromosome 17 • 50% are new mutations
Neurofibromatosis type II	• Acoustic neuromas	• Defect located on chromosome 22
Rendu-Osler-Weber syndrome	• Telangiectasias • Arteriovenous malformations • Gastrointestinal bleeding	
Treacher-Collins syndrome	• Small chin • Conductive hearing loss • Lower eyelid anomalies (coloboma) • Normal intelligence	• Often confused with Pierre Robin syndrome
Tuberous sclerosis	• Hamartoma of brain (tubers) • Ash leaf spots (present at birth, better visualized using Wood lamp) • Shagreen patches (usually over lumbar spine) • Adenoma sebaceum (appears in adolescence) • Periungual fibromas	• Associated with infantile spasms • Giant cell astrocytoma • Renal cysts
Waardenburg syndrome	• White forelock • Hearing loss • Heterochromia of the iris • Cleft lip/palate • Lateral displacement of inner canthi	

Autosomal Recessive Disorders

Individuals with autosomal recessive disorders have two altered copies of the mutated gene. If a person has only one defective copy, she/he is called a "carrier." Carriers do not express the disease, but are capable of passing the gene on to their offspring. If two carrier parents have a child, the chances of having an affected offspring is 25%; 50% of the offspring will be carriers, and 25% of the offspring will have a normal chromosomal complement (i.e., neither affected nor a carrier). These disorders occur more frequently in families with consanguinity. Autosomal recessive disorders are usually limited to a single generation. Most inborn errors of metabolism and enzymatic defects (except for X-linked ornithine transcarbamylase deficiency [OTC] and Hunter disease) are inherited in an autosomal recessive fashion.

TABLE 16-2	*AUTOSOMAL RECESSIVE DISORDERS*	
CONDITION	**CLINICAL FEATURES**	**NOTES**
Alpha 1-antitrypsin deficiency	• Obstructive lung disease • Cirrhosis • Hepatitis • Jaundice	• PIZZ phenotype most common
Ataxia-telangiectasia	• Cerebellar ataxia • Oculocutaneous telangiectasias • Recurrent infection • Malignancies	• ↓ T cells • ↓ IgA and/or IgE levels • Defect located on chromosome 11 • ↑ Serum alpha-fetoprotein • Chromosomal breakage syndrome • Bone marrow transplantation is curative
Bloom syndrome	• Symmetric intrauterine growth retardation • Malar hypoplasia • Telangiectatic erythematous rash • Malignancies	• Defect located on chromosome 15 • More frequent in Ashkenazi Jews • Butterfly distribution of rash on face • Chromosomal breakage syndrome
Cockayne syndrome	• Photosensitivity • Microcephaly • Mental retardation • Cataracts • Retinitis pigmentosa	• Premature aging syndrome • Genetic heterogeneity • Chromosomal breakage syndrome

(Continued)

TABLE 16-2	AUTOSOMAL RECESSIVE DISORDERS (CONTINUED)	
CONDITION	**CLINICAL FEATURES**	**NOTES**
Fanconi anemia	• Pancytopenia • Bone marrow hypoplasia • Radius, thumb hypoplasia • Abnormal facies • Short stature	• Defect located on chromosome 16 • Chromosomal breakage syndrome • Most common heritable aplastic anemia
Hurler syndrome	• Corneal clouding • Umbilical hernias • Recurrent pneumonias • Skeletal dysplasia • Cardiomyopathy • Psychomotor retardation	• Mucopolysaccharidosis disorder (all of which are autosomal recessive except for Hunter syndrome, which is X-linked)
Kartagener syndrome	• Sinusitis • Situs inversus • Bronchiectasis	• Defective cilia motility
Smith-Lemli-Opitz syndrome	• Short stature • Microcephaly • Ptosis • Mental retardation • Behavioral problems • Hypospadias	• Disorder of cholesterol metabolism • Defect located on chromosome 11
Thrombocytopenia absent radius (TAR) syndrome	• Thrombocytopenia • Absent radius • Normal thumbs • Heart defects	• Thrombocytopenic episodes may be precipitated by cow's milk allergy, stress, and infection
Walker-Warburg syndrome	• Hydrocephalus • Agyria • Retinal dysplasia • Encephalocele	• Mnemonic HARD +/- E

(Continued)

TABLE 16-2	AUTOSOMAL RECESSIVE DISORDERS (CONTINUED)	
CONDITION	**CLINICAL FEATURES**	**NOTES**
Wilson disease (hepatolenticular degeneration)	• Kayser-Fleisher rings • Basal ganglia defects • Liver disease • Hemolytic anemia • Psychiatric disease	• Disorder of copper metabolism • Copper-induced cell injury • ↓ Serum ceruloplasmin • Increased urinary copper excretion • Treat with D-penicillamine • Defect located on chromosome 13
Xeroderma pigmentosum	• Photosensitivity • Photophobia • Pigment changes of the skin • Neurologic symptoms • Malignancies	• Defect in nucleotide excision repair • Genetic heterogeneity • Chromosomal breakage syndrome

X-LINKED RECESSIVE DISORDERS

X-linked disorders are single gene disorders. Males are more commonly affected than females. The defective gene is transmitted from an affected father through his daughters, who are rarely affected (X-chromosome inactivation). Each daughter is an obligatory carrier. There is a 50% chance that a female carrier will transmit the disease to her son. No male-to-male transmission occurs. Although rare, an affected male and a female carrier have a 25% chance of having an affected female offspring.

TABLE 16-3.   X- LINKED RECESSIVE DISORDERS

	TABLE 16-3	*X- LINKED RECESSIVE DISORDERS*

CONDITION	CLINICAL FEATURES	NOTES
Alport syndrome	• Hematuria • Proteinuria • Deafness	
Aicardi syndrome	• Agenesis of the corpus callosum • Blindness • Myoclonic seizures • Mental retardation	• Affects only females as the condition is fatal in the male fetus
Duchenne muscular dystrophy	• Proximal muscle weakness • Gower sign • Pseudohypertrophy of calf muscles • Cardiomyopathy	• Defect in dystrophin • Fatty infiltration of calf muscles • 40% of cases have sudden cardiac death secondary to atrial conduction defects
Fragile-X syndrome	• Mental retardation • Macro-orchidism • Long face • Large everted ears • High arched palate	• The most common cause of mental retardation in males • The second most common genetic cause of mental retardation, following Down syndrome • The mutation is characterized by a repeating sequence of three nucleotides (trinucleotide repeats) • Approximately 50% of carrier females are affected with some degree of developmental delay
G6PD deficiency	• Risk for severe hemolysis	• Oxidant drugs or stress can precipitate - Sulfa drugs (TMP/SMP, furosemide) - Fava beans, moth balls
Hemophilia A/B	• Factor VIII deficiency (A) • Factor IX deficiency (B) • Hemarthrosis • Severe hemorrhage	• Hemophilia A accounts for 80%-85% of hemophilia • Hemophilia B = Christmas disease • Often picked up following circumcision • Prenatal diagnosis is available

(Continued)

TABLE 16-3	X- LINKED RECESSIVE DISORDERS (CONTINUED)	
CONDITION	**CLINICAL FEATURES**	**NOTES**
Hunter syndrome	• Coarse facies • Severe mental retardation • Skeletal abnormalities	• The only X-linked mucopolysaccharide disorder • Absent corneal clouding
Lesch-Nyhan syndrome	• Self-mutilation • Hyperuricemia • Severe mental retardation • Choreiform movements	• Orange crystals in diaper
Lowe syndrome	• Cataracts • Mental retardation • Hypotonia • Renal tubular dysfunction	• "Oculocerebrorenal" syndrome
Menkes syndrome	• Sparse, kinky hair • Seizures • Hypotonia • Hypothermia • Mental retardation	• "Menkes kinky hair" syndrome • Defect in copper metabolism
Wiskott-Aldrich syndrome	• Combined immune deficiency • Eczema • Eosinophilia • Thrombocytopenia, small platelets • Malignancies	• Bone marrow transplant is curative
X-linked alpha-thalassemia	• Severe mental retardation • Seizures • Genital abnormalities	• Mild thalassemia

TRISOMY SYNDROMES

These disorders are a substantial cause of fetal loss and mental retardation. The most common autosomal chromosome syndromes are summarized in Table 16-4.

TABLE 16-4	TRISOMY SYNDROMES	
CONDITION	**CLINICAL FEATURES**	**NOTES**

Trisomy 21
(Down syndrome)
	• Mental retardation
	• Hypotonia
	• Congenital heart disease (endocardial cushion defect)
	• Duodenal atresia
	• Brushfield spots
	• Simian crease
	• Early Alzheimer disease
		• Occurs in 1/800 infants
		• Nondisjunction during meiosis yields extra copy of chromosome 21
		• Associated with advanced maternal age
		  • Maternal age 40 = 1/40 risk
		• Increased risk for acute leukemias
		• Prenatal diagnosis is available
		  - Increased nuchal folds on ultrasound
		  - ↓ MSAFP

Trisomy 18 **(Edward syndrome)**	• Mental retardation • Rocker bottom feet • Horseshoe kidneys • Clenched fists with overlapping fingers • Congenital heart disease	• Occurs in 1/6,000 infants • Associated with advanced maternal age • Prenatal diagnosis is available - ↓ MSAFP • 90% mortality by age 1 y
Trisomy 13 **(Patau syndrome)**	• Mental retardation • Cleft lip/palate • Polydactyly • Congenital heart disease • Holoprosencephaly	• Occurs in 1/10,000 infants • Associated with advanced maternal age • Prenatal diagnosis is available - ↓ MSAFP

MASP, maternal serum alpha-fetoprotein.

MITOCHONDRIAL DISORDERS

Mitochondrial DNA, located outside of the cell nucleus in the cytoplasm, encodes primarily for enzymes involved in cellular energy production (oxidative phosphorylation). Mitochondrial disorders can be caused by deletions, duplications, or point mutations affecting mitochondrial DNA. These disorders are maternally transmitted, as sperm contains little to no mitochondria. Most mitochondrial disorders present with neuromuscular and central nervous system abnormalities. The most frequently encountered syndromes are summarized in Table 16-5.

TABLE 16-5. MITOCHONDRIAL DISORDERS

TABLE 16-5	*MITOCHONDRIAL DISORDERS*	
CONDITION	**CLINICAL FEATURES**	**NOTES**
Kearns-Sayre syndrome	• Ataxia • Ophthalmoplegia • Myopathy • Hypotonia	
Leber hereditary optic neuropathy	• Progressive vision loss	• Typically presents in teenagers with painless bilateral central vision loss
Leigh disease (subacute necrotizing encephalopathy)	• Ataxia • Cranial nerve dysfunction • Encephalopathy • Hypotonia • Optic atrophy	• Elevated lactate
Mitochondrial encephalopathy, lactic acidosis, and stroke-like episodes (MELAS)	• Ataxia • Progressive myopathy • Strokes • Seizures	• Elevated lactate
Myoclonic epilepsy, ragged red fibers (MERRF)	• Ataxia • Myopathy • External ophthalmoplegia	
Pearson syndrome	• Anemia • Neutropenia • Myopathy • Pancreatic dysfunction	• Elevated lactate

MICRODELETION SYNDROMES

Chromosomal deletions occur when a small fragment of a chromosome is missing. *Microdeletions* are chromosome deletions that are too small to be identified reliably by standard cytogenetic methods, and require molecular methods for detection (i.e., fluorescence in situ hybridization [FISH]). These disorders follow no specific pattern of inheritance.

TABLE 16-6	MICRODELETION SYNDROMES	
CONDITION	**CHARACTERISTICS**	**NOTES**
Angelman syndrome	• Mental retardation • Seizures • Unprovoked laughter • Wide mouth, protruding tongue	• "Happy puppet" syndrome • Maternal chromosome 15 deletion • Angelman syndrome and Prader-Willi syndrome are examples of genetic "imprinting," where a single genotype is responsible for more than one phenotype

DiGeorge syndrome	• "CATCH 22"
	  - **C**ongenital heart disease (aortic arch disease)
	  - **A**bnormal ears
	  - **T**hymic aplasia
	  - **C**left palate
	  - **H**ypocalcemia
	• *Candida* and *Pneumocystis* infections
	• Profoundly decreased T cells
		• Abnormal development of the 3rd and 4th pharyngeal pouch, with resultant thymic aplasia
		• T-cell deficiency
		• Chromosome 22 deletion

Miller-Dieker syndrome	• Lissencephaly • Severe mental retardation • Seizures	• Chromosome 17 deletion
Prader-Willi syndrome	• Hypotonia • Hypogonadism • Obesity • Mental retardation	• Feeding problems/failure to thrive at birth followed by obesity in childhood • Paternal chromosome 15 deletion
Rubinstein-Taybi syndrome	• Broad thumbs and toes • Cryptorchidism • Mental retardation • Congenital heart disease	• Chromosome 16 deletion
Velocardiofacial (Shprintzen) syndrome	• Cleft palate • Micrognathia • Cardiac defect • Developmental delay • Psychiatric disease	• Chromosome 22 deletion • Often confused with DiGeorge syndrome

(Continued)

TABLE 16-6   *MICRODELETION SYNDROMES (CONTINUED)*

CONDITION	CHARACTERISTICS	NOTES
Williams syndrome	• Mental retardation • Blue irises with stellate pattern • Supravalvular aortic stenosis • Renal artery stenosis • "Cocktail party personality"	• Hypercalcemia at birth

CHAPTER 17

RHEUMATOLOGY

TABLE 17-1   *COMMON SIGNS AND SYMPTOMS OF RHEUMATOLOGIC DISEASE*

SIGNS/SYMPTOMS	MOST COMMON ASSOCIATED ILLNESSES
Fever	• Acute rheumatic fever • Infection—septic joint; osteomyelitis • Systemic JRA • Malignancy—leukemia, lymphoma • SLE • Familial Mediterranean Fever
Weight loss, poor growth, delayed puberty	• Inflammatory bowel disease • Any chronic disease • Hypothyroidism • Malignancy • Infectious/postinfectious disease
Hypertension, tachycardia	• SLE, PAN, HSP • Myocardial disease
Fatigue	• All inflammatory rheumatic diseases • Fibromyalgia
Alopecia	• SLE, dermatomyositis
Red eyes	• Conjunctival injection: Kawasaki syndrome; Stevens-Johnson syndrome; Reiter syndrome

(Continued)

TABLE 17-1	*COMMON SIGNS AND SYMPTOMS OF RHEUMATOLOGIC DISEASE (CONTINUED)*
SIGNS/SYMPTOMS	**MOST COMMON ASSOCIATED ILLNESSES**
Painful eyes	• Iritis: sarcoidosis; spondyloarthropathies; Behçet disease; inflammatory bowel diseases; JRA (rarely symptomatic)
Mouth sores	• SLE • Inflammatory bowel disease • Behçet disease • Reiter syndrome (painless)
Red lips/tongue	• Kawasaki syndrome • Stevens-Johnson syndrome
Headache	• SLE • Fibromyalgia • Central nervous system vasculitis • Lyme disease • Psychosomatic condition
Trouble swallowing	• Dermatomyositis • Scleroderma • Mixed connective tissue diseases
Chest pain	• Pericarditis/carditis; systemic-onset JRA
Friction rubs	• SLE • Acute rheumatic fever • Histoplasmosis
Chest wall tenderness	• Chest wall pain/costochondritis; fibromyalgia; JRA; spondyloarthropathies
Shortness of breath	• Scleroderma • Dermatomyositis • SLE • JRA

TABLE 17-1 *COMMON SIGNS AND SYMPTOMS OF RHEUMATOLOGIC DISEASE (CONTINUED)*

SIGNS/SYMPTOMS	MOST COMMON ASSOCIATED ILLNESSES
Abdominal symptoms: pain; diarrhea; vomiting	• Inflammatory bowel disease • Dermatomyositis • Pancreatitis • SLE • Fibromyalgia • Medication-induced illness • Henoch-Schönlein purpura • Hepatitis • Psychosomatic condition
Genital lesions	• Behçet disease; Reiter syndrome; gonococcal infection
Rash:	
Photosensitivity	• SLE (may be photosensitive) • Dermatomyositis (may be photosensitive) • Infectious (parvovirus B19 is photosensitive)
Evanescent	• Systemic-onset JRA
Psoriasis	• Psoriatic arthritis
Livedo reticularis	• Vasculitis (Kawasaki syndrome)
Palpable purpura	• Henoch-Schönlein purpura; polyarteritis nodosa
Urticaria	• Serum sickness—urticaria
Erythema marginatum	• Acute rheumatic fever
Erythema migrans	• Lyme disease
Erythema nodosum	• Sarcoidosis; inflammatory bowel disease; histoplasmosis; streptoccal infection
Raynaud phenomenon	• Scleroderma (systemic sclerosis) • SLE • Mixed connective tissue disease
Vasomotor instability	• Reflex sympathetic dystrophy

HSP, Henoch-Schönlein purpura; JRA, juvenile rheumatoid arthritis; PAN, polyarthritis nodosa; SLE, systemic lupus erythematosus.

Source: Rudolph CD, Rudolph AM, Hostetter MK, Lister G, Siegel NJ, eds. Rudolph's Pediatrics. 21st ed. New York: McGraw-Hill, 2002, p. 834.

ARTHRITIS

JUVENILE RHEUMATOID ARTHRITIS (JRA)

JRA is an immune-mediated disease characterized by nonmigratory arthritis and systemic manifestations. Pathology reveals chronic synovitis and pannus formation (invasion of cartilage by synovium). There are five classes of disease, grouped by number of joints involved, systemic manifestations, and associated laboratory findings: pauciarticular types I and II, polyarticular rheumatoid factor (RF) positive and negative, and systemic JRA.

TABLE 17-2.   *JUVENILE RHEUMATOID ARTHRITIS (JRA)*

TABLE 17-3.   *MISCELLANEOUS CHILDHOOD ARTHRITIDES*

TABLE 17-4.   *SYNOVIAL FLUID CHARACTERISTICS*

TABLE 17-2   *JUVENILE RHEUMATOID ARTHRITIS (JRA)*

TYPE	CLINICAL	EVALUATION	TREATMENT/NOTES

Pauciarticular	• ≤4 joints involved for first 6 mo of disease
	• Primarily asymmetric large joint involvement
	• Morning stiffness
	• Pain usually limited to movement
	• Untreated cases present with leg length discrepancy (involved side is longer)
		• ↑ ESR
		• Mild anemia
			• NSAIDs
			• Slit lamp examinations
			  - ANA+: q 3 mo
			  - ANA−: q 6 mo

Type I (**most common type of JRA**)	• Females >> males • Blond girl aged 2-4 y with inflamed joints is a common presentation • ANA-positive patients are at high risk of iridocyclitis	• RF negative • Usually ANA positive	
Type II	• Males >> females • Onset later in childhood • Associated with sacroiliitis, hip girdle disease	• RF negative • ANA negative • Associated with HLA B27	

TABLE 17-2 *JUVENILE RHEUMATOID ARTHRITIS (JRA) (CONTINUED)*

TYPE	CLINICAL	EVALUATION	TREATMENT/NOTES
Polyarticular	• Females > males • ≥5 joints for first 6 mo of disease • Symmetric joint involvement (small and large joints) • Hip disease major cause of disability in late disease	• Leukocytosis • ↑ ESR	• NSAIDs • Methotrexate • TNF-alpha inhibitors
RF positive	• More severe than RF-negative disease, with high incidence of joint deformities, rheumatoid nodules	• RF positive • 75% ANA positive	• NSAIDs • Slit lamp exams at least once/year, more often if ANA positive • Joint deformities may require surgical intervention
RF negative	• Severe arthritis less common than in RF-positive disease	• RF negative • 25% ANA positive	
Systemic-onset "Still's disease")	• Females = males • Variable number of joints • Daily fever spikes • Systemic signs may precede the arthritis by many years (may present as fever of unknown origin) • Salmon-colored evanescent rash during fever • Hepatosplenomegaly • Lymphadenopathy • Serositis • Anemia • *Definitive* diagnosis requires joint symptoms for more than 6 consecutive wk	• Leukocytosis • ↑ ESR • Anemia • Thrombocytosis • Transaminitis • Chest radiograph may show pleural effusion • Echocardiogram may show pericardial effusion • RF negative • ANA negative	• NSAIDs • Methotrexate • TNF-alpha inhibitors

ANA, antinuclear antibody; ESR, erythrocyte sedimentation factor; NSAIDs, nonsteroidal anti-inflammatory drugs; TNF, tumor necrosis factor; RF, rheumatoid factor.

TABLE 17-3　　　*MISCELLANEOUS CHILDHOOD ARTHRITIDES*

TYPE	CLINICAL	EVALUATION	TREATMENT/NOTES
Psoriatic arthritis	• Family/personal history of psoriasis • Females > males • Asymmetric joint involvement, variable in number • Dactylitis • Nail pitting	• Elevated to normal ESR	• NSAIDs • Methotrexate • TNF-alpha inhibitors
Gout	• Rarely seen in children without associated malignancy, or metabolic or renal disease	• Birefringent urate crystals in synovial fluid • Serum uric acid	• NSAIDs • Colchicine • Allopurinol
Inflammatory bowel disease (IBD)–associated arthritis	• Arthritis may be the first presenting symptom of ulcerative colitis or Crohn's disease • ~10% of patients with IBD develop joint symptoms • Pauciarticular, large joints (including sacroiliac) • Usually waxes and wanes with bowel symptoms	• ↑ ESR • Anemia • ANCA positive • HLA B27 may be positive in patients with sacroiliitis	• Treatment of underlying IBD • NSAIDs • Physical therapy for sacroiliitis
Celiac disease–associated arthritis	• Polyarticular • Weight loss	• Antiendomysial antibody positive	• Gluten-free diet
Ankylosing spondylitis–associated arthritis	• Males > females • Pauciarticular, large joints • Sacroiliac joint, hips, knees, heels commonly affected • Enthesopathy: inflammation of tendon insertions	• HLA-B27 positive in large majority • ↑ ESR • Anemia • ANA negative • RF negative	• NSAIDs • Physical therapy

TABLE 17-3	*MISCELLANEOUS CHILDHOOD ARTHRITIDES (CONTINUED)*		
TYPE	**CLINICAL**	**EVALUATION**	**TREATMENT/NOTES**

Reiter syndrome	• Males > females
	Classic triad*:
	  - Arthritis
	  - Sterile urethritis
	  - Uveitis
	*Rarely see all 3
	  simultaneously
	• Preceding gastrointestinal illness (i.e., *Yersinia, Shigella, Campylobacter*)
	• *Neisseria gonorrhoeae*
	• *Chlamydia trachomatis*
		• ↑ ESR
		• Pyuria
		• Strong association with HLA B27
		• Screen for sexually transmitted diseases if appropriate
		• Stool culture if appropriate
			• Antibiotics for infection
			• NSAIDs for symptoms
			• Physical therapy

Toxic synovitis	• Females = males • Age <5 y • Usually involves hip joint • History of preceding upper respiratory infection • Low-grade fever • Limp • Hip held in adduction/ external rotation • Nontoxic appearing	• Diagnosis of exclusion • Joint usually has minimal limits in range of motion • ESR, WBC, joint fluid cell count, culture/Gram stain are all normal • Rule out septic joint	• NSAIDs for hip pain • Self-limited, resolves within 1 wk
Reactive arthritis	• Pauciarticular • Usually transient • History of preceding infection (i.e., *Salmonella, Yersinia, Shigella, Neisseria, Streptococcus*)	• Stool studies if appropriate • Serology for suspected pathogen if cause uncertain	• Poststreptococcal etiology requires prophylactic antibiotics similar to those for rheumatic fever
Growing pains	• Usually bilateral leg/thigh pain • Pain *only* at night	• Diagnosed by history and physical examination	• Massaging the legs may help • NSAIDs if severe

ANCA, antineutrophil cytoplasmic antibody; ESR, erythrocyte sedimentation rate; HLA, human leukocyte antigen, NSAID, non-steroidal anti-inflammatory drug; WBC, white blood cell.

TABLE 17-4   *SYNOVIAL FLUID CHARACTERISTICS*

TYPE	WBC	PROTEIN	GLUCOSE	GRAM STAIN/ CULTURE
Normal	< 200	Normal	Equal to serum	Negative
Septic arthritis	50,000-500,000 ↑ Neutrophils	↑	↓	• Gram stain + • Culture 25%-50% +
Juvenile rheumatoid arthritis	15,000-100,000 ↑ Neutrophils	Normal	Normal	Negative
Toxic synovitis	Normal	Normal	Normal	Negative
Lyme arthritis	50,000-150,000	↑	↓	Negative

CONNECTIVE TISSUE DISORDERS

SYSTEMIC LUPUS ERYTHEMATOSUS

TABLE 17-5   *THE LUPUS SPECTRUM*

TYPE	CLINICAL	EVALUATION	TREATMENT/NOTES
Systemic lupus erythematosus (SLE)	• 11 clinical criteria: 1) Malar rash (spares nasolabial folds) 2) Discoid rash 3) Photosensitivity 4) Arthritis 5) Oral ulcers 6) Serositis 7) Renal disease 8) Neurologic: 　-Cerebritis 　-Seizures 　-Psychosis	• Diagnosis requires 4 of 11 criteria • One criteria *must* be ANA positivity • Positive anti–double-stranded DNA is specific for SLE • C3 and C4 decrease with disease flares, and are a useful marker of disease course • Anti-Ro, Smith, La, and ribonucleic protein anti-bodies may also be present, but are not specific for SLE	• NSAIDs • Steroids • Antimalarials • Chemotherapeutic agents

TABLE 17-5 *THE LUPUS SPECTRUM (CONTINUED)*

TYPE	CLINICAL	EVALUATION	TREATMENT/NOTES

Systemic lupus erythematosus (SLE) (Cont.)	9) Hematologic:
	  - Anemia
	  - Lymphopenia
	  - Thrombocytopenia
	10) ANA positive
	11) Immunologic:
	  - ↓ Complement
	  - False-positive syphilis test
	  - Coombs positive
	• Alopecia common but not one of the 11 criteria		

Drug-induced lupus	• Lupus-like syndrome caused by common drugs:
	  - Procainamide
	  - Quinidine
	  - Hydralazine
	  - Sulfonamides
	  - Isoniazid
	  - Phenytoin
	  - Oral contraceptives
		• +/- Antihistone antibody
		• Immune complexes
			• Resolves after discontinuation of offending agent

Discoid lupus	• Scaly rash in sun-exposed areas • No systemic signs	• Anti-Ro positive	• Avoid sunlight • Anti-malarials

(Continued)

TABLE 17-5	*THE LUPUS SPECTRUM (CONTINUED)*		
TYPE	**CLINICAL**	**EVALUATION**	**TREATMENT/NOTES**
Neonatal lupus	• 3rd-degree heart block • Fetal bradycardia • Fetal congestive heart failure • Rash common • Photosensitivity • Thrombocytopenia • Transaminitis	• Anti-Ro positive • Anti-La positive • Thrombocytopenia • Hemolytic anemia • Leukopenia	• Serial fetal echocardio-grams • Supportive care • Consider maternal steroids • Test mother for Sjögren's syndrome and SLE (maternal Sjögren's more common cause of neonatal lupus than maternal SLE)
Antiphospholipid antibody (APLA) syndrome (lupus anticoagulant)	• Recurrent fetal loss • Unexplained venous and arterial thrombosis • Strokes • Pulmonary embolus • Avascular bone necrosis • Myocardial infarcts (young age) • Menorrhagia	• APLA positive • Prolonged PT/PTT that does not correct with fresh frozen plasma administration (APLA causes thrombosis *in vivo*, but is an anticoag-ulant *in vitro*)	• Lifelong anticoagulation following thrombotic event

ANA, antinuclear antibody; PT, prothrombin time; PTT, partial thromboplastin time.

SCLERODERMA

Scleroderma is a chronic disease of connective tissue, causing fibrosis and the characteristic "hard, tight, shiny skin" described with the disease. The skin feels indurated and may be discolored. Lesions are located proximal to the wrist. Disease may be localized (involving only skin) or systemic (involving skin, as well as viscera). Localized disease may in turn be broken down further into morphea or linear disease, depending on the morphology of the lesions. Systemic disease may also be further subcategorized into either diffuse or limited disease, depending on the severity of disease and laboratory findings. Females are affected more often than males.

TABLE 17-6   *THE SCLERODERMA SPECTRUM*

TYPE	CLINICAL	EVALUATION	TREATMENT/ NOTES
Localized scleroderma	• Morphea: plaques and /or drops ("guttate" pattern) • Linear: affects single dermatome • *En coup de sabre*: involvement of scalp	• +/- RF • +/- ANA • Increased immunoglobulins • Skin biopsy	• Severe disease may adhere skin to underlying structures, causing contractures that require splinting or surgical intervention • Disease is usually self-limited, but may be permanently disfiguring
Systemic scleroderma	Limited (CREST syndrome): • **C**alcinosis (calcium deposits in the skin) • **R**aynaud phenomenon • **E**sophageal disease • **S**clerodactyly • **T**elangiectasias • Pulmonary lesion similar to primary pulmonary hypertension	• Anti-centromere antibodies • +/- ANA • +/- RF • Skin biopsy	• Pulmonary function testing • Physical therapy • Aggressive treatment of complications (i.e., hypertension)
	Diffuse (progressive): • May have all of above plus: • Pulmonary fibrosis, secondary pulmonary hypertension • Hypertension, renal failure may occur • Cardiac disease main cause of death in children (heart block, congestive heart disease, pericardial effusion)	• Antiscleroderma 70 antibody • Anti-RNP antibody • +/- ANA • +/- RF • Skin biopsy	
Raynaud phenomenon	• Vasospastic attacks preceded by cold exposure or emotion • Fingers/involved digits show a 3-phase color change: White→blue→red • Numbness/pain	• +/- ANA	• Calcium-channel blockers

ANA, antinuclear antibody; RF, rheumatoid factor; RNP, ribonuclear protein.

VASCULITIDES OF CHILDHOOD

KAWASAKI SYNDROME

TABLE 17-7   *KAWASAKI SYNDROME*

DEFINITION	ETIOLOGY	CLINICAL	DIAGNOSIS	TREATMENT/NOTES

• Mucocutaneous lymph node syndrome
• Coronary artery vasculitis
• Most common cause of acquired heart disease in children
	• Unknown	• Males ≥ females
		• Peak incidence age 18-24 mo
		• Increased incidence in Japanese/Asian children
		• Diagnosis requires fever for more than 5 d *and* 4/5 of the following:
		  1. Nonexudative conjunctivitis (spares limbus)
		  2. Mucosal changes: reddened oropharynx, cracked lips, strawberry tongue
		  3. Extremity changes: induration/swelling of hands/feet
		  4. Rash (any type)
		  5. Cervical lymphadenopathy >1.5 cm
		• Fever, 3/5 criteria, and evidence of coronary artery disease also acceptable for diagnosis
			• Clinical
			• Echocardiogram to rule out coronary artery disease (aneurysms)
			• Increased acute-phase reactants
			• Thrombocytosis occurs >10 d into illness
				• IVIG at time of diagnosis, most useful for preventing cardiac sequelae when given in first 10 d of disease
				• Echocardiogram at diagnosis and again at 6-8 wk
				• Aspirin: high dose (anti-inflammation), then low dose (antiplatelet)
				• Corticosteroids are controversial
				• Hold aspirin if patient has chickenpox or influenza to help prevent Reye syndrome
				• Associated findings:
				  - Irritability
				  - Gallbladder hydrops
				  - Sterile pyuria
				  - Aseptic meningitis
				  - Transaminitis

IVIG, intravenous immunoglobulin.

HENOCH-SCHÖNLEIN PURPURA (HSP)

TABLE 17-8   *HENOCH-SCHÖNLEIN PURPURA*

DEFINITION	ETIOLOGY	CLINICAL	DIAGNOSIS	TREATMENT/NOTES
• "Anaphylactoid purpura" • Small-vessel vasculitis primarily involving gastrointestinal tract, skin, and kidneys • Most common small-vessel vasculitis in childhood	• Idiopathic IgA-mediated inflammation and destruction of arterioles, capillaries, and venules • May have history of preceding upper respiratory infection	• Boys > girls • Peak age 2-5 y • Classic triad: 1. Palpable purpura (usually on lower extremities, may be widespread in younger patients) 2. Colicky abdominal pain 3. Arthritis • Nephritis (IgA nephropathy) is present in 25%-50% at time of onset • Testicular torsion in males is a possible presentation and complication • Intussusception may occur in up to 15% as a result of bowel hemorrhage and edema	• Clinical history and presentation • ↑ ESR • Normal platelets • Normal coagulation studies • Guaiac + stools • Urinalysis may show evidence of nephritis: hematuria, proteinuria, cell casts	• Supportive • Corticosteroids in severe cases • Avoid NSAIDs due to risk for bleeding • Nephrology should evaluate all suspected cases. IgA nephropathy may present after resolution of the acute episode. Renal failure is number one cause of mortality

ESR, erythrocyte sedimentation rate; NSAID, nonsteroidal anti-inflammatory drug.

DERMATOMYOSITIS

TABLE 17-9   *DERMATOMYOSITIS*

DEFINITION	ETIOLOGY	CLINICAL	DIAGNOSIS	TREATMENT/NOTES
• Chronic multi-organ disease with inflammation of skin and striated muscle	• Unknown	• Symmetric trunk and proximal muscle weakness • Dysphagia or respiratory difficulties may be present • Classic "heliotrope" rash (violet-colored eyelids +/- periorbital edema) • The rash does *not* spare the nasolabial folds (vs. SLE, which does) • Gottron papules (scaly rash of extensor surfaces and knuckles) • Nailfold capillary changes	• ↑ CPK, aldolase, lactate dehydrogenase, or transaminases (from muscle breakdown) • MRI reveals edematous areas proximal to affected muscles • Electromyography reveals small-amplitude spike and waves • Muscle biopsy reveals perifascicular inflammation	• Corticosteroids • Physical therapy • Monitoring of respiratory and swallowing function • Methotrexate • Immune globulin

CPK, creatinine phosphokinase; SLE, systemic lupus erythematosus.

RHEUMATIC HEART DISEASE

FIGURE 17-1.   ACUTE RHEUMATIC FEVER.

TABLE 17-10.   MISCELLANEOUS RHEUMATOLOGIC DISORDERS

Diagnosis: Evidence of a preceding Strep infection: (positive throat culture, rapid antigen, elevation of anti-streptolysin O, anti-hyaluronidase, or anti-DNAase B antibody, or history of scarlet fever) AND

2 major OR 1 major and 2 minor Jones criteria or Sydenham's Chorea alone

JONES CRITERIA:	**MAJOR**	**MINOR**
	-Carditis	-Fever
	-Polyarthritis (migratory)	-Arthralgia (NOT ARTHRITIS!)
	-Erythema Marginatum	-Prolonged P-R interval
	-Sydenham's Chorea	-Elevated acute phase reactants
	-Subcutaneous nodules	

Most Common Cardiac Lesion: Mitral Regurgitation
Treatment : Salicylates for arthritis, mild carditis
　　　　　　　Consider steroids for severe carditis
　　　　　　　Benzodiazapines/haloperidol for chorea
　　　　　　　Lifelong prophylaxis to prevent further streptococcal infections, usually penicillin

— FIGURE 17-1 — Acute rheumatic fever.

TABLE 17-10   MISCELLANEOUS RHEUMATOLOGIC DISORDERS

TYPE	FACTS
Sarcoidosis	• Systemic, chronic, granulomatous disease
	• Rare in childhood
	• Noncaseating granulomas, usually in the lung
	• Hilar/peripheral adenopathy
	• Labs may show hypercalcemia, increased levels of ACE, increased ESR
	• Diagnosis made by biopsy of granuloma

(Continued)

TABLE 17-10   *MISCELLANEOUS RHEUMATOLOGIC DISORDERS (CONTINUED)*

TYPE	FACTS
Wegener granulomatosis	• Vasculitis of lungs and kidney • Granulomas of upper respiratory tract and kidneys • Hemoptysis and renal failure common clinical features • P-ANCA/C-ANCA positive • Diagnose by biopsy
Behçet syndrome	• Recurrent painful genital and oral ulcers, and uveitis • Commonly seen associated features include: arthritis, colitis, rash, and fever
Sjögren syndrome	• Xerostomia (dry mouth), dry eyes, and connective tissue disorder • Parotid swelling • May occur in conjunction with JRA • Increased risk of lymphoma • Labs: positive anti-Sm and anti-Ro

ACE, angiotensin-converting enzyme; ANCA, antineutrophil cytoplasmic antibody; ESR, erythrocyte sedimentation rate; JRA, juvenile rheumatoid arthritis.

CHAPTER 18

SPORTS MEDICINE/ ORTHOPEDICS

PREPARTICIPATION PHYSICAL EXAMINATION

The goal of the preparticipation physical examination is to identify conditions which may interfere with participation in sports or may worsen as a result of physical activity. The main components include a review of any past injuries, current existing conditions, family history (focusing on cardiac disease), and full physical examination (focusing especially on the musculoskeletal and cardiovascular systems). Patients should also be asked about use of performance-enhancing agents (including but not limited to steroids and ephedrine).

SPORTS INJURIES

HEAT CRAMPS, HEAT EXHAUSTION, AND HEAT STROKE

This spectrum of disorders is caused by overheating and dehydration. They can be largely avoided by ensuring adequate hydration (before, during, and after training) and by avoiding strenuous exercise during hot weather.

TABLE 18-1.   HEAT CRAMPS, HEAT EXHAUSTION, AND HEAT STROKE

CONCUSSION

A concussion is defined as minor head trauma that causes confusion or loss of consciousness (<1 minute). Seizures, vomiting, confusion, headaches, or lethargy may accompany the injury. Mechanical force predisposes the patient to diffuse brain injury. Most minor concussions resolve with time. Repetitive concussions may result in permanent deficits including cognitive disabilities.

Concussions are generally graded on a scale from 1 to 3, with 1 being mild and 3 most severe. Although a child may seem well shortly after sustaining a head injury, subtle late findings such as persistent headache, memory problems, irritability, behavioral changes, or deterioration of school performance may be present, and should prompt further evaluation. Management guidelines for concussions are shown in Table 18-2.

TABLE 18-1   *HEAT CRAMPS, HEAT EXHAUSTION, AND HEAT STROKE*

DISEASE	PRESENTATION	DIAGNOSIS	TREATMENT
Heat cramps	• Fatigue, muscle cramps	• Clinical history and presentation	• Fluid replacement
Heat exhaustion	• Elevated core temperature (38-40°C), dizziness, visual disturbances, cramps, syncope, nausea, vomiting	• Clinical history and presentation	• Cooling (ice packs, fanning), IV fluids
Heat stroke	• Elevated core temperature (>40°C), • Delirium, seizures, coma • Sweating and flushing may be absent • May present with multisystem organ failure	• Clinical history and presentation	• Ice packing to head, neck, groin; IV fluids; hospital observation

SPRAINS AND STRAINS

- **Sprains**: Injury to a ligament or joint capsule.
- **Strains**: Injury to a muscle or tendon.

    Most minor injuries can be treated with RICE: **R**est, **I**ce, **C**ompression, and **E**levation, and with nonsteroidal anti-inflammatories, such as ibuprofen. More severe injuries may require further treatment, as shown in Table 18-3.

TABLE 18-2   *CONCUSSION MANAGEMENT*

GRADE OF INJURY	CLINICAL	MANAGEMENT	RETURN TO PLAY
Grade 1	• No loss of consciousness • May experience transient confusion • Symptoms resolve in <15 min	• Examine at 5-min intervals • May return to play if asymptomatic after 15 min	• Second grade 1 concussion in same game eliminates player for the day • After second grade 1 concussion, may return to play if asymptomatic for 1 wk both at rest and with exercise
Grade 2	• No loss of consciousness • Transient confusion • Symptoms last >15 min	• Examine frequently on site • Remove from play that day	• Return to play if asymptomatic for 1 wk both at rest and with exercise • Following a second grade 2 concussion, may return to play when asymptomatic for 2 wk both at rest and with exercise • Obtain CT or MRI if symptoms persist >1 wk • Any abnormality on CT or MRI terminates season
Grade 3	• Any loss of consciousness, regardless of duration	• Remove from play that day • Perform thorough neurologic evaluation • Consider immediate imaging (depending on severity of signs and symptoms)	• Brief loss of consciousness: return to play when symptom-free for 1 wk both at rest and with exercise • Prolonged loss of consciousness: return to play when symptom-free for 2 wk both at rest and with exercise • Following a second grade 3 concussion: return to play when symptom-free for 1 mo both at rest and with exercise • Obtain CT or MRI if symptoms last >1 wk • Any abnormality on CT or MRI terminates season

TABLE 18-3 COMMON SPORTS INJURIES

LOCATION	FREQUENT DIAGNOSIS	PRESENTATION	DIAGNOSIS	TREATMENT	RETURN TO PLAY
Back	• Strains	• Pain • Loss of flexibility	• Clinical diagnosis	• Stretching	• Full range of motion • Resolution of symptoms
Shoulder	• Glenohumeral dislocation	• Pain	• Radiograph	• Sling • Reduction, possible surgical intervention	• Full range of motion • Resolution of symptoms (minimum 8 wk)
Fingers	• Sprain • "Jammed finger"	• Pain • Swelling • Limitation of motion	• X-ray if high suspicion of a fracture	• Buddy taping	• Full range of motion • Resolution of symptoms
Knee	• Medial collateral ligament (MCL) sprains	• Trauma to lateral knee (valgus stress) • "Pop" is often heard in football players hit from the side • Limited range of motion	• Decreased range of motion • Point tenderness over MCL	• Bracing	• Full range of motion • Resolution of symptoms (minimum 8-12 wk)
	• Anterior collateral ligament (ACL) tear - More severe than MCL strain - More common in females	• Twisting motion of knee with planted foot • "Pop" is often heard (~70% of patients) • Usually unable to continue activity • Common in gymnastics, soccer, skiing	• Severe pain • Limited range of motion • Large effusion within hours • Positive anterior drawer and Lachman tests • MRI	• Physical therapy • Bracing • May require surgical intervention	• Full range of motion • Resolution of symptoms

Hip	• Apophyseal avulsion of anterior superior iliac spine	• Forceful flexion of hip joint, such as a strong kick • Patient feels a "pop" in hip • Seen in soccer players, cheerleaders	• Radiograph	• Supportive care • Weight bearing as tolerated	• Full range of motion • Resolution of symptoms
Ankle	• Sprains - Most common: anterior talofibular ligament	• Twisting, eversion, or inversion injury	• Swelling • Limited range of motion • Point tenderness over ligaments • Lack of bony pain • X-ray all bone pain and significant swelling	• Assistive devices: cane or crutches	• Full range of motion • Resolution of symptoms

PERFORMANCE-ENHANCING DRUGS

Agents such as anabolic steroids, ephedrine, creatine, diuretics, and erythropoetin are used by athletes to increase muscle mass and/or enhance performance. They are used by athletes of all ages and both sexes. Education and counseling beginning at the grade-school level is important. Selected agents are discussed below:

- **Anabolic Steroids**: Used to increase muscle mass. Side effects include acne, hirsutism, and mood changes. Complications include gynecomastia, testicular atrophy, and sterility in males. In females, menstrual abnormalities and voice changes are common. There is an increased risk of hepatitis and hepatocellular carcinoma in both sexes.
- **Ephedrine**: Used to suppress appetite and encourage weight loss. It is chemically similar to amphetamine. Side effects include palpitations, irregular heartbeat, hypertension, nervousness, insomnia, and weight loss. Its use has been linked to strokes, myocardial infarctions, and death.
- **Diuretics**: Used by some athletes in an attempt to lose weight. They are most commonly used in sports where a low weight is desirable, i.e., wrestlers, jockeys, and gymnasts. Side effects are secondary to dehydration: tachycardia, weakness, and fatigue. Electrolyte abnormalities, including fatal hypokalemia, may also occur.

ORTHOPEDICS

This section should be studied along with an atlas that demonstrates the radiographic images associated with this group of disorders. When a radiograph is shown in the picture section of the pediatric board exam, it is NOT likely to be a normal film, and clues to the diagnosis will likely be present in the accompanying clinical vignette.

Fractures

Definitions: the *diaphysis* refers to the bone shaft, the *epiphysis* refers to the ends of the bone, the *physis* is the growth plate, and the *metaphysis* is the widened area of long bone between the physis and the diaphysis.

FRACTURE TYPES

- **Buckle Fracture (Torus Fracture)**: A common injury of childhood. The bone buckles and the bone is compressed rather than broken, usually at the diaphysis.
- **Greenstick Fracture**: The bone is incompletely fractured, with a portion of the cortex and periosteum remaining intact, although deformed, on the compressed side.
- **Complete Fracture**: These fractures propagate completely through the bone. They are further classified by descriptions of the fracture line. The most common types include:

- *Transverse fracture*: The fracture line is at a right angle to the long axis.
- *Spiral fracture*: The fracture line is oblique and encircles a portion of the shaft.
- *Oblique fracture*: The fracture line is at an angle to the long axis.
- *Comminuted fracture*: The fracture site involves more than two fragments.

FIGURE 18-1. *TYPES OF FRACTURES COMMON IN CHILDREN.*

COMMON FRACTURES

- *Clavicle*: Most commonly fractured bone in childhood. Occurs secondary to fall onto shoulder or outstretched arm, or from direct blow to area. Usual site of fracture is midshaft. Treated with simple sling. Figure-of-eight bandage no longer recommended.
- *Supracondylar fracture of the humerus*: Most common elbow fracture. Occurs from fall onto outstretched arm. The patient may have secondary neurovascular (especially ulnar nerve) injury.

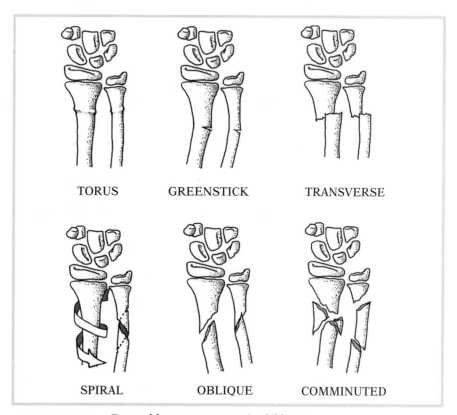

TORUS   GREENSTICK   TRANSVERSE

SPIRAL   OBLIQUE   COMMINUTED

— **FIGURE 18-1** — Types of fractures common in children.

- *Toddler fracture*: Spiral or oblique fracture of the tibia. Often results from a fall associated with a twisting motion (common scenario is falling with foot entrapped in playground equipment). Child presents with limp and refusal to walk. Radiographs may be normal.
- *Metatarsal fracture ("march fracture")*: Stress fracture of head of the second and/or third metatarsal. Commonly seen in runners and soldiers. Presents with pain while walking.
- *Metacarpal fracture ("boxer's fracture")*: Fracture of the fifth metacarpal, usually as a result of a direct blow (such as punching a wall with a closed fist).

COMPARTMENT SYNDROME

Compartment syndromes are most common with supracondylar fractures of the humerus and in forearm fractures. The patient presents with pain, pallor, paralysis, and pulselessness. Compartment pressures should be measured and fasciotomy performed in true cases.

Salter Harris Classification

This system is used to describe the relationship of fractures to the physis. It is useful for predicting long-term deformity resulting from damage to the growth plate.

- *Type I*: Fracture through the physis only, may or may not be displaced; if undisplaced, the radiographs may appear normal. Prognosis is good.
- *Type II*: Fracture involving the physis and the metaphysis on the side opposite to the instigating force. Prognosis is good.
- *Type III*: Fracture involving the physis and the epiphysis. Permanent deformity may occur.
- *Type IV*: Fracture involving the metaphysis, physis, and epiphysis. Permanent deformity may occur.
- *Type V*: Crush injury of the physis. Radiographs are nonrevealing, and diagnosis is clinical. Poor prognosis.

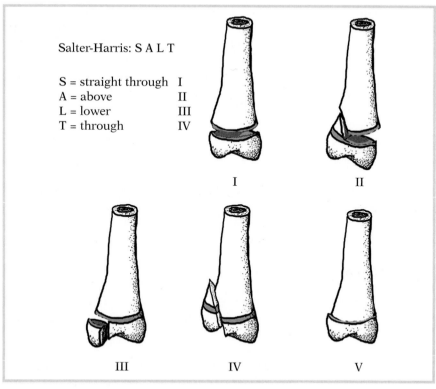

Salter-Harris: S A L T

S = straight through I
A = above II
L = lower III
T = through IV

– FIGURE 18-2 – Salter Harris classification.

Common Orthopedic Disorders in Children

TABLE 18-4.   *COMMON NEONATAL ORTHOPEDIC DISORDERS*
TABLE 18-5.   *COMMON PEDIATRIC ORTHOPEDIC DISORDERS*

COMMON CAUSES OF INTOEING AND OUT-TOEING

- **Valgus**: Distal portion of limb is displaced laterally in comparison to proximal portion.
- **Varus**: Distal portion of limb is displaced medially in comparison to proximal portion.
- **Metatarsus Adductus**: Adducted and inverted forefoot that is present at birth. Occurs secondary to intrauterine compression. Treatment consists of passive range of motion exercises. Casting is required in severe cases that do not correct by age 3 to 4 months.
- **Talipes Equinovarus (Clubfoot)**: The etiology is multifactorial, including genetic predisposition and intrauterine compression. May be unilateral or bilateral.

(Text continues on page 354.)

TABLE 18-4   COMMON NEONATAL ORTHOPEDIC DISORDERS

DISORDER	DEFINITION	ETIOLOGY	PRESENTATION	DIAGNOSIS	TREATMENT
Torticollis	• Positional abnormality of neck resulting in head tilt and rotation	• In infants: congenital injury to SCM muscle • In children: Klippel-Feil syndrome/other cervical vertebral anomalies, intracranial masses, cervical adenitis, retropharyngeal abscess	• SCM injury: chin points away from side of injury • With other causes, history and physical will often vary	• SCM injury may often present with palpable "mass" in muscle body, which is area of fibrosis within muscle • 20% of congenital cases will have associated developmental dysplasia of the hip • Cases diagnosed later in disease may have craniofacial abnormalities (ipsilateral flattening)	• Active physical therapy • Surgery may be indicated to release muscle if physical therapy does not work
Developmental dysplasia of the hip (DDH)	• Abnormal development of the relationship between the acetabulum and the femoral head	• Intrauterine mechanical forces	• 1-2/1000 births • Female > male • First born • Unilateral more common than bilateral	• Barlow test (adduction of hip) may dislocate hip • Ortolani test (abduction of hip) may relocate displaced hip	• Pavlik harness to properly position hips for proper development • Surgical management may be necessary in children who fail treatment with harnesses, or who are diagnosed late in disease

- Physical exam:
  - Leg is held adducted and externally rotated.
  - If unilateral, affected leg may appear shorter, and gluteal fold may be asymmetric

- Ultrasound exam

- Associated with increased incidence of torticollis, clubfoot, and scoliosis

SCM, sternocleidomastoid.

TABLE 18-5   COMMON PEDIATRIC ORTHOPEDIC DISORDERS

DISORDER	DEFINITION	ETIOLOGY	PRESENTATION	DIAGNOSIS	TREATMENT
Klippel-Feil disease	• Congenital malformation of the neck	• Failure of cervical vertebrae segmentation	• Short, broad neck (may appear webbed) • May have secondary torticollis • Associated anomalies include: Sprengel's deformity; scoliosis; cardiac, renal, or pulmonary disease	• X-ray of cervical vertebrae	• Physical therapy • Bracing
Sprengel deformity	• Congenital malformation of the scapula	• Possibly familial	• Small, high-riding, medially rotated scapula • Inability to fully extend/abduct arm • Asymmetry of neck • Associated with scoliosis, torticollis, and Klippel-Feil	• X-ray of cervical vertebrae and chest	• Surgical correction
Nursemaids elbow	• Subluxation of the radial head from the annular ligament	• Sudden traction to an extended arm (such as when a caretaker pulls a child by the arm, or an infant rolls over extended arm)	• Refusal to use arm • Arm held with elbow flexed and forearm pronated • No bony pain or swelling	• Clinical	• Gentle supination and flexion of the elbow • Resolution of symptoms within minutes • High recurrence rate
Legg-Calvé-Perthes disease	• Ischemic necrosis of the proximal femoral epiphysis	• Unknown	• Males > females • Age 4-10 y • 15% bilateral • Painless limp	• X-ray findings range from normal in early disease to narrow	• Earlier cases may require only observation and curtailment of activities

Disease	Definition	Etiology/Pathophysiology	Clinical Features	Diagnosis	Treatment
Slipped capital femoral epiphysis (SCFE)	• Displacement of the femoral head from the femoral neck	• It is postulated that the combination of shearing stresses and increased hormone levels during puberty may compromise the growth plate	• Males > females • Age 8-14 y (pubertal) • Patient often obese • May present incidentally after a fall • Pain*ful* limp • May complain of hip, knee, or thigh pain • May complain of hip, knee, or thigh pain • Pain with passive adduction and internal rotation	• X-ray reveals femoral head displaced inferiorly and posteriorly on the proximal femur ("ice cream falling off the cone") • femoral epiphysis and collapse of the femoral head in late disease	• Surgical intervention (in situ pinning) • Later cases will require bracing and/or surgical intervention to reposition femoral head within the acetabulum
Osgood-Schlatter disease	• Apophysitis (inflammation at site of tendon insertion) of the tibial tubercle	• Stress at apophysis from: - Vigorous activity at joint - Differential growth between bony and soft tissue structures (occurs during growth spurts)	• Pain over tibial tubercle, especially with bending or jumping • Point tenderness and swelling • Usually bilateral • Prominent tibial tubercle	• In long-standing cases, X-ray may show fragmentation of apophysis	• Temporary cessation of aggravating activity • NSAIDs • Bracing in severe cases • Self-limiting
Blount disease	• Varus deformity of proximal tibia	• Growth disturbance and collapse of medial tibial epiphysis	• Unilateral or bilateral • May appear "knock-kneed," but deformation is localized to proximal tibia (physiologic genu varum has diffuse angularity) • Thighs are straight (not bowed)	• X-ray of tibia reveals collapse of proximal tibial epiphysis and "beaking" of tibia	• Bracing • Surgical intervention in severe cases

NSAID, nonsteroidal anti-inflammatory drug.

The foot is plantar flexed, the hind foot is in a varus position, and the forefoot is adducted and sometimes supinated. The underlying cause is a rotational deformity of the subtalar joint. Associated with arthrogryposis and developmental dysplasia of the hip. Treatment consists of physical therapy and casting. Severe, unresponsive, or cases diagnosed at later stages may require surgical intervention.

- **Internal Tibial Torsion**: A normal developmental inward twisting of the tibiofibular axis, which results in clinical intoeing. Clinically, knees face forward, and lower legs rotate inward. Diagnosed early in life, usually *before* age 3 years. Spontaneous resolution is common. Corrective shoes and leg braces no longer in common practice.

- **Femoral Anteversion**: Inward twisting of the femur resulting in inturning of entire leg and intoeing. Diagnosed *after* age 3 years. Spontaneous resolution is common.

- **Physiologic Genu Varum ("Bowlegs")**: Presents between 1 and 3 years of age. Considered a normal variant. Spontaneous resolution is common. Differential diagnosis includes rickets, dwarfism, and Blount disease.

- **Physiologic Genu Valgum ("Knock Knees")**: Presents between 3 and 5 years of age. Also considered a normal variant. Spontaneous resolution is common. Differential diagnosis includes rickets and renal disease.

SCOLIOSIS

DEFINITION: Scoliosis is a deformity of the spine resulting from curving in the lateral plane, as well as rotation along the sagittal axis.

ETIOLOGY: Scoliosis may be structural (resulting from a fixed spine curvature) or nonstructural, as a secondary result of deformity elsewhere (i.e., leg-length discrepancy, or splinting from pneumonia). Syndromes associated with scoliosis include: Marfan syndrome, neurofibromatosis, Klippel-Feil, Sprengel deformity, and the VATER association.

CLINICAL PRESENTATION: Clinical presentation can range from asymptomatic to severe deformities with compression of internal organs. The disease may involve any portion of the vertebral column, including the sacrum.

DIAGNOSIS: Screening for scoliosis should be conducted at all well child exams, either by physical inspection, or, in children who are old enough to cooperate, by the Adam's forward-bending test. Findings on physical exam may include asymmetric prominence of the posterior ribs or flank, or asymmetric shoulders or pelvis. Pain is an unusual finding. The diagnosis of scoliosis is made via radiograph, by measuring the Cobb angle.

TREATMENT: Complete resolution of nonstructural scoliosis requires that the underlying cause be treated. Treatment options for scoliosis include observation, bracing, and surgical correction. Bracing is useful to prevent progression; it is not intended as a corrective measure. Not all curvatures need to be completely corrected in order to be considered successfully treated. Only surgery will completely correct scoliosis.

TABLE 18-6   *SCOLIOSIS*

TYPE	ETIOLOGY	PRESENTATION	TREATMENT

Congenital scoliosis (5%)	• Incomplete segmentation *and/or*
	• Incomplete formation of vertebrae during the first trimester
		• Presents at birth or shortly thereafter
		• Genitourinary abnormalities are present in 20% (most common lesion is solitary kidney)
		• Spinal cord defects are present in 20% (most common lesion is spina bifida)
			• Depends on type of vertebral defect:
			  - Observation if mild curvature and no progression
			  - Surgery if curvature is severe or progressive

Neuromuscular scoliosis (10%)	• Asymmetric muscular forces of the trunk and paraspinal muscles cause curvature of the spinal column	• May present at any age • Associated with cerebral palsy, muscular dystrophy, and arthrogryposis • Disease more severe in wheelchair-bound patients • May have secondary respiratory compromise	• Bracing usually not helpful • Surgical intervention usually necessary • Goal is improved sitting ability and ambulation, and preservation of pulmonary function
Idiopathic scoliosis (80%); may be further divided by age groups: **• Infantile: 0-3 y** **• Juvenile: 4-10 y** **• Adolescent: 11+ y**	• 20% familial • Occurs in otherwise healthy children • Females > males	• Usually diagnosed via screening exam • Curvature is usually to the right • Scoliosis associated with pain and left-sided curvatures has increased incidence of underlying disease (i.e., tumors) • Risk of progression is higher in prepubertal girls than in postpubertal girls	• If curve is <20° at diagnosis: follow with serial X-rays • If curve progresses past 20°, or is >25° at diagnosis: bracing • If curve progresses past 45°, or is >40° at diagnosis: surgical intervention

Inherited Disorders of Bone

OSTEOGENESIS IMPERFECTA (OI)

DEFINITION: An inherited group of disorders involving abnormal type I collagen resulting in osteopenia and excessive bone fragility. There is a wide spectrum of disease severity classified by four types.

DIAGNOSIS: The diagnosis is clinical, although bone biopsy will show osteopenia, disorganized osteoid, and a reduced number of osteoblasts.

TREATMENT: Management consists of prevention of fractures and aggressive management of fractures if they occur. Minimization of deformities is an important goal. Genetic counseling should be offered to affected families.

TABLE 18-7	OSTEOGENESIS IMPERFECTA	
TYPE	**GENETIC CHARACTERISTICS**	**FEATURES/NOTES**
Type I • **Most common type** • **Two subtypes: IA and IB**	• Autosomal dominant	• Usually do not have fractures until preschool age • Blue sclera • Wormian skull bones • Ligamentous laxity • Mildly short stature • Type IB patients have abnormal teeth (dentinogenesis imperfecta); Type IA patients have normal teeth • Hearing loss in adulthood common • Can have normal life span • Frequency of fractures tends to decrease with increased age
Type II • **Most severe form**	• Usually new mutation, but may may be autosomal recessive	• Intrauterine growth retardation • Multiple fractures present at birth • Blue sclera • Dysmorphic facies (triangular face, beaked nose) and "bag of bones" skull • Small chest, short limbs • Fatal in-utero (50%) or shortly after birth from respiratory insufficiency

TABLE 18-7   *OSTEOGENESIS IMPERFECTA (CONTINUED)*

TYPE	GENETIC CHARACTERISTICS	FEATURES/NOTES
Type III	• Usually new mutation, but may be autosomal recessive	• Multiple fractures present at birth • May have either blue or normal sclerae • Wormian skull bones • Extreme short stature from long bone deformities • Kyphoscoliosis leads to cardiopulmonary compromise • Dentinogenesis imperfecta present in 50% • Majority do not reach adulthood
Type IV • **Rarest form** • **Two subtypes: IVA and IVB**	• Autosomal dominant	• Majority do NOT have fractures at birth • Fractures usually occur by school age • May have either blue or normal sclerae • Wormian skull bones in majority • Short stature • Type IVB patients have dentinogenesis imperfecta; Type IVA patients have normal teeth • Can have normal life span • Frequency of fractures tends to decrease with increased age

CHAPTER 19

CHILD ABUSE AND NEGLECT

- Two-thirds of victims are under age 3 years.
- The leading cause of death in children aged 6 months to 1 year.
- Siblings of abused children are at increased risk of abuse.
- Other forms of domestic violence are frequently associated with child abuse.

TABLE 19-1   *RISKS FACTORS FOR CHILD ABUSE*

CARETAKER	CHILD
• Abused as a child	• Majority are aged <3 y
• Depression	• Prematurity
• Poverty	• Multiple births
• Family discord	• Chronic illness
• Difficulty coping with stress and anger	• Perceived as "different" by the caretaker
• History of alcohol and drug use	• Foster children
• Members of sects/cults	

PHYSICAL ABUSE

BRUISES

Ninety percent of physically abused children have cutaneous injuries.

TABLE 19-2   *SITES OF INFLICTED BRUISES*

Buttocks

Lower back

Ribs

Scapula

Genitals

Inner thigh

Cheeks (slap marks)

Ear lobes (pinch marks)

Upper lip (frenulum)

Neck (choke marks)

TABLE 19-3   *CHARACTERISTICS OF INFLICTED BRUISES*

Human hand marks

Bite marks

- >3 cm between incisors = adults
- <3 cm between incisors = child

Strap marks

Gag marks

Multiple bruises at different stages

TABLE 19-4   *CHARACTERISTICS OF NONINFLICTED BRUISES*

Mongolian spots are often mistaken for bruises.

Pretibial bruises (toddlers)

Forehead bruises (infants)

The injury is appropriate for developmental age

| TABLE 19-5 | STAGES OF BRUISES |

TIME SINCE INJURY	COLOR
0-3 d	Blue, purple
4-7 d	Green
7-10 d	Brown
10-14 d	Yellow
14-30 d	Clear

BURNS

Burns make up 10% of all child abuse. Burn degrees are defined as:

- 1st degree: Epidermis only; painful
- 2nd degree: Epidermis plus dermis; blisters present; painful
- 3rd degree: Full thickness; painless

TABLE 19-6.	COMMON NONACCIDENTAL BURNS
TABLE 19-7.	COMMON ACCIDENTAL BURNS
TABLE 19-8.	COMMON CONDITIONS CONFUSED WITH BURNS

| TABLE 19-6 | COMMON NONACCIDENTAL BURNS |

BURN TYPE	EXAMPLE
Flame burns	• Cigarette burns
Contact burns	• Heating grates
	• Electric hot plates
	• Radiators
	- These burns are found in suspicious locations (back, abdomen)
Immersion burns	• Dunking burns
	• Glove and stocking burns
	- May be found on buttocks and genitalia
	- Symmetric involvement of the extremities

TABLE 19-7	*COMMON ACCIDENTAL BURNS*

Splash burns

Bathtub accidents (asymmetric involvement of the extremities)

Car seat burns (motor vehicle accidents, contact burns)

Frostbite

TABLE 19-8	*COMMON CONDITIONS CONFUSED WITH BURNS*

CONDITION	EXAMPLE
Infection	• Bullous impetigo
	• Diaper rash
Dermatitis	• Photodermatitis
Inherited disorders	• Epidermolysis bullosa
Drug reactions	• Stevens-Johnson syndrome

HEAD INJURY

Head injury is the most common cause of death from child abuse. Types of head injury are:

- Anoxic head injuries
- Traumatic head injuries

SHAKEN BABY SYNDROME (SHAKEN IMPACT SYNDROME)

Caused by repetitive shaking with considerable force or by blunt trauma. The patient presents with an acute history of irritability, lethargy, fever, vomiting, or seizures. There is usually no recent history of illness and no explanation for the symptoms. The child is usually less than 6 months of age.

TABLE 19-9. *SIGNS OF SHAKEN BABY SYNDROME*

ABDOMINAL INJURIES

Abdominal injuries are the second most common cause of death in child abuse.

TABLE 19-10. *PHYSICAL SIGNS OF ABDOMINAL INJURIES*

TABLE 19-9 *PHYSICAL SIGNS OF SHAKEN BABY SYNDROME*

Intraparenchymal hemorrhage
Subdural hematoma
Subarachnoid hemorrhage
Cerebral contusions
Retinal hemorrhage

TABLE 19-10 *PHYSICAL SIGNS OF ABDOMINAL INJURIES*

Ruptured liver
Ruptured spleen
Intestinal perforation
Small bowel hematoma
Pancreatic injury

ORTHOPEDIC INJURIES

Fractures in abused children are very common. It is important to recognize suspicious fractures in order to identify potential cases of child abuse. A high-suspicion fracture in a child less than 3 years of age warrants a retinal exam and a skeletal survey to rule out the possibility of old injuries.

TABLE 19-11. *LEVEL OF SUSPICION FOR ORTHOPEDIC FRACTURES*

TABLE 19-11 *LEVEL OF SUSPICION FOR ORTHOPEDIC FRACTURES*

HIGH SUSPICION	MODERATE SUSPICION	LOW SUSPICION
• Bucket-handle fracture	• Multiple fractures	• Clavicular fracture
• Posterior rib fracture	• Fractures of different ages	• Long bone fracture
• Spiral fracture in a nonambulating child	• Vertebral body fracture	• Spiral fractures in an ambulating child
• Scapular fracture	• Digital fracture	• Linear skull fracture
• Sternal fracture		
• Vertebral process fracture		
• Nonlinear skull fracture		

CHILD NEGLECT

Any disregard to safety or medical care constitutes child neglect. A suspected case of child neglect warrants an investigation by a social worker and/or child protective services. Physicians have a legal responsibility to report cases of suspected neglect.

TABLE 19-12. *SYMPTOMS OF CHILD NEGLECT*

SEXUAL ABUSE

Sexual abuse has reached epidemic proportions in the United States. Recognize that most cases of sexual abuse occur with a person the child knows. This may include a family member, friend, or neighbor. The history is the most important component of the evaluation. Most physical exams will be normal. The child is always telling the truth until proven otherwise.

TABLE 19-13. *PHYSICAL SIGNS OF SEXUAL ABUSE*

TABLE 19-14. *SEXUALLY TRANSMITTED DISEASES ASSOCIATED WITH SEXUAL ABUSE*

TABLE 19-15. *PHYSICAL SIGNS OFTEN CONFUSED WITH SEXUAL ABUSE*

TABLE 19-12	SYMPTOMS OF CHILD NEGLECT
Excessive quietness	
Social withdrawal	
Lack of bonding behavior	
Difficult behavior	
Failure to thrive	

TABLE 19-13	PHYSICAL SIGNS OF SEXUAL ABUSE
Vaginal lacerations	
Anal lacerations	
Transected hymen	
Dilatation of the anal sphincter	
Vesicular lesions of the genital tract	
Bruising of the posterior fourchette	
Bruising on the inner thigh	

TABLE 19-14	*SEXUALLY TRANSMITTED DISEASES ASSOCIATED WITH SEXUAL ABUSE*

*Chlamydia**
*Trichomonas**
Gonorrhea
Human papilloma virus
Human immunodeficiency virus
Herpes simplex I/II
Syphilis

*The most suspicious organisms associated with sexual abuse.

TABLE 19-15	*PHYSICAL SIGNS OFTEN CONFUSED WITH SEXUAL ABUSE*

Nonintact hymen
Labial adhesions
Vulvar erythema
Anal tags
Lichen sclerosis
Molluscum contagiosum
Diaper rashes

MUNCHAUSEN BY PROXY

This term is best applied to cases of child abuse in which a caregiver, usually the child's mother, fabricates symptoms or induces illness in a dependent child. The guilty parent often has an unusually good grasp of medical terminology. The child will present for medical assessment and care resulting in multiple procedures and diagnostic tests. The caretaker will deny any knowledge about the etiology of the child's illness. A diagnosis is often made by observing the resolution of the symptoms when the child is separated from the parent.

< 1yr & 20 lbs (9kg) → middle back seat
                           rear-facing

>1yr & >20lbs → forward facing

>40 lbs → booster seat

>4'9" → Ø booster seat
          ⊕ back seat

>12yo → may sit in front seat

CHAPTER 20

PREVENTION PEARLS

BICYCLES

Riders of all ages should always wear helmets. Laws vary by state. Most injuries are sustained by children under 15 years of age. Head injury is the most common cause of death in bicycle-related incidents. Bicycles should have front and rear reflectors, and helmets should meet federal safety standards.

CAR SEATS

All infants should ride in rear-facing car seats, in the middle of the back seat, at a 45° angle. The seat should remain in that position until the infant is 1 year of age *and* weighs 20 pounds (9 kg). The car seat may face forward at that point, but should remain in the back seat. Children over 1 year of age (20 to 40 pounds) should then be placed in convertible, forward-facing seats. Children over 40 pounds (4 to 8 years old) should be placed in a belt-positioning booster seat until they are at least 4 feet, 9 inches tall. All safety seats should meet federal standards (i.e., five-point harness, shock-absorbing material). Children under 12 years of age should never ride in the front seat, regardless of airbag placement. Side airbags are no safer for children than front airbags.

SUN EXPOSURE

Most sun exposure occurs during the first two decades of life. Therefore, the safest advice is to use of sunscreen that has a sun protection factor (SPF) of at least 15 and is active against both UVA and UVB radiation. Parents should be reminded to apply sunscreen at least 20 minutes before exposure, to use an adequate amount (2 mL/cm of body surface area), and to reapply regularly, especially after swimming or prolonged sweating. Additional preventive measures include protective clothing and sun avoidance during peak hours (i.e., between 10 A.M. and 4 P.M.).

POOLS

A locked gate is the best prevention against drowning. Swim lessons are useful, but are not a substitute for adequate adult supervision when children are in the water. Additionally, if a child falls in the water accidentally and becomes unconscious, he will not be able to swim. A fence that a child cannot climb over, crawl under, or unlock is the best method of drowning prevention.

LEAD POISONING

Baseline screening should be performed between 12 and 24 months of age, via venous blood lead levels. Lead lines in bones, anemia, and gingival appearances are nonspecific and may be absent early in lead poisoning. Fingerstick samples may be contaminated by lead on the skin, resulting in falsely elevated levels. Classic risk factors for chronic exposure include living in or exposure to houses built before 1960, friends or siblings treated for lead exposure, or occupational/recreational exposure. Other possible sources include lead pottery, lead soldering in pipes, soil near roadways (from gasoline fumes), and home remedies (especially in some Hispanic families). Lead levels more than 10 μg/dL require further investigation and treatment.

CARDIOVASCULAR DISEASE

Risk factors for coronary artery disease include smoking, hypertension, diabetes mellitus, elevated total cholesterol, increased levels of low-density lipoprotein (LDL) cholesterol, and decreased levels of high-density lipoprotein (HDL) cholesterol. Universal testing of all patients is *not* currently recommended. Children should be screened if a parent has an elevated cholesterol level, or if a parent or grandparent had evidence of cerebrovascular disease, peripheral vascular disease, or coronary atherosclerosis (i.e., stroke, myocardial infarction, angina, coronary bypass surgery, angioplasty, or sudden cardiac death) on or before the age of 55.

CHAPTER 21

ADOLESCENT MEDICINE

The goal of adolescent medicine is to provide support during the period of biological, psychosocial, and sexual maturation that bridges the period from childhood to adulthood. A gradual separation from parental influence and an increased importance placed on peer groups are characteristic of this age group. This increased reliability on peer groups and desire for independence can result in many positive, healthy lifelong habits, or may provide an environment for accidents, drug use, and suicide. (The leading causes of death among teens are accidents, homicide, and suicide.)

THE ADOLESCENT INTERVIEW

Health care encounters between physicians and adolescents are an opportunity to advise, promote, and encourage positive health habits and lifestyles. Adolescents should be interviewed with their parents and alone during each maintenance health visit. It should be explained that all information the adolescent discloses privately to the health care provider is confidential. Although specific laws vary from state to state, adolescents generally may seek treatment for sexual and drug-related matters without permission from a parent. Examples include birth control, sexually transmitted disease testing and treatment, tobacco cessation, and addiction counseling. Confidentiality may be broken if the teen discloses a danger of harming themselves (suicidal ideation) or if he/she is being abused. In cases of potential suicide or abuse, the teen should be informed about the practitioner's plan to disclose sensitive information.

A useful mnemonic for remembering the general areas that should be covered during the adolescent interview is HEADSSS:

1. **H**ome environment
2. **E**ducation (school) and **E**mployment
3. **A**ctivity
4. **D**rugs
5. **S**exual activity

6. Suicide (depression)
7. Safety

Conditions that legally emancipate a minor, allowing him or her to consent for and/or refuse medical treatments, include:

- Marriage
- Parenthood
- Military service
- Evidence of self-support

EATING DISORDERS

Eating disorders mainly affect adolescent Caucasian females. Adolescents that participate in activities that stress low body weight (i.e., gymnastics, cheerleading, wrestling) are especially at risk. The etiology of eating disorders is unknown, but is thought to be multifactorial. A family history of eating disorders may be elicited. Onset of disease is often traced to times of stress, such as during the development of body changes associated with puberty, or upon starting college.

ANOREXIA NERVOSA

DEFINITION: A condition characterized by insufficient caloric intake (as demonstrated by either failure to gain weight in a normal fashion and/or weight loss) combined with an intense fear of being fat and desire to be thinner.

CLINICAL PRESENTATION: Anorexia affects approximately 1% of the adolescent population. Affected patients have a distorted body image, imagining themselves to be overweight even though they are quite thin. A history of "dieting" may be elicited. Amenorrhea, a diagnostic criterion, may occur before significant weight loss. The physical exam may reveal bradycardia, hypothermia, lanugo (fine, downy body and facial hair), and symptoms of malnutrition. The medical consequences include electrolyte disturbances, cardiac dysrhythmias, prolonged Q-T interval, osteoporosis, anemia, pancreatitis, hypercholesterolemia, and a low white blood cell count. Common comorbid conditions include obsessive-compulsive disorder, depression, and bulimia nervosa.

DIAGNOSIS: There are four diagnostic criteria of anorexia nervosa:

1. Refusal to maintain or gain a weight that is more than 85% of ideal
2. Amenorrhea for three cycles
3. Intense fear of becoming fat
4. Distortion of body image

BULIMIA NERVOSA

DEFINITION: The most distinctive feature of bulimia is recurrent binge eating. Binges are followed by an inappropriate compensatory attempt at weight loss. The patient feels they are not in control during binges. Compensatory measures include purging (i.e., vomiting, laxative and diuretic use, exercise) or fasting.

CLINICAL PRESENTATION: Patients with bulimia are often of normal weight or slightly overweight. Physical examination may reveal salivary gland enlargement (especially parotid and submandibular), dental enamel erosion (especially the lingual surface) from recurrent vomiting, and peripheral edema from fluid shifts. Laboratory findings include electrolyte disturbances (i.e., hypokalemic alkalosis from vomiting, or metabolic acidosis from laxative use). Comorbid conditions are more frequently associated with bulimia than anorexia, including depression, drug and alcohol abuse, delinquency, and personality disorders. Anorexia nervosa may also be present.

DIAGNOSIS: Diagnostic criteria of bulimia include:

1. Recurrent episodes of binge eating, with a feeling of loss of control during episodes
2. Recurrent inappropriate compensatory behavior, at least twice a week for 3 months
3. Sense of self disproportionately influenced by weight

Treatment of Eating Disorders

Nutritional rehabilitation is the most important goal in providing care and support for patients with eating disorders. Family and patient counseling are important to help educate and prevent progression of the disease. Antidepressant therapy may help patients with associated psychiatric illness. For patients with moderate to severe symptoms, or who have failed outpatient therapy (i.e., patients with syncope, evidence of electrolyte imbalance, or severe bradycardia), hospitalization should be considered.

ABNORMAL VAGINAL BLEEDING

In any patient with abnormal vaginal bleeding, the hemodynamic stability of the patient should be assessed, a pelvic exam performed, and the presence of a possible bleeding disorder entertained.

DYSFUNCTIONAL UTERINE BLEEDING

Defined as heavy or irregular menstrual bleeding not caused by underlying anatomic pathology. The fundamental cause is unopposed estrogen action due to decreased progesterone production from anovulation. Most patients present within the first 2 years of menarche, when anovulatory cycles are common. Depending on the stability of the patient, treatment options include medroxyprogesterone or oral contraceptives, and iron supplementation. More symptomatic patients (hemodynamically unstable, severely anemic) may require transfusion and/or hospitalization.

DYSMENORRHEA (PRIMARY OR SECONDARY)

Primary dysmenorrhea consists of crampy abdominal, back, thigh and/or pelvic pain with no other pelvic pathology, and is secondary to excess prostaglandin production. Secondary dysmenorrhea is associated with the same symptoms as primary dysmenorrhea, but is associated with pelvic pathology (endometriosis is the most common associated condition). Treatment options include nonsteroidal anti-inflammatory medications to decrease prostaglandin production, and possibly oral contraceptive agents. Patients who do not respond to these initial interventions should undergo more extensive evaluation (i.e., radiologic imaging) to evaluate for underlying disease.

AMENORRHEA (PRIMARY OR SECONDARY)

Primary amenorrhea is defined as the absence of menarche by age 16 in the presence of normal secondary sexual characteristics, or by the age of 14 when there is no visible secondary sexual characteristic development; *secondary* amenorrhea is the absence of 3 consecutive menstrual cycles, or 6 months of amenorrhea in patients who have had previously established regular menses.

Patients with amenorrhea should be assessed for other signs of puberty, as this will help guide the ultimate diagnosis. Treatment is based on the underlying cause. In patients with abnormal pubertal development, the causes of amenorrhea include:

- Hypergonadotropic hypogonadism (ovarian failure with resultant low estrogen levels and *high* FSH levels)
  - Chromosomal abnormalities (XY gonadal dysgenesis)
  - Turner syndrome

- Pituitary pathology (*low* FSH/LH production and resultant low estrogen)
  - Craniopharyngioma
  - Prolactinomas

- Hypothalamic disorders
  - Stress
  - Malnutrition associated with illness or anorexia nervosa
  - Genetic syndromes: Laurence-Moon-Biedl, Prader-Willi, and Kallmann syndromes

The causes of amenorrhea in patients with otherwise normal pubertal development include:

- Pregnancy
- Polycystic ovarian syndrome
- Testicular feminization
- Imperforate hymen
- Acquired ovarian failure (i.e., damage from chemotherapy)

- Acquired pituitary pathology (prolactinoma and infiltration)
- Hyperthyroidism
- Hypothalamic pathology (similar to that seen in primary disease)
- Hormonal contraceptive use
- Mayer-Rokitansky sequence: agenesis of the proximal two-thirds of the vagina, resulting in normal external genitalia, and a blind vaginal pouch

POLYCYSTIC OVARIAN SYNDROME (STEIN-LEVENTHAL SYNDROME)

A constellation of symptoms, the most prominent of which are irregular menses, anovulation, and hyperandrogenism. Affected patients are classically obese, hirsute, virilized, and infertile. The ovaries are usually, but not invariably, cystic. Hyperinsulinism, lipid abnormalities, and increased levels of leutinizing hormone are associated laboratory findings. Acanthosis nigricans is often present in insulin-resistant patients. Treatment consists of oral contraceptives, antiandrogen agents (spironolactone), and metformin.

ADOLESCENT PREGNANCY AND CONTRACEPTION

A large proportion of adolescent females are sexually experienced. There are approximately 1 million adolescent pregnancies in the United States each year. Adolescents often engage in risky sexual behavior because they fail to appreciate the potential consequences of their actions (sexually transmitted diseases). Contraception should be addressed during each adolescent health visit, even if the patient is not currently sexually active. Safer sex options should be outlined and explained in a clear, age-appropriate manner, along with the associated risks and benefits. Abstinence remains the best method of prevention of both pregnancy and sexually transmitted diseases. Sexually active patients should be instructed to use methods that protect against both pregnancy and sexually transmitted diseases; this usually requires the consistent use of two birth control methods.

TABLE 21-1. *OPTIONS FOR CONTRACEPTION*

EMERGENCY POSTCOITAL CONTRACEPTION

This form of contraception is often requested after unprotected consensual intercourse or rape has occurred. Treatment options include the "morning-after pill" and mifepristone. The morning-after pill is administered as two doses of combined oral contraceptives taken 12 hours apart and within 72 hours of unprotected intercourse. Mifepristone (a progesterone inhibitor) may be administered after a longer waiting period and is more effective.

TABLE 21-1   *OPTIONS FOR CONTRACEPTION*

METHOD	MECHANISM	PRO	CON	NOTES
Hormonal methods: act by suppressing ovulation, increasing cervical mucus (making penetration of sperm difficult), and thinning the endometrial lining (making implantation difficult).				
Oral contraceptives ("the pill")	• A combination of estrogen and/or progesterone	• Ease of use • Nonsexual benefits include regularity of menses and decreased incidence of gonorrhea, anemia, and ovarian cancers	• No protection against *Chlamydia*, herpes, or HIV • Requires physician visit and prescription to obtain • Can be expensive • Teenagers tend to have suboptimal compliance, making efficacy low in this age group	• Most common form of birth control amongst adolescents • Complications include thrombophlebitis, thromboembolic disease, cholestatic jaundice and hepatic adenomas • Absolute contraindications include: pregnancy, liver disease, thrombophlebitis, hyperlipidemia, and cerebrovascular and coronary artery disease • Relative contraindications for use include hypertension, sickle cell disease, depression, and migraine headaches • Many drugs, including some antibiotics, sedative hypnotics, and antiepileptics, interfere with the effectiveness of the pill

TABLE 21-1	*OPTIONS FOR CONTRACEPTION (CONTINUED)*			
METHOD	**MECHANISM**	**PRO**	**CON**	**NOTES**
"The patch"	• Same formulation as oral contraceptives: a combination of estrogen and/or progesterone	• Increasing popularity amongst teens • Patch is placed once/wk on arm, abdomen, or back • Possible increased compliance when compared to the pill	• Same as the pill	• Complications, contraindications, and drug interactions are identical to the pill
Depot medroxy-progesterone acetate (DMPA)	• Long-acting, highly effective progestin-only contraceptive	• Failure rate of less than 0.3% when used consistently • Requires little patient effort (other than office visits) • Can be used in patients who cannot take estrogen	• Irregular menstrual bleeding/amenorrhea is common side effect • Low continuation rates among teenagers • No protection against STDs • Requires physician visit and prescription to obtain	• Weight gain, headaches, bloating, mood changes, and depression • Can take as long as 18 mo for full fertility to return after discontinuation
Barrier methods: physically prevent the passage of sperm into the cervix				
Male condom	• Latex or animal skin sheath placed over the penis	• Decreases the transmission of STDs when used correctly and consistently • Readily available • Low cost • No prescription needed	• Requires interruption of activity to put on condom • Often used incorrectly by adolescents, decreasing efficacy • Requires replacement with each sexual act	• Should be used in conjunction with spermicide • Latex condoms provide better protection than animal skin condoms

(Continued)

TABLE 21-1	OPTIONS FOR CONTRACEPTION (CONTINUED)			
METHOD	**MECHANISM**	**PRO**	**CON**	**NOTES**
Diaphragm/ cervical cap	• Dome-shaped rubber cup that fits over the cervix offering a physical barrier to conception	• Can be placed up to 6 h (diaphragm) and 72 h (cap) prior to inter-course	• Can be difficult to place initially • Does not protect against STDs • Requires physician for fittin, and prescription	• Not particularly popular among teenagers
Other methods				
Intrauterine device	• A device inserted into the uterus, creating a chronic inflam-matory response in the uterus interfering with conception	• Little patient effort required after insertion complete	• Does not protect against STDs • Associated with an increased risk of PID, ectopic pregnancy, and infertility	
Coitus interruptus	• Withdrawal of the penis prior to ejaculation		• *Highly* ineffective, as pre-ejaculatory fluids can contain semen	

PID, pelvic inflammatory disease; STDs, sexually transmitted diseases.

ADOLESCENT SUBSTANCE ABUSE

Over one-fifth of middle school and one-half of high school students have used illicit substances. Over one-third of high school students use tobacco. The most commonly abused illicit drug in adolescence is marijuana. Patients may *abuse* drugs (use in a manner that is different from the intended use), become *dependent* on drugs (lifestyle is adapted to use of substance, even in presence of persistent/recurrent adverse consequences), or develop *tolerance* to a substance (requiring escalating dosages of medications to experience same effect). Frequent comorbidities include depression, attention deficit-hyperactivity disorder, and personality disorders. Additional risk factors for drug abuse include physical and/or sexual abuse, family history of drug use, and association with peers who use drugs.

It is unethical to test an adolescent for drugs without his or her consent (except in the emergency setting, i.e., acute overdose). Parental request is not a sufficient reason to perform clandestine screening. Most screening tests are performed on urine.

A review of commonly abused substances is provided in Table 21-2. Toxic ingestions of these substances are covered in Chapter 8.

TABLE 21-2   *REVIEW OF ABUSED SUBSTANCES IN ADOLESCENCE*

SUBSTANCE	HOW USED/EFFECT	NOTES
Tobacco	• Smoked, chewed (snuff) • Nicotine causes alertness, muscle relaxation, increased memory and attention, and decreased appetite • Most smokers start smoking in adolescence • Cigarette smoking has been linked to early cardiovascular disease, chronic lung disease, ulcers, and cancer	• Potential nicotine replacement modalities include nicotine gum, patches, and inhalers • Anticipatory guidance in prepubescents is important to prevent initiation of smoking
Marijuana (delta-9-tetrahydrocannbinol [THC] and cannabinoids)	• Smoked or orally ingested • Causes feelings of euphoria, relaxation, and well-being	• Physiologic addiction is possible

(Continued)

TABLE 21-2	REVIEW OF ABUSED SUBSTANCES IN ADOLESCENCE (CONTINUED)	
SUBSTANCE	**HOW USED/EFFECT**	**NOTES**
Cocaine/amphetamines	• Cocaine may be smoked or injected (intranasal or intravenous; "crack-cocaine") • Other amphetamines may be orally ingested, or crushed and taken intranasally • Stimulates release and inhibits reuptake of dopamine and norepinephrine, causing feelings of euphoria and sympathomimetic effects	• "Ecstasy" (MDMA) is a derivative of methamphetamine • Phenylpropanolamine, ephedrine, ma-huang, and caffeine all can cause a similar effect if taken in large enough quantities • Nasal septal damage, sinus infections, and nosebleeds can all be consequences of intranasal snorting
Opiates	• Can be taken intranasally (i.e., heroin), intravenously (morphine, heroin), orally (oxycodone, codeine), subcutaneously (morphine), transdermally (fentanyl), or smoked (opium) • Effects include analgesia, sedation, and decreased anxiety	• Dependency can develop quickly (~2 wk) with use of short-acting opiates • Route of administration may pose its own risks (i.e., infectious endocarditis from intravenous injection, HIV from shared needles)
Hallucinogens	• Orally ingested • Cause alteration of perception (especially visually), and altered sense of time • Disinhibition, euphoria, and psychosis may also occur	• This group includes hallucinogenic mushrooms, lysergic acid diethylamide (LSD), ketamine (special-K), and phencyclidine (PCP) • "Ecstasy" (MDMA) also has hallucinogenic properties • "Flashbacks" are possible
Inhalants	• Substance is poured or sprayed into container or on cloth and then inhaled ("huffing") • Causes rapid onset of euphoria, and alteration of mental status	• Commonly used household substances include glue, gasoline, markers, aerosolized products, and cleaning fluid • More commonly used by younger adolescents

CHAPTER 22

BASIC STATISTICS

The general purpose of laboratory tests is to screen, diagnose, and monitor people with disease. Disease *screening* takes place in asymptomatic persons in the general population (example: testing for PKU in newborns). Screening tests are generally developed for diseases that have a high prevalence in the population at risk *and* have associated morbidity and mortality. Additionally, the test and the therapy must be cost-effective and available. Tests that aid in the *diagnosis* of disease are reserved for the symptomatic patient in the office setting or hospital (example: sweat test to rule out cystic fibrosis). Tests that help *monitor* disease after diagnosis has been made (example: hemoglobin A1C measurement in diabetics) have an important role in preventing disease-associated morbidity and mortality.

On the boards, questions about statistics will generally ask you to evaluate a laboratory test or to interpret the results of a simple study. The following terms and formulas will be helpful to you.

- **True Positive**: A patient tests positive for a specific disease, and actually has that disease.

- **True Negative**: A patient tests negative for a specific disease, and actually does not have that disease.

- **False Positive**: A patient tests positive for a specific disease, but actually does not have that disease.

- **False Negative**: A patient tests negative for a specific disease, but actually has that disease.

TABLE 22-1   *BASIC STATISTICAL DEFINITIONS*

	POSITIVE TEST	NEGATIVE TEST
Patient has disease	True positive (TP)	False negative (FN)
Patient does NOT have disease	False positive (FP)	True negative (TN)

- **Positive Predictive Value (PPV):** The probability that a positive test result for a disease means the patient truly has the disease. Calculated as: $TP / (TP + FP) \times 100$.
- **Negative Predictive Value (NPV):** The probability that a negative test result for a disease means the patient truly does not have the disease (i.e., is a true negative). Calculated as: $TN / (TN + FN) \times 100$.
- **Sensitivity:** The probability that patients who have a disease will test positive for the disease. The greater the sensitivity of the test, the more likely the test will detect a person with the disease. A highly sensitive test is helpful to *screen* for the disease. Calculated as: $TP / (TP + FN) \times 100$.
- **Specificity:** The probability that patients without a disease will test negative for the disease. The greater the specificity, the more likely that a person without the disease will be excluded by the test. A highly specific test is helpful to *confirm* disease. Calculated as: $TN / (TN + FP) \times 100$.

Example: Test X is used to detect Lyme disease in 100 people. Forty people have a positive test, indicating Lyme disease. Of those 40 people, only 35 actually have Lyme disease. The other 60 people test negative for Lyme disease. Of those 60 people, 3 actually have Lyme disease. This data is charted in Table 22-2.

TABLE 22-2	*EXAMPLE*

For the data below:

PPV = 35 / (35 + 5) = 87.5% of people with a positive test have Lyme disease.

NPV = 57 / (57 + 3) = 95% of people with a negative test do not have Lyme disease.

Sensitivity = 35 / (35 + 3) = 92% of people with Lyme disease had a positive test.

Specificity = 57 / (57 + 5) = 91.9% of people who do not have Lyme disease had a negative test.

	POSITIVE TEST	**NEGATIVE TEST**
Patient has Lyme disease	True positive = 35	False negative = 3
Patient does NOT have Lyme disease	False positive = 5	True negative = 57

- **Mean**: The average of all the values given.

TABLE 22-3	CALCULATING THE MEAN

Data: 4, 4, 5, 5, 6, 6

Mean: 4 + 4 + 5 + 5 + 6 + 6 = 30

    30/6 = 5

- **Mode**: The most common of all the values given.

TABLE 22-4	DETERMINING THE MODE

Data: 4, 4, 4, 5, 5, 6, 6

Mode = 4

- **Median**: When a set of values is sorted from highest to lowest, the number in the middle is the median. For example, if a set of 15 numbers is sorted, the eighth number is the median value: 7 numbers are higher and 7 numbers are lower.

TABLE 22-5	DETERMINING THE MEDIAN

Data: 1, 3, 5, 7, 9, 11, 13, 15, 17, 19, 21, 23, 25, 27, 29

Median = 15

- **Range**: The difference between the greatest and least value in a set or distribution $(x - y)$. For example, if a set of hemoglobin levels are given in an anemia study and the lowest value is 5.4 and the highest value is 14.3, the range is $(14.3 - 5.4) = 8.9$.

- **Null Hypothesis**: The null hypothesis generally states that there is no difference between research groups. The purpose of a clinical trial is to disprove the null hypothesis. The null hypothesis can only be rejected (disproved); it is never accepted (proven). A failure to disprove the null hypothesis does not prove the null hypothesis. For example: If a study proposing that breast-fed infants given supplement X suffer from eczema less often than breast-fed infants who are not supplemented, the null hypothesis states there is no difference between the two groups (as opposed to the researcher's hypothesis that supplemented babies get eczema less often).

- **Type I Error**: Rejecting the null hypothesis, when the null hypothesis is true. For example, the researcher concludes there is a difference in the incidence of eczema between supplemented and nonsupplemented infants, when in fact no difference exists. A type I error may occur when a study is conducted in an unblinded fashion, leading to bias in the results.

- **Type II Error**: A failure to reject the null hypothesis when it is actually false. For example, the researcher concludes there is no difference in the incidence of eczema between supplemented and nonsupplemented infants, when in fact a difference exists. A type II error is likely to occur when the sample sizes are too small.

- **P-value**: Measures the probability that a type I error is being committed. For example, if the researcher states that study drug X significantly ($P = 0.02$) decreases eczema, that means there is a 2% chance that study drug X does *not* decrease eczema and that the findings were purely coincidental (i.e., there is a 2% chance of type I error). Conversely, there is a 98% chance that supplement X truly decreases eczema. The condition $P \leq 0.05$ is considered significant. You likely will *not* have to calculate this number in a board exam question; it will be given to you to interpret.

CHAPTER 23

DERMATOLOGY

Note: This chapter is best studied in conjunction with a pediatric picture atlas.

NEONATAL DERMATOLOGY

Benign Neonatal Lesions

- **Milia**: Multiple, small 1-to-2 mm papules found on the nose, chin, and cheeks. Papules are clear/yellow in color, and arise from the epithelial lining of hair follicles. The rash usually regresses by 2 to 3 weeks of life. No treatment is necessary.

- **Neonatal Acne**: Comedones, papules, and pustules usually found on the cheek, nose, and forehead. Lesions may be apparent at the time of birth or develop within a few months of age. Maternal and fetal androgens are the suspected etiology. These lesions closely resemble adolescent acne. They are generally self-limited and require no treatment.

- **Erythema Toxicum**: Yellow-white pustules surrounded by a ring of erythema, occurring mainly on the trunk and extremities. These lesions occur in up to 60% of term newborns. The onset is usually within 48 hours of life. Wright stain of pustule contents reveals a high number of eosinophils. They are generally self-limited and require no treatment.

- **Transient Neonatal Pustular Melanosis**: This disorder consists of noninflammatory pustules/vesicles that erupt on the face, hands, and feet at the time of birth. They often regress or rupture within 24 to 48 hours of onset, leaving behind hyperpigmented, scaling macules (often described as having a "collarette of scale"). The hyperpigmentation may remain visible for up to 3 months. It is more common in black infants. Staining of pustule contents reveals neutrophils. The course is generally self-limited and requires no treatment.

- **Infantile Acropustulosis**: Often confused with scabies, these are crops of pruritic pustules that appear on the hands and feet of a young infant. The cause is unknown. The lesions are sterile, tend to recur every 2 to 3 weeks, and generally remit after 1 to 2 years.

- **Subcutaneous Fat Necrosis**: This eruption consists of hard, nontender, irregular, lumpy lesions present in the subcutaneous tissue. They are usually noticed shortly after birth while in the nursery, and are most likely due to pressure or trauma during the birth process. They are most common on the cheeks, buttocks, back, arms, and thighs, and generally resolve within a few months. No treatment is required.

Birth Marks

- **Mongolian Spots**: A skin discoloration characterized by blue-gray and blue-green areas of dermal hyperpigmentation. They usually occur on the buttocks and lumbosacral areas, and have often been confused with bruises resembling child abuse. They are present in up to 80% to 90% of Asian and African American newborns. These lesions usually resolve by age 5 years.
- **Ash Leaf Spots**: These lesions are described as hypopigmented white macules resembling an oval or an "ash leaf." They are usually found on the trunk, arms, or legs. Detection is aided by use of a Wood's lamp. Ash leaf spots are the earliest cutaneous manifestations of tuberous sclerosis.
- **Café-au-Lait Spots**: Light brown macules of various shapes and sizes. They can be a normal finding, or can be associated with neurofibromatosis. The presence of more than six of these lesions measuring at least 0.5 cm each is considered cutaneous evidence of neurofibromatosis.
- **Port-Wine Stain (Nevus Flammeus)**: These lesions are dark red or purple congenital vascular malformations formed from dilated capillaries. They may occur anywhere on the body, although they are seen most commonly on the face. Infants with port-wine stains are at risk for associated vascular malformations of the central nervous system. Port-wine stains in the trigeminal nerve are highly associated with Sturge-Weber syndrome. They do not regress, but may be reduced with pulsed dye laser therapy.

PEDIATRIC DERMATOLOGY

TABLE 23-1 *VERRUCOUS LESIONS*

LESION	ETIOLOGY	CLINICAL	DIAGNOSIS	TREATMENT/ NOTES
Common wart	• Benign skin tumor produced by HPV • Transmitted via direct contact or autoinoculation • Common wart: HPV 2, 3, and 4 • Plantar wart: HPV 1	• 5%-10% of all children affected • Several types: raised, round papules with a rough surface (verruca vulgaris); small flat, hyperpigmented lesions (verruca plana); and painful scaly lesions on feet (plantar warts) • Fingers, dorsum of hands, elbows, and knees are commonly involved sites • Spread by scratching and direct inoculation	• Clinical • Plantar warts interrupt the normal skin lines of the foot	• 50% spontaneously resolve within 1-2 y • Electrodesiccation and curettage • Liquid nitrogen • Daily use of 10%-17% salicylic acid • Occlusive tape
Genital wart (Condylomata acuminata)	• Genital wart: HPV 6 and 11 (benign genital lesions) • Anogenital neoplasia: HPV 16,18,31,33,35	• Soft, flesh-colored lesions that can become pedunculated (cauliflower-like) • Perineum, vagina, anus, penis, mouth • The virus can be transmitted to a newborn through the birth canal	• Clinical	• Liquid nitrogen • CO$_2$ laser therapy • Weekly applications of 25% podophyllin • Sexual abuse should be suspected in school age-children presenting with new onset genital warts • There is an increased risk of cervical carcinoma with anogenital neoplasia (HPV 16,18, 31, 33, 35)
Molluscum contagiosum	• Pox virus • Transmitted via direct contact, fomite, or autoinoculation	• Small, round, skin-colored papules; may be umbilicated • Clusters of lesions common (spread by scratching) • School-age and immunosuppressed children most common host • Contagious	• Clinical • Microscopic examination of expressed core reveals molluscum bodies	• Most are self-limited • Curettage • Liquid nitrogen • Topical retinoic acid

HPV, human papilloma virus.

TABLE 23-2 VASCULAR LESIONS

Hemangiomas are the most common tumor of infancy; almost 10% of all children are affected. Girls are affected more often than boys. Premature infants weighing less than 1500 gm have an increased incidence (~25%). These lesions are usually not present at birth; most appear within the first month of life. The head and neck are the most frequently involved sites. They are usually solitary, although some children will have multiple lesions. Almost all hemangiomas resolve spontaneously. There are three types: capillary, cavernous, and mixed. Mixed hemangiomas have characteristics of each type.

LESION	ETIOLOGY	CLINICAL	DIAGNOSIS	TREATMENT/ NOTES
Capillary hemangioma	• Densely packed endothelial cells forming capillaries	• Accounts for 50% of all hemangiomas • Size can range from a few millimeters to several centimeters • Starts as macule, followed by period of rapid growth to bright red raised nodule or plaque, then slow involution	• Clinical • MRI is helpful for tumors that invade the airway or cranium, or involve vital organs	• Usually do not require therapy • 30% regress by 3 y, 50% by 5 y, 90% by 9 y • Treatment indicated for lesions that compromise vision, the airway, spinal cord, or the brain • Pulse dye laser, interferon, and surgical resection are controversial • Corticosteroids can aid involution; reserved for large tumors or complicated cases • Most common complication is ulceration
Cavernous hemangioma	• Similar to capillary hemangioma, although the vessels are larger in size	• Deeper location (beneath the skin) • Bluish in color • Indistinct mass below skin		
Pyogenic granuloma	• Post-traumatic reaction resulting in vessel hyperplasia	• Solitary dark red/ purple nodular lesion • Fast growing • Usually occur in areas of previous trauma • They are very friable and bleed easily with trauma	• Clinical	• Surgical excision

TABLE 23-3   *DISORDERS OF PIGMENTATION*

LESION	ETIOLOGY	CLINICAL	DIAGNOSIS	TREATMENT / NOTES
Congenital melanocytic nevi	• Groups of melanocytes clustered at the dermis, forming a plaque	• 1%-2% of newborns • May be very small or extremely large in size, and have associated hypertrichosis • Darken with age to brown-black color	• Clinical • Biopsy required for lesions that are suspect for malignancy*	• Surgical removal of entire mass is controversial • Large lesions have increased risk of transformation to malignant melanoma over time, and should be removed if possible

Acquired melanocytic nevi (pigmented/ common mole)	• Groups of melanocytes initially clustered in dermal epidermal junction (*junctional nevi*), with eventual progression to involve the dermis (*compound nevi*)
	• Occasionally, the skin around a mole becomes hypopigmented; these are called *halo nevi*)
		• First appear at age ~ 1 y, peaking in number during late adolescence
		• More common in fair-skinned persons
		• Brown or black in color
		• Round, smooth shapes with regular borders (those with irregular borders are called *dysplastic nevi*)
		• Occur mainly in sun-exposed areas
				• Observation
				• Signs of malignant transformation requiring biopsy or removal:
				  • Irregular/change in color
				  • Irregular/change in shape
				  • Irregular/change in border
				  • Irregular/change in size
				  • Painful, pruritic
				• Sun exposure during early childhood may contribute to the number of acquired melanocytic nevi and increases the risk for developing malignant melanoma (use sunscreen!)

Acanthosis nigricans	• Hyperplasia and pigmentation of the epidermis	• Velvety, thickened, darkened skin over antecubital area, back of neck, inner thighs, anogenital area		• Strong association with obesity, insulin resistance, and type II diabetes

(Continued)

TABLE 23-3   DISORDERS OF PIGMENTATION (CONTINUED)

LESION	ETIOLOGY	CLINICAL	DIAGNOSIS	TREATMENT/ NOTES

Cutaneous mastocytosis	• Dermal infiltration of mast cells
	• Two most common forms:
	  1. Mastocytoma (these are isolated lesions)
	  2. Urticaria pigmentosa (these are multiple lesions)
		• Light brown macules or plaques, present in infancy
		• Stroking lesion produces histamine release and wheal-and-flare response (Darier sign)
		• Usually resolves by adolescence
		• Most common in sun-exposed areas
			• Clinical
			• Biopsy required for lesions that are suspect for malignancy*
				• Excessive histamine release can cause diarrhea, flushing, and bronchospasm

Phytophotoder-matitis	• Light-sensitizing substances in plants or fruit make the skin photosensitive • Citrus fruits are most common (lemons, limes, oranges, tomatoes)	• Hyperpigmented, erythematous lesions • Lesions may blister or burn • May resemble bruising or hand marks on a child		• Phytophotodermatitis is an important differential diagnosis when evaluating the etiology of bruising in children • Self-limited
Vitiligo	• Autoimmune disease of melanocytes	• Well-demarcated areas of hypopigmentation • Perioral area, genitals, elbows, hands and feet often affected	• Clinical • Will appear purple under Wood lamp • Often seen in association with other autoimmune diseases (especially Addison disease)	• Supportive • Treatment of underlying disease

*Risk factors for the development of malignant melanoma include: (1) a new or changing mole; (2) increasing age; (3) family history of melanoma; (4) dysplastic nevus syndrome; (5) large congenital nevus (>20 cm); (6) multiple nevi; (7) Caucasian race; (8) severe childhood sunburns; and (9) immunosuppression.

TABLE 23-4   HYPERSENSITIVITY SYNDROMES

LESION	ETIOLOGY	CLINICAL	DIAGNOSIS	TREATMENT/NOTES
Rhus dermatitis (poison ivy, poison oak, poison sumac)	• T-cell-mediated hyper-sensitivity • Antigen-mediated immune reaction • The antigen is contained in the sap of the plant	• Linear streaks of vesicles and/or blisters (where the plant has touched the skin) • The lesions may occur many days after the initial contact (delayed hypersensitivity) • Pruritus is prominent • Spread is by antigen which may be present on the skin and fingernails, *not* by vesicular fluid • Patient may appear very uncomfortable	• Clinical	• Wash the hands and skin as quickly as possible after suspected exposure • Topical antihistamines • Topical corticosteroids • If large amounts of body surface area are involved, or the reaction is severe, systemic antihistamines and corticosteroids are indicated
Urticaria (hives)	• Mediated by several factors, including IgE, complement, and vasoactive amines • Type I hypersensitivity (IgE) is the most frequent cause • Common inciting agents include: foods, drugs, contact allergy, insect bites, and infections (strep and mono) • In most cases of urticaria, the cause is unknown	• Extremely pruritic, slightly raised lesions (wheals) that appear suddenly • May be red with white halo, or white with red halo • Not vesicular • The lesions will last 2-12 h before resolving, changing shape and/or shifting to new sites (migrating) • If involves subcutaneous tissue: angioedema • Chronic urticaria (>6 wk) can be sign of chronic infection (hepatitis, sinusitis) or connective tissue disorder	• Clinical	• Antipruritics • Antihistamines • In angioedema: consider epinephrine • Corticosteroids not proven to be beneficial

(Continued)

389

TABLE 23-4   *HYPERSENSITIVITY SYNDROMES (CONTINUED)*

LESION	ETIOLOGY	CLINICAL	DIAGNOSIS	TREATMENT/NOTES
Fixed drug eruption	• Unknown	• Reaction occurs in same site every time after exposure to offending agent • May be macular, papular, vesicular, or target lesion	• Clinical	• Avoidance of offending agent

Erythema multiforme (EM)
 	
Minor
	• Possible autoimmune syndrome triggered by an organism
	• Common triggers include
	  - Medications (especially sulfas and anticonvulsants)
	  - Bacteria (*Mycoplasma*)
		• Classic "target lesions": Erythematous rash with central clearing. May be macular, papular, and vesicular. Usually located on extremities
		• Lesions last 5-7 d, recur every 2-4 wk, resolve spontaneously
		• May be preceded by mild flu-like symptoms
			• Clinical
			• The diverse morphology of the rash is diagnostic
				Supportive

Major **(Stevens–Johnson)**	- Viruses (HSV) - Connective tissue disorders	• Lesions are identical to EM minor, the only difference being they often become necrotic and slough • Mucous membranes involved: oral, genital, and conjunctiva; less commonly genitourinary, gastrointestinal, and respiratory tracts are involved as well • Systemic illness: fever, fluid and electrolyte imbalance, vomiting, diarrhea, arthralgias		• Supportive • Steroids are controversial • Aggressive fluid and electrolyte management • Ophthalmology to evaluate for corneal scarring • 5%-25% of cases are fatal

Toxic epidermal necrolysis (TEN)	• Possible autoimmune syndrome triggered by an organism or medication • Drug reactions are most common suspected etiology (sulfonamides, penicillin, phenytoin)	• An acute inflammatory condition that involves injury to the skin, mucous membrane, bowel, and respiratory epithelium • Full-thickness epidermal necrosis of more than 30% of the body surface • Lesions begin on the face and upper extremity and spread to the lower body • Lesions resemble 2nd-degree burns • Conjunctivitis • Diarrhea, bowel obstruction • Respiratory failure	• Clinical • Biopsy of active lesions will reveal a separation at the dermal-epidermal junction • Presence of Nikolsky sign: sloughing of skin with rubbing/light trauma	• Supportive • Steroids are controversial • Aggressive fluid and electrolyte management

TABLE 23-5   *SCALING LESIONS*

LESION	ETIOLOGY	CLINICAL	DIAGNOSIS	TREATMENT/NOTES
Atopic dermatitis	• Allergic disorder	• Affects 5% of children aged 1-5 y • Face and extensor surfaces are commonly affected in infants • Flexural surfaces are commonly involved in older children • Erythematous, crusted, weeping, scaly rash • Often pruritic in quality • Chronic irritation results in lichenification and pigment changes • Superinfection with *S. aureus* or HSV (eczema herpeticum) is common	• Clinical	• Avoidance of suspected allergens • Emollients • Steroid creams • Antihistamines • 80%-90% resolve by puberty • More than 50% of patients with atopic skin disease develop allergic rhinitis and/or asthma
Psoriasis	• Unknown • Genetic predisposition • Role of antecedent infections, T-cell mediation unclear	• Red, elevated papules or plaques with central thick adherent scale • Removal of scale results in punctate hemorrhages (Auspitz sign) • Scalp, ears, elbows, knees, umbilicus, and gluteal cleft are commonly involved sites • Koebner phenomenon: lesions occurring at sites of trauma • Guttate psoriasis: lesions appear in "drop-like" distribution on trunk and upper extremities; associated with streptococcal infections • May see pitting of nail or separation of nails from nail bed • Arthritis	• Clinical	• Emollients • Topical corticosteroids • Tar-based solutions • Topical immunotherapy in severe cases

Acrodermatitis enteropathica	• Zinc deficiency • Can be acquired (poor intake) or inherited as a autosomal recessive defect resulting in abnormal zinc metabolism	• Dry, scaly, crusted lesions with sharp borders • Affects perioral, periorbital, and perineal areas • Resembles a severe diaper rash • Superinfection with *Candida* spp is common • Alopecia, diarrhea, and failure to thrive may be present
	• Clinical • Serum zinc levels	• Although this condition is inherited, consider it in children with chronic total parenteral nutrition administration, chronic malnutrition, and premature infants • Treat with oral zinc supplementation (1mg/kg/d elemental) for 5 d
Ichthyosis vulgaris	• Autosomal dominant disorder of keratinocytes	• Onset after age 3 mo • Affects 1:250 people • Scaling dry, lesions (resembling fish scales) with pasted-on appearance most commonly found on the legs • Flexural creases spared • Thickening of the palms and soles
	• Clinical	• Often confused with atopic dermatitis • Emollients containing lactic acid will help • Other more severe forms of ichthyosis include lamellar ichthyosis (colloidion baby) and hyperkeratosis (thick scales and blistering)
Seborrheic dermatitis	• Unknown	• Affects young infants and adolescents • Greasy, yellow, scaling lesion begins on the scalp and spreads to hair-bearing and intertriginous areas of the body • Nonpruritic in quality • Facial hypopigmentation • Superinfection with *Candida* spp is common
	• Clinical	• Tar-based shampoo • Ketoconazole-based shampoo or skin treatments if *Candida* suspected • Mild topical corticosteroids • Histiocytosis X should be considered in severe or persistent cases

(Continued)

TABLE 23-5   *SCALING LESIONS (CONTINUED)*

LESION	ETIOLOGY	CLINICAL	DIAGNOSIS	TREATMENT/NOTES
Pityriasis rosea ("rose-colored scale")	• Unknown	• Begins with a "herald patch," a large oval-shaped erythematous lesion on the trunk • Multiple oval-shaped, salmon-colored, dry, scaling lesions follow a few weeks later • Often pruritic in quality • Distribution of lesions is often described as resembling a "Christmas tree"	• Clinical	• The "Christmas tree" distribution is usually the key to diagnosis • The herald patch may be confused with tinea corporis or nummular eczema • Benign, self-limited disease • Antihistamines for pruritus • Send serologic studies to rule out syphilis, which can present with a similar rash

TABLE 23-6   *DERMATOPHYTE LESIONS*

LESION	ETIOLOGY	CLINICAL	DIAGNOSIS	TREATMENT/NOTES
Tinea corporis ("ringworm of the body")	• *Microsporum* spp • *Trichophyton* spp	• Affects any age group • Erythematous, annular, scaling lesion with a central clearing "ring" • Found anywhere on the body • Often pruritic in quality	• Clinical • Wood light examination • Fungal culture	• Treatment depends on the severity • Local lesions may only require topical antifungal treatment • More extensive infections or infections involving scalp and nails require oral griseofulvin, itraconazole, or fluconazole
Tinea capitis ("ringworm of the scalp")	• *Microsporum* spp • *Trichophyton* spp • *Epidermophyton* spp	• Scaling scalp lesions • Alopecia • Multiple "black dots" are visible on the surface of the scalp as a result of broken hair shafts	• Clinical • Fungal culture • The lesion can be scraped and placed in a dermatophyte test medium, which changes color within 1 mo if dermatophytes are present	• A *kerion* is a hypersensitivity reaction to the dermatophyte infection. It is NOT a superinfection. It is characterized by a boggy, firm swelling of the scalp. • Associated cervical lymphadenopathy may be present • Treatment depends on the severity of symptoms • Treat with oral griseofulvin, itraconazole, or fluconazole
Tinea cruris ("jock itch")	• *Trichophyton* spp	• Affects adolescents and adults • Pruritic rash of the genital area	• Clinical	• Topical antifungal treatment is usually sufficient • Wear loose clothing
Tinea versicolor (pityriasis versicolor)	• *Pityrosporum orbiculare* • *Malassezia furfur*	• Hypopigmented, oval, scaling lesions • Most noticeable on sun-exposed areas • Nonpruritic in quality • Common areas include the neck, chest, and back	• Clinical • Wood light examination • Microscopic examination of lesions reveal a "spaghetti and meatballs" pattern	• Topical 2.5% selenium sulfide

TABLE 23-7   LESIONS OF THE SCALP

LESION	ETIOLOGY	CLINICAL	DIAGNOSIS	TREATMENT/NOTES
Alopecia areata	• Unknown • Possible autoimmune mechanism	• Smooth, shiny, round, hairless patch present on the scalp • Nail pitting may be present • Alopecia *totalis* is the loss of all body hair as well as eyelashes • Nails may have "Scotch plaid pitting"	• Clinical • Scalp biopsy reveals peribulbar lymphocytic infiltrate "swarm of bees"	• Topical corticosteroids • Intralesional injections of corticosteroids • Variable clinical course • "Traction alopecia" occurs at sites of scalp stress (i.e., tightly braided hair)
Trichotillomania	• Disorder of impulse control	• Patchy, irregular bald spots on the scalp • Hair may be chewed and swallowed forming a trichobezoar in the esophagus or stomach	• History is important • Broken hair shafts are present on microscopic examination	• Supportive
Telogen effluvium	• Stress • Illness	• Stress shifts hair shafts into the resting (telogen) phase of growth • The resting hair is shed when the hair reenters the growing phase (several weeks after precipitating event)	• Clinical	• Supportive • Hair usually spontaneously grows back within a few weeks • Anagen effluvium: sudden loss of growing hair, such as that seen in patients receiving chemotherapy
Nevus sebaceous of Jadassohn	• Hamartomatous nevi made up of variable epidermal components	• Hairless, well-circumscribed, flat, yellowish patch presenting in early childhood • May become raised and verrucous during adolescence	• Clinical	• Regular observation or prophylactic excision, as 10%–15% will become malignant

TABLE 23-8   INHERITED DISORDERS

LESION	ETIOLOGY	CLINICAL	DIAGNOSIS	TREATMENT/NOTES
Epidermolysis bullosa (three types: simplex, junctional, and dystrophic)	• **Simplex**: blister formation in epidermis • Autosomal dominant	• Blisters occur in areas of trauma and pressure points (hands, elbows) • Nonscarring	• Clinical • Histopathology • Electron microscopy	• Supportive • Treatment of superinfection
	• **Junctional**: blister formation at dermal-epidermal junction • Autosomal recessive	• Presents at birth with extensive blistering • Death usually occurs in infancy secondary to fluid imbalances and sepsis		
	• **Dystrophic**: blister formation in dermis • Autosomal dominant or recessive	• Presents at birth with blistering and milia • In more severe forms, scarring of blisters can result in syndactyly, nail loss, and growth retardation • Oral blisters may also occur		
Incontinentia pigmenti (IP)	• X-linked dominant • Excessive melanin deposition	• Affects mostly females (lethal in males) • Three phases: 1. Truncal vesicles/bullae; *followed by* 2. Irregular warty papules; these resolve, *followed by* 3. The appearance of brownish-gray swirls which persist for life • Unusual patterns of hyperpigmented skin seen in mothers of patients • Associated symptoms include absent teeth, strabismus, seizures		• The hyperpigmentation changes of IP usually fade over time • Neurologic manifestations may persist • Corrective lenses for visual loss • Seizure prophylaxis

(Continued)

TABLE 23-8   INHERITED DISORDERS (CONTINUED)

LESION	ETIOLOGY	CLINICAL	DIAGNOSIS	TREATMENT/NOTES
Albinism	• Two types: X-linked ocular albinism, and autosomal recessive oculocutaneous albinism (OCA) • Results in hypopigmentation of hair, skin, and/or eyes	• OCA: Children are born without *any* pigmentation; associated with various ophthalmologic pathologies, including strabismus, and nystagmus • Ocular: Children have normal skin pigmentation, but no eye pigmentation (the iris appears pink)	• Clinical exam • Hair from OCA patients can be incubated in tyrosine to determine if they are tyrosine positive or tyrosine negative (Children who are tyrosine positive may develop more pigmentation as they get older)	• There is a high risk of skin cancer (OCA) and retinal damage (both types), requiring the use of sunscreen and sunglasses; patients should be assessed regularly for these complications

TABLE 23-9 *COMMON NAIL FINDINGS AND ASSOCIATIONS*

FINDING	ASSOCIATION
Nail pitting	Psoriasis
"Scotch-plaid" pitting	Alopecia areata
Spoon nails	Iron deficiency anemia
Clubbing	Chronic hypoxemia
Telangiectasias of nail bed	Dermatomyositis, scleroderma
Splinter hemorrhages	Endocarditis
Onycholysis (thickening and splitting of nail bed)	Fungal disease, rheumatic disease
Horizontal nail grooves, discoloration of nail base ("half-and-half nails")	Acute illness
Darkened discoloration of the nail bed	Acute trauma (hematoma), melanoma

REFERENCES AND SELECTED READINGS

When studying for the boards, we suggest reviewing a general pediatric picture atlas, as well as an atlas of inherited disorders. For topics on which additional information is needed, a general pediatric textbook should be on hand. The *Pediatrics in Review* series from the American Academy of Pediatrics has detailed discussions of selected topics covered in this book; particularly helpful references from the series are noted in the lists below.

Suggested general review books include:

American Academy of Pediatrics. *2000 Red Book: Report of the Committee on Infectious Diseases*. 25th ed. Elk Grove Village, IL: American Academy of Pediatrics, 2000.

Behrman RE, Kliegman RM, Jenson HB. *Nelson Textbook of Pediatrics*. 16th ed. Philadelphia: WB Saunders, 2000.

Jones KL. *Smith's Recognizable Patterns of Human Development*. 5th ed. Philadelphia: WB Saunders, 1997.

McMillan JA, Deangelis CD, Warshaw JB, Oski FA. *Oski's Pediatrics: Principles and Practice*. 3rd ed. Philadelphia: Lippincott Williams & Wilkins, 1999.

Rudolph CD, Rudolph AM, Hostetter MK, Lister G, Siegel NJ. *Rudolph's Pediatrics*. 21st ed. New York: McGraw-Hill, 2002.

Zitelli BJ, Davis HW. *Atlas of Pediatric Physical Diagnosis*. 4th ed. St. Louis: Mosby, 2002.

For additional chapter-specific information, we recommend the following resources.

NEONATOLOGY

American Academy of Pediatrics and American College of Obstetricians and Gynecologists. *Guidelines for Perinatal Care*. 4th ed. Elk Grove Village, IL: American Academy of Pediatrics, 1997.

American Academy of Pediatrics, Work Group on Breastfeeding. Breastfeeding and the use of human milk. *Pediatrics* 1997;100:1035.

American Academy of Pediatrics, Provisional Committee for Quality Improvement and Subcommittee on Hyperbilirubinemia. Practice parameter: management of hyperbilirubinemia in the healthy term newborn. *Pediatrics* 1994;94:558.

NEURODEVELOPMENTAL

American Academy of Pediatrics, Committee on Quality Improvement, Subcommittee on Attention-Deficit/Hyperactivity Disorder. Diagnosis and evaluation of the child with attention-deficit/hyperactivity disorder. *Pediatrics* 2000;105:1158.

American Academy of Pediatrics. Practice guideline endorsement: practice parameter: screening and diagnosis of autism. *Neurology* 2000;55:468.

American Psychiatric Association. *Diagnostic and Statistical Manual of Mental Disorders.* 4th ed. (*DSM-IV*). Washington, DC: American Psychiatric Association, 1994.

Colson ER, Dworkin PH. Toddler development. *Pediatr Rev* 1997;18:255.

Johnson CP, Blasco PA. Infant growth and development. *Pediatr Rev* 1997;18:224.

Miller KJ, Castellanos FX. Attention deficit/hyperactivity disorders. *Pediatr Rev* 1998;19:373.

Parker S, Zuckerman B. *Behavioral and Developmental Pediatrics.* Boston: Little, Brown, 1995.

Simms MD, Schum RL. Preschool children who have atypical patterns of development. *Pediatr Rev* 2000;21:147.

Zinner SH. Tourette disorder. *Pediatr Rev* 2000;21:372.

NUTRITION

Groff JL, Gropper SS. *Advanced Nutrition and Human Metabolism.* 3rd ed. Belmont, CA: Wadsworth, 2000.

Klish WJ. Childhood obesity. *Pediatr Rev* 1998;19:312.

Zenel JA: Failure to thrive: a general pediatrician's perspective. *Pediatr Rev* 1997;18:371.

GASTROENTEROLOGY

American Academy of Pediatrics. Practice guideline endorsement: guidelines for evaluation and treatment of gastroesophageal reflux in infants and children. *J Pediatr Gastroenterol Nutr* 2001; 32 (suppl 2).

Hyams JS: Inflammatory bowel disease. *Pediatr Rev* 2000;21:291.

PULMONOLOGY

American Academy of Pediatrics. Practice guideline endorsement: National Asthma Education and Prevention Program Expert Panel Report 2: guidelines for the diagnosis and management of asthma. NIH Publication 97-4051.

Davis PB. Cystic fibrosis. *Pediatr Rev* 2001;22:257.

CARDIOLOGY

Artman A, Mahoney L, Teitel D. *Neonatal Cardiology*. New York: McGraw-Hill, 2002.

Chang AC, Hanley FL, Wernovsky G, Wessel DL. *Pediatric Cardiac Intensive Care*. Philadelphia: Lippincott Williams & Wilkins, 1998.

ACUTE/CRITICAL CARE

American Academy of Pediatrics and American Heart Association. *PALS Provider Manual*. Dallas, TX: American Heart Association, 2002.

Crain EF, Gershel JC. *Clinical Manual of Emergency Pediatrics*. 4th ed. New York: McGraw-Hill, 2002.

Fuhrman BP, Zimmerman JJ. *Pediatric Critical Care*. 2nd ed. St. Louis: Mosby, 1998.

Goldfrank L, Flomenbaum N, Lewin N, et al. *Goldfrank's Toxicologic Emergencies*. 5th ed. New York: McGraw-Hill, 2002.

NEPHROLOGY

Chan JCM, Scheinman, JI, Roth, KS. Consultation with the specialist: renal tubular acidosis. *Pediatr Rev* 2001;22:277.

Elder JS, Peters CA, Arant BS Jr, et al. Pediatric Vesicoureteral Reflux Guidelines Panel summary report on the management of primary vesicoureteral reflux in children. *J Urol* 1997;157:1846.

Hogg RJ, Portman, RJ, Milliner D, et al. Evaluation and management of proteinuria and nephrotic syndrome in children: recommendations from a pediatric nephrology panel established at the National Kidney Foundation Conference on Proteinuria, Albuminuria, Risk, Assessment, Detection, and Elimination (PARADE). *Pediatrics* 2000;105:1242.

Roy S. Consultation with the specialist: hematuria. *Pediatr Rev* 1998;19:209.

NEUROLOGY

American Academy of Pediatrics, Committee on Quality Improvement, Subcommittee on Febrile Seizures. The neurodiagnostic evaluation of a child with a first simple febrile seizure. *Pediatrics* 1996;97:769.

American Academy of Pediatrics, Committee on Quality Improvement, Subcommittee on Febrile Seizures. Long-term treatment of the child with simple febrile seizures. *Pediatrics* 1999;103:1307.

American Academy of Pediatrics. Practice guideline endorsement: practice parameter: evaluating a first non febrile seizure in children. Report on the Quality Standards Subcommittee of the American Academy of Neurology, the Child Neurology Society, and the American Epilepsy Society. *Neurology* 2000;55:616.

Greenlee JDW, Donovan KA, Hasan DM, Menezes AH. Chiari I malformation in the very young child: the spectrum of presentations and experience in 31 children under age 6 years. *Pediatrics* 2002;110:1212.

Liptak GS, Serletti, J: Consultation with the specialist: pediatric approach to craniosynostosis. *Pediatr Rev* 1998;19:352.

ALLERGY/IMMUNOLOGY

Austen KF, Frank MM, Atkinson JP et al: *Samter's Immunologic Diseases*. 6th ed. New York: Lippincott Williams & Wilkins, 2001.

Knoell KA, Greer KE. Atopic dermatitis. *Pediatr Rev* 1999;20:46.

Lasley MV, Shapiro GG. Testing for allergy. *Pediatr Rev* 2000;21:39.

Nimmagadda SR, Evans R. Allergy: etiology and epidemiology. *Pediatr Rev* 1999;20:110.

INFECTIOUS DISEASES

American Academy of Pediatrics: Committee on Quality Improvement. Subcommittee on Urinary Tract Infection. The diagnosis, treatment, and evaluation of the initial urinary tract infection in febrile infants and young children. *Pediatrics* 1999;103:843.

Centers for Disease Control and Prevention. 1994 revised classification system for human immunodeficiency virus infection in children less than 13 years of age: official authorized addenda: human immunodeficiency virus infection codes and official guidelines for coding and reporting ICD-9CM. *MMWR Morb Mortal Wkly Rep* 1994;43(RR-12):1.

HEMATOLOGY

Giardina PJ, Hilgartner MW. Update on thalassemia. *Pediatr Rev* 1992;13:55.

Goodnight SH, Hathaway WE. *Disorders of Hemostasis and Thrombosis: A Clinical Guide*. 2nd ed. New York: McGraw-Hill, 2001.

Nathan DG, Orkin SH, Ginsburg D et al: *Hematology of Infancy and Childhood*. Philadelphia: W.B. Saunders Company, 1998.

Segel GB, Hirsh MG, Feig SA. Managing anemia in a pediatric office practice: part 1. *Pediatr Rev* 2002;23:75.

Segel GB, Hirsh MG, Feig SA. Managing anemia in a pediatric office practice: part 2. *Pediatr Rev* 2002;23;111.

ONCOLOGY

Pizzo PA. Poplack DG. *Principles and Practice of Pediatric Oncology*. 4th ed. New York: Lippincott, Williams & Wilkins, 2001.

ENDOCRINOLOGY

Joiner TA, Foster C, Shope T. The many faces of vitamin D deficiency rickets. *Pediatr Rev* 2000;21:296.

Lifshitz FA. *Pediatric Endocrinology.* 4th ed. New York: Marcel Dekker, 2003.

Root AW. Precocious puberty. *Pediatr Rev* 2000;21:10.

Vogiatzi MG, Copeland KC. The short child. *Pediatr Rev* 1998;19:92.

RHEUMATOLOGY

Schaller JG. Juvenile rheumatoid arthritis. *Pediatr Rev* 1997;18:337.

SPORTS MEDICINE/ORTHOPEDICS

American Academy of Pediatrics, Committee on Quality Improvement. The management of minor closed head injury in children. *Pediatrics* 1999;104:1407.

Bull RC. *Handbook of Sports Injuries.* New York: McGraw-Hill, 1999.

Metzl JD. Preparticipation examination of the adolescent athlete: part 1. *Pediatr Rev* 2001;22:199.

Metzl JD. Preparticipation examination of the adolescent athlete: part 2. *Pediatr Rev* 2001;22:227.

PREVENTION PEARLS

American Academy of Pediatrics, Committee on Injury and Poison Prevention. Policy statement: bicycle helmets. *Pediatrics* 2001;108:1030.

Child Passenger Safety Laws and Recommendations. Available at: National Highway Traffic Safety Administration Website: http://www.nhtsa.dot.gov/people/injury/childps/.

Markowitz, M. Lead poisoning. *Pediatr Rev* 2000;21:327.

ADOLESCENT MEDICINE

American Academy of Pediatrics, Committee on Adolescence. Policy statement: adolescent pregnancy, current trends and issues: 1998. *Pediatrics* 1999;103:516.

Braverman PK, Sondheimer SJ. Menstrual disorders. *Pediatr Rev* 1997;18:17.

Kreipe RE, Dukarm CP. Eating Disorders in adolescents and older children. *Pediatr Rev* 1999;20:410.

BASIC STATISTICS

Greenburg RS, Daniels SR, Flanders D, Eley JW, Boring JR. *Medical Epidemiology*. 2nd ed. Stamford, CT: Appleton & Lange, 2000.

DERMATOLOGY

Kane K, Bissonette J, Baden HP, Johnson RA, Stratigos A. *Color Atlas and Synopsis of Pediatric Dermatology*. New York: McGraw-Hill, 2002.

INDEX